CHALLENGING ISSUES ON PARANASAL SINUSES

Edited by **Tang-Chuan Wang**

Challenging Issues on Paranasal Sinuses
http://dx.doi.org/10.5772/intechopen.74308
Edited by Tang-Chuan Wang

Contributors

Silviya Nikolova, Diana Toneva, Ivan Georgiev, Nikolai Lazarov, Deepti Sharma, Neha Sharma, Vivek Sharma, Alper Sindel, Mehmet Mustafa Özarslan, Öznur Özalp, Berkem Atalay, Lizette Mowatt, Mehmet Şentürk

First published in London, United Kingdom, 2019 by IntechOpen
IntechOpen is the global imprint of INTECHOPEN LIMITED, registered in England and Wales, registration number: 11086078, The Shard, 25th floor, 32 London Bridge Street
London, SE19SG – United Kingdom
Printed in Croatia

British Library Cataloguing-in-Publication Data
A catalogue record for this book is available from the British Library

Additional hard copies can be obtained from orders@intechopen.com

Challenging Issues on Paranasal Sinuses, Edited by Tang-Chuan Wang
p. cm.
Print ISBN 978-1-78985-401-5
Online ISBN 978-1-78985-402-2

For EU product safety concerns:
IN TECH d.o.o., Prolaz Marije Krucifikse Kozulić 3, 51000 Rijeka, Croatia,
info@intechopen.com or visit our website at intechopen.com.

Meet the editor

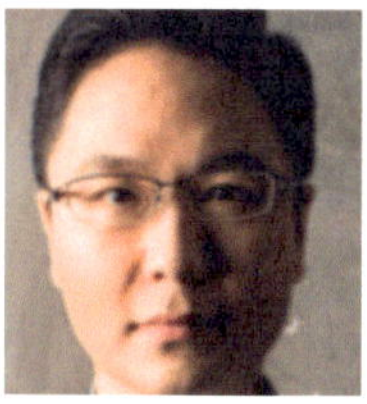

Dr Tang-Chuan Wang is an excellent otolaryngologist – head and neck surgeon in Taiwan. He is also a research scholar of Harvard Medical School and the University of Iowa Hospitals. During his Fulbright experience, he worked in the Hospital of the University of Pennsylvania, Boston Children's Hospital, and Massachusetts Eye and Ear. He is not only working hard on clinical and basic medicine but also launching out into public health in Taiwan. In recent years, he has devoted himself to innovation. He always says that "in theoretical or practical aspects, no innovation is a step backward". Due to his contribution to biomedical engineering, he was invited onto the executive committee of HIWIN-CMU Joint R & D Center in Taiwan.

Contents

Preface

Management of paranasal sinus disorders is not only a test of knowledge but it is also an art form. Great progress has been made on endoscopic sinus surgery in recent decades and this technique lets us look into the remote corners of sinuses. However, we still have a lot of challenging issues, such as frontal sinus, sinus lifting, and sinonasal cancers. The only way to solve these problems is to face them. Based on these concepts, this book incorporates new clinical and research developments as well as future perspectives in the ever-expanding field of rhinology. The book is a comprehensive reference for ENT residents and practicing otolaryngologists who wish to expand their expertise, develop a broader armamentarium of techniques, and successfully manage their patients with sinonasal disorders.

In this book, there are sections on the challenges of today, such as the development of frontal sinuses, complications of sinus augmentation, managements of rhinosinusitis and sinonasal Neoplasms. I hope this book helps readers explore the mystery of paranasal sinuses.

In the section of the Challenging Issue on Frontal Sinuses, *Dr. Nikolova Silviya et all.* will discuss the frontal bone development and maturation, from the viewpoint of the frontal sinus pneumatization in relation to the metopic craniosynostosis and failed closure of the metopic suture. Furthermore, the persistent metopic suture is frequently associated with a frontal sinus underdevelopment. In the section of Challenging Issue on Sinus Augmentation, *Dr. Sindel Alper et all.* will review the contemporary methods for maxillary sinus augmentation and presents both recommendations for prevention and management of the sinus lifting associated complications. Then *Dr. Atalay Berkem* will present his application of Platelet-rich fibrin (PRF) in sinus augmentation and the clinical and radiological findings that have shown good results regarding new bone formation. In the section of Challenging Issue on Rhinosinusitis and Sinonasal Neoplasms, *Dr. Şentürk Mehmet* will talk about medical management of rhinosinusitis, which includes antibiotics, antihistamines, nasal decongestants, corticosteroids, mucolytics, leukotriene antagonists, and nasal irrigations. Each patient must have the appropriate treatment option selected for them and prescriptions must be tailored according to the patient need. Then *Dr. Mowatt Lizette* will review the epidemiology of orbital cellulitis, pathogenesis, causative organisms, investigations, and treatment. Prognostic factors will be also presented. At the end, *Dr. Sharma Deepti et all.* discusses why the management of sinonasal cancers remains a major challenge in oncology due to highly advanced cancer stage at the time of diagnosis.

I appreciate everyone's contributions to this book. They made great efforts to do it resulting in the success of academic work. I would like to thank Marijana Francetic, the Author Service Manager, and Mirena Calmic, the Commissioning Editor, for their wonderful assistance.

Besides, the technical editors are also indispensable to the uniform format in this book. At last, I am always full of gratitude towards the people that helped me mature, including my family, teachers, and colleagues.

Tang-Chuan Wang (Vincent Wang)
Chairman of Otolaryngology-Head and Neck Surgery
China Medical University Hsinchu Hospital, Taiwan

School of Medicine, China Medical University, Taiwan

Department of Public Health, China Medical University, Taiwan

Research Scholar of Harvard Medical School, USA

Research Scholar of University of Iowa Hospitals and Clinics, USA

Fellows of the American College of Surgeons
Member of American Academy of Otolaryngology-Head and Neck Surgery

Section 1

Challenging Issue on Frontal Sinuses

Relation between Metopic Suture Persistence and Frontal Sinus Development

Silviya Nikolova, Diana Toneva, Ivan Georgiev and
Nikolai Lazarov

Additional information is available at the end of the chapter

http://dx.doi.org/10.5772/intechopen.79376

Abstract

The frontal bone develops as two halves, which further unite in a single bone by the closure of the mid-sagittal metopic suture, typically by the end of the first postnatal year. The frontal sinus begins to expand into the orbital and vertical plates of the frontal bone postnatally and reaches the level of the *nasion* by the fourth year of age. At this time, the metopic suture is usually entirely closed. However, in the cases of failed closure of the metopic suture, its relationship to the frontal sinus development is still obscure. Here, we review the relevant literature and discuss the frontal bone development and maturation, from the viewpoint of the frontal sinus pneumatization in relation to the metopic craniosynostosis and failed closure of the metopic suture. The peculiar to the metopic skulls frontal bone configuration is rather an expression of the underlying neural mass demands than a consequence of the metopic suture persistence. Furthermore, the persistent metopic suture is frequently associated with a frontal sinus underdevelopment. It seems that the metopic suture does not inhibit the frontal sinus pneumatization itself, but rather both traits are an expression or an aftereffect of a certain condition during the early development.

Keywords: frontal bone, frontal sinus, persistent metopic suture, *metopism*, metopic craniosynostosis

1. Introduction

The different partitions and layers of the frontal bone develop and maturate simultaneously, but independently from one another in accordance with the functional demands of the related soft tissues/cavities [1]. It has been observed that in cases of persistent metopic suture (MS), the frontal sinus (FS) develops separately on either side of the suture, as well as the MS precludes the likelihood of development of the sinus beyond the median plane [2–4]. Nevertheless, the supposed influence of *metopism* on the FS development has not been synonymous. Some authors did not find a significant correlation between *metopism* and the underdevelopment of the FS [5–8], which leads to the assertion that the association of these variations is rather random. Other studies, however, revealed a tendency of MS persistence to be significantly related to the FS underdevelopment, including both FS aplasia and hypoplasia [4, 9–14]. Both the MS persistence and FS underdevelopment are not exceptional variations, but the correlation between them is intricate. There are many congenital disorders characterized by an underdevelopment of the nasomaxillary complex accompanied with diminished pneumatization of the FS such as Hajdu-Cheney syndrome, Down syndrome (DS), cleidocranial dysostosis and pyknodysostosis [11], which also feature a preservation of the MS [15–17]. In healthy adults, this correlation is still misunderstood. An adequate assessment of the relation between the frontal sinus development and metopic suture persistence requires a precise study of the events during their formation, development and maturation. In this study, we review the extant literature and discuss the frontal bone development and maturation, from the viewpoint of the frontal sinus pneumatization in relation to the metopic craniosynostosis and failed closure of the metopic suture. We aimed to reveal the possible underlying factors causing a delayed MS closure along with FS underdevelopment.

2. Frontal bone as a functional unit

The functional matrix concept of Moss [1, 18] considers the adult human frontal bone as a single morphological structure, which by no means is a single functional unit. In fact, the form of the frontal bone accurately reflects the functional demands of the protected and supported soft tissues/cavities. Furthermore, each of the three bone layers is functionally independent and responds to different functional demands. The inner table of the frontal bone is functionally associated with the development of the frontal lobe of the cerebral cortex and is exquisitely sensitive to alterations in the cerebral morphology throughout life [18]. The intimate dependence of endocranial form upon the state of adjacent soft tissues could be traced in examples like an extensive compensatory pneumatization and inward displacement of the frontal endocranial plate followed by an atrophy of the frontal cerebral lobe/cerebral hemiatrophy [18, 19]. The differentiation of the outer table is correlated with the increasing demands of the scalp tissues in general and of calvarial muscles in particular [1, 20], as well as with the growing nasomaxillary facial complex [11]. The diploë has several simultaneous functions, including hematopoiesis, weight reduction and pneumatization, functionally responsive to the respiratory system. Even the MS is far from being a simple, intrinsically regulated entity, being greatly influenced by related soft tissues, dura and cranial base [18].

3. Frontal sinus

3.1. Anatomy and development

The FS is one of the four paranasal sinuses and represents a space of variable shape and size between the inner and outer tables of the frontal bone. In adults, the FS appears as two irregularly shaped cavities separated from each other by a thin septum commonly deviated from the mid-sagittal plane. Usually, the FS lobes extend vertically upwards into the frontal bone squama, but could also expand horizontally backwards between the two tables of the orbital plate [21] and sometimes into the crista galli of the ethmoid bone [11]. Not infrequently, the FS does not invade far into the vertical portion, but grows extensively into the horizontal one and forms large air spaces over the orbits [2]. In cases of the so-called ethmofrontal, orbital or infantile FS [2], it adheres closely to the ethmoidal labyrinth and extends only into the horizontal portion of the frontal bone. In rare cases, the pneumatization could be so profuse to extend beyond the frontal bone into the lesser and greater wings of the sphenoid, the parietal, the temporal, the nasal bone and even into the frontal process of the maxilla [11]. Furthermore, many other variations such as single midline sinus, due to a lack of septum, or supernumerary septa forming additional chambers in a variable pattern, have been reported [2, 11, 22].

Unlike the other sinuses, the FS is practically absent at birth. It could be recognized during the fourth fetal month as diverticula from the lateral nasal wall following the development of the frontal recess. The FS may also arise from the laterally placed anterior ethmoidal cells, the anterior part of the frontal recess or from the frontal furrow [23], but does not pneumatize the frontal bone until the postnatal period. The pneumatization begins in the horizontal (orbital) plate during the first year of life, whereas the pneumatization of the vertical plate commences during the latter half of the second postnatal year and progresses slowly to reach the level of the *nasion* by the fourth year of age [11]. Both lobes of the FS develop independently, and therefore they are often highly asymmetrical due to more rapid pneumatization on one side at the expense of the other [21]. The main period of enlargement coincides with the pubertal growth spurt, but may go on increasing into the fourth decade of life [24].

From the viewpoint of the functional matrix concept, the FS develops through resorption of the diploë, which is housed between the two functionally independent bone tables. The internal table is the intrinsic part of the cerebral capsule, since its periosteum is the outer layer of the dura and is functionally related to the configuration of the frontal lobes. The outer table is related with the increasing demands of the scalp tissues, calvarial muscles [1] and nasomaxillary facial complex [11]. During the first few years of life, the inner table drifts anteriorly in response to the growing frontal lobes. Since there is no significant diploë at this time, the inner table carries the contiguous outer table along with it. After the frontal lobes have undergone their major development at the age of 6–7 years, growing of the inner table ceases and adopts the general shape of the brain. However, the functionally independent outer table continues to drift anteriorly in response to the stimulus of the growing nasomaxillary facial complex, which during puberty is intensively remodeled and displaced more anteriorly and inferiorly. This results in a progressive separation of both tables of the frontal bone, resorption of the diploë and formation of the FS cavities [11].

3.2. Function

Currently, the insight into the biological and functional significance of the paranasal sinuses is speculative rather than known. It has been suggested that the FS contributes to the ventilation and air-conditioning (heating and humidifying the inspired air), the increase in the olfactory membrane area, the lightening of the skull, voice resonance, protection and thermal insulation of the cerebrum and orbits, shock absorption, an adjustment to the growth and development of the cranium. Finally, the FS has been supposed to be an evolutionary residual space [25, 26].

3.3. Factors affecting the FS development and morphology

The factors modifying the FS development and morphology are heterogeneous and are of genetic, environmental or pathological origin. Factors related to the final shaping of the FS and responsible for the wide variations are supposed to be a craniofacial configuration, frontal bone thickness, extent of the supraorbital ridges [27], hormonal growth factors, *metopism*, [11], sex [28, 29], cranial indices and ancestry [30], climatic factors [26, 28, 31], a varying degree of resorption of the diploë, an ambient air pressure and breathing [32]. According to Arnaud et al. [33], both craniofacial configuration and frontal bone width related to the intracranial pressure influence the frontal pneumatization. Heterogeneous pathological condition such as trauma, infection, tumors, mucoceles and various congenital disorders have also been reported as factors affecting the frontal sinus size and morphology in a different way [11].

3.4. FS aplasia

The FS is topographically ethmoidal before it becomes a frontal through pneumatization of the frontal bone, and in this way, it is conspicuously present at birth in all cases [2]. A total agenesis of the FS or the lack of any pneumatization of the frontal bone in healthy adults is very rare [2, 21]. The FS aplasia has been reported to vary from 0.7 to 62% in different population groups [4, 21, 23, 28, 31, 34–39]. The unilateral aplasia of the FS has been found to be more common than the considerably rarer bilateral one [4, 21, 40]. The side prevalence varies in different population groups, but right-sided aplasia seems to be more frequent [4, 8, 21]. There have also been reported cases of agenetic FS, where the contralateral sinus expands and crosses the midline towards the agenetic side and mimics the presence of bilateral frontal sinuses [41]. Sex differences in the frequency of the FS aplasia have been established as well and it tends to be more common in females [21, 35, 38].

3.5. Relation between FS development and definite pathological conditions

Abnormal pneumatization of the FS has been a concomitant finding in a number of heterogeneous disorders. It has been noted that in patients with cerebral hypoplasia, the FS is larger in size while in hypoplasia of the midface, it is smaller [11].

3.5.1. FS hyperpneumatization

The etiology of an excessive sinus aeration and growth resulting in a condition known as "pneumosinus dilatans" is unclear [42]. Pneumosinus dilatans is a generalized or partial enlargement of the paranasal sinuses containing only air. Pneumosinus dilatans occurs as an idiopathic disorder as well as in association with other disorders, including cerebral hemiatrophy [19]. Furthermore, the extreme sinus pneumatization has been associated with heterogeneous disorders such as osteogenesis imperfecta tarda, Turner syndrome, Klinefelter syndrome and acromegaly [11].

3.5.2. FS underdevelopment

The *FS underdevelopment* usually occurs in patients with craniofacial abnormalities. There are many congenital disorders characterized by an underdevelopment of the nasomaxillary complex. According to Shapiro and Schorr [11], the hypoplasia of the midface blocks one of the major stimuli for the FS pneumatization, i.e. the need to provide a structural bridge between the cranium and the face. Such disorders like Hajdu-Cheney syndrome, cleidocranial dysostosis and pyknodysostosis exhibit diminished pneumatization of the FS [11, 43] and also feature a preservation of the MS [15–17]. Aplasia/hypoplasia of the FS has also been associated with Down syndrome, Apert syndrome, maxillofacial dysplasia, osteodysplasia (Melnick-Needles), Treacher-Collins syndrome [11], cystic fibrosis [44], etc.

3.6. FS in forensic medicine for identification in medico-legal cases

The FS has been considered to be unique in each person [45, 46]. Its shape differs significantly even in monozygotic twins [47]. Being an internal skull structure between the plates of the frontal bone, the FS is well protected from injuries and taphonomic processes. Thus, due to its uniqueness, relatively constant morphology, protected location and frequent radiological documentation, the FS is particularly useful for the identification of human remains [48–52]. The FS has also been used as a feature for sex prediction [53].

3.7. Neurosurgery and endoscopic surgery

The FS morphology has an impact in neurosurgical and endoscopic nasal interventions because of its proximity to the orbit and the anterior cranial base [41, 54]. The possibility to identify the internally located FS through superficial anatomical landmarks is essential for neurosurgery to avoid injury of the FS during intervention, which could lead to postoperative complications [54].

3.8. Methods for FS investigation

As an internal skull structure, the FS has been investigated using different destructive and non-destructive methods with specific advantages and shortcomings which are briefly considered. It has to be noted that when comparing data of the FS agenesis, development, morphology and morphometry, the examining techniques and equipment should be carefully taken into account.

3.8.1. Destructive methods

The FS has been investigated directly through sectioning of dry macerated skulls [7, 55] or by cadaveric dissections [2, 41, 54, 56]. These approaches are applicable for FS investigation on osteological material and in forensic aspect in medico-legal cases.

3.8.2. Non-destructive methods

3.8.2.1. Transillumination

It is the technique of illumination by the transmission of light through a sample/body part. Transillimination of the FS with electric lamp and permanent mapping of its outlines by drawing of the illuminated area with a pencil has been used for FS investigation and measurement in healthy living persons, patients with chronic suppuration, cadavers and macerated skulls in the beginning of the twentieth century [21]. The method has many limitations and is not widely used thereafter.

3.8.2.2. Radiological investigation

With the discovery of the X-rays in 1895 by Wilhelm Röntgen and the subsequent fast development of the radiography, computed tomography (CT) and their application in the clinical practice, the non-invasive diagnostic has been significantly improved. *Radiography (projectional radiography)* is an imaging technique using X-rays to visualize the internal structure of an object. Basically, a beam of X-rays, produced by an X-ray generator, is transmitted through the specimen. The X-rays are absorbed in different amounts by the object they pass through, depending on its density and composition. The unabsorbed X-rays, passed through the object, are recorded on an X-ray sensitive film or a digital detector. The first radiographic signs of FS development are detected between the ages of 4 and 11, with an average of 8.3 years [57]. It is well known that the investigation of a complex 3D structure like FS on 2D radiographs has some inherent limitations. The superimposition of anatomical structures beyond the plain of interest complicates the interpretation of the FS morphology. Furthermore, the estimation of the FS depth, area and volume is complicated and rude [50]. In radiograph-based measurements of the FS, the magnification, positioning and angulation of the skull are crucial for a reliable morphometry [4, 58]. Therefore, in radiographic FS investigations, a definite head/skull orientation is indispensable. Caldwell's view is recommendable, since it provides the clearest FS silhouette and the least chance for error in the interpretation [22]. In Caldwell's view, the skull is inclined 20° from the Frankfurt horizontal plane (FH), the one determined by both landmarks of *porion* and the left *orbitale*. An inclination of 45° from the FH or the so-called Waters' view is also acceptable, but a little bit incorrect for FS measurements [58]. On the plain radiography, the orbital pneumatization is hardly recognizable and is commonly reported as FS aplasia, which unavoidably increases the frequency of FS agenesis [30]. *Conventional plain radiography* has been widely used for FS investigation due to its accessibility. Until now, the conventional plain radiography has been used as a frequent method for diagnostic imaging and documentation of the head including the dentition. Thus, many investigations of the FS in different contexts have been carried out on such datasets of patients' archives. The conventional plain radiography has also been purposefully used for FS investigation on osteological material [26, 30]. In *digital radiography,* the X-ray film/plaque is replaced by a digital X-ray detector. Digital radiography performed on industrial CT systems has been termed an *industrial digital radiography*. Its application as a modality for FS investigation and morphometry in dry skulls has been discussed by Nikolova et al. [4, 14, 58]. Industrial digital radiography allows a precise orientation at the appropriated position, a real-time inspection with optimal X-ray parameters and storage of the captured projections in image file formats. The high resolution of the flat panel detector ensures perfect image quality, precise scaling of the pixel size and reliable readings of the linear FS measurements (**Figure 1**).

3.8.2.3. Volumetric imaging (3D)

It has many advantages and enables the examination of the inner structure of the scanned object into the three orthogonal plains. The volumetric imaging allows the selection of a definite structure as a "region of interest" and its further segmentation. After segmentation,

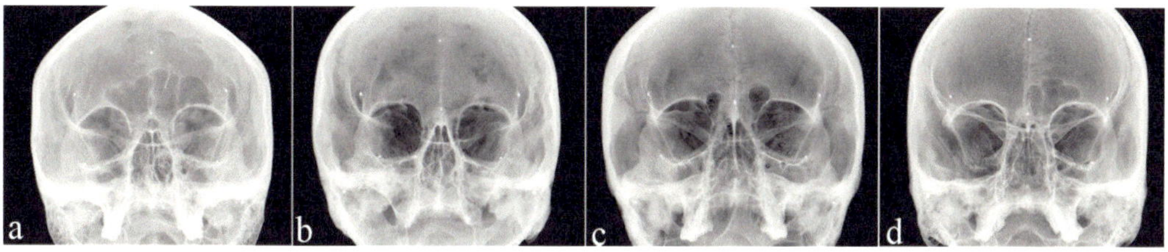

Figure 1. Industrial digital radiographs of dry adult male skulls oriented in Caldwell's view: (a) frontal sinus of normal size; (b) bilateral aplasia of the frontal sinus; (c) underdeveloped frontal sinus of the orbital type in a metopic skull; and (d) right-sided frontal sinus aplasia in a metopic skull.

a representation of the FS cavities could be generated as a separate 3D object, the so-called virtual endocast (**Figure 2**). The virtual endocasts ensure precise metric analyses, storage and further verification of the obtained results, as well as visualization of the real object by 3D printing (**Figure 3**). However, both the resolution and segmentation algorithm are essential for the endocasts reliability (**Figure 4**). In principle, medical and industrial CT systems use different scanning process and algorithms for the calculation and reconstruction

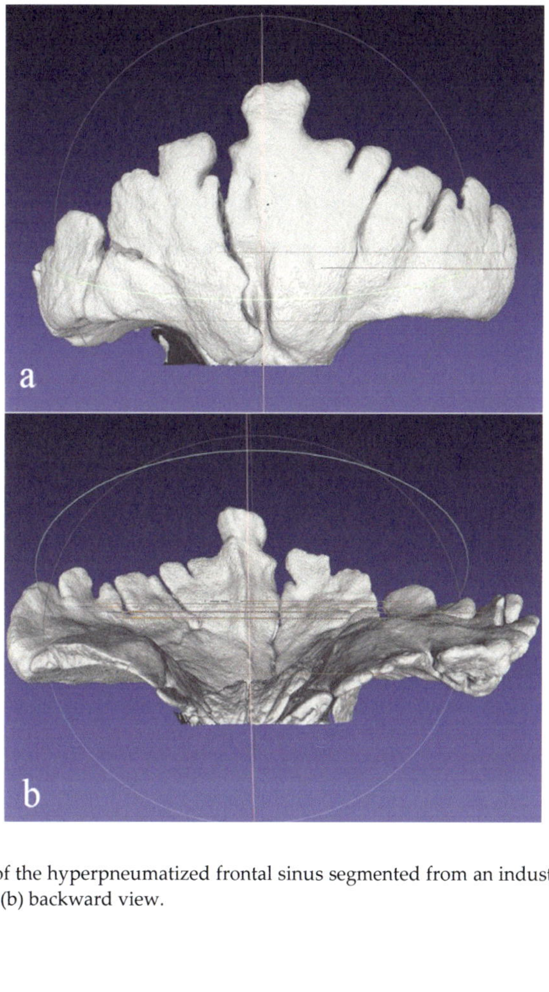

Figure 2. Virtual endocast of the hyperpneumatized frontal sinus segmented from an industrial μCT dataset above the *nasion*: (a) frontal view and (b) backward view.

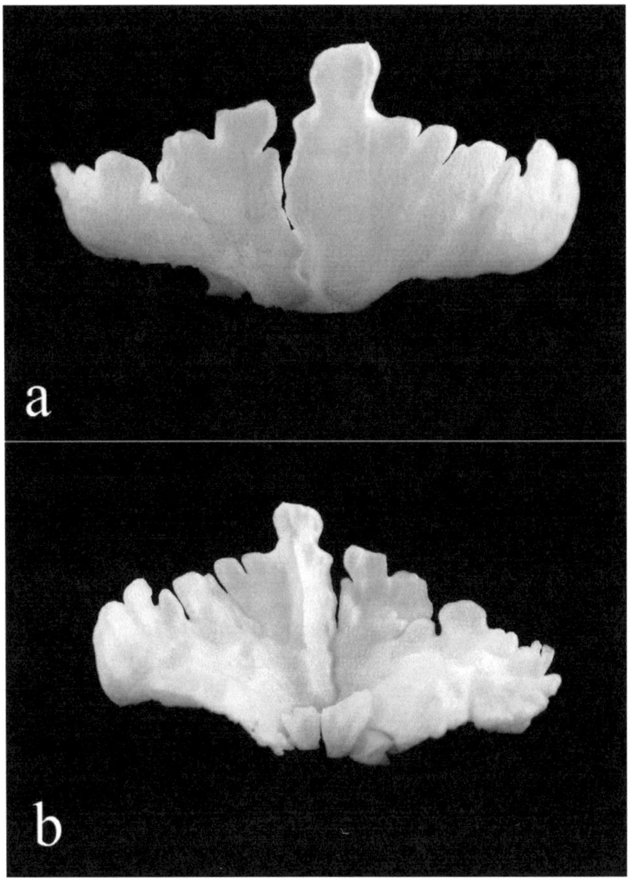

Figure 3. A 3D printed representation of the same hyperpneumatized frontal sinus in real size: (a) frontal view and (b) backward view.

of the volume of the object. Both types of CT systems have their advantages and limitations. For instance, medical CT systems are able to perform fast scan of a large object such as the human body. Limitations are the short exposure time with minimal radiation doses; hence, the images have relatively low resolution. On the other hand, the diagnostic imaging of patients enables the accumulation of large databases which could be used for various investigations on the contemporary populations. Industrial μCT systems are highly versatile and generate images with a high resolution, which allow qualitative observation [59] and quantitative calculation of stereological parameters and degree of anisotropy for porous materials like bone tissue directly from the datasets [60]. Besides, the virtual endocasts of the FS generated from μCT data are very reliable. However, the dimensions of the scan object are too limited, the generated files are large and the modality is entirely inapplicable *in vivo*.

http://dx.doi.org/10.5772/intechopen.79376

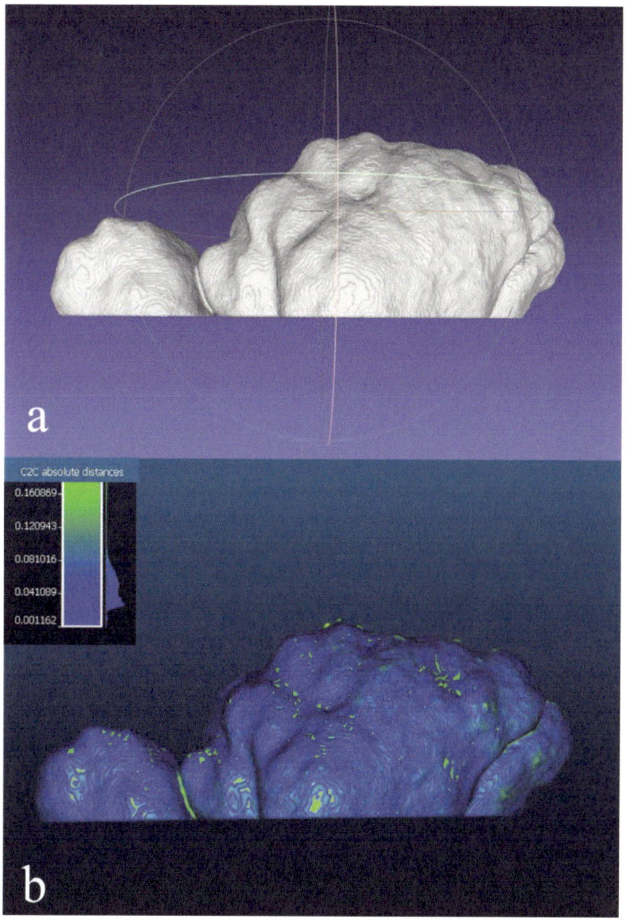

Figure 4. Comparison of frontal sinus virtual endocasts for the establishment of their reliability: (a) virtual endocast and (b) superimposition of two virtual endocasts of the same frontal sinus.

4. Metopic suture, metopic craniosynostosis and *metopism*, definitions and causative factors

The MS is considered an anterior continuation of the sagittal suture. It runs from *nasion* to the anterior border of the anterior fontanelle and is responsible for the growth of the anterior part of the calvaria in width. During the fetal life, the frontal bones undergo intramembranous ossification from a single primary centre located in each halve. The halves are separated by the sutural space [61]. At the ninth gestational week, a small ossification centre is visible in the middle of each supraorbital part of the frontal bones, and subsequently the ossification spreads. The frontal bones reach the midline at the nasal area at the 11th gestational week. The gap between the two frontal bones in the midline starts closing from the nasal region at around the 16th intrauterine week and moves superiorly towards the anterior fontanelle by the 28th week. At the 32nd week of gestation, there is apparent closure of the MS at the supranasal region, and subsequently, the closure moves superiorly towards the anterior fontanelle [62].

The metopic sutural area, i.e. the adjacent frontal bone edges along with the intervening soft tissues, tends to have a simple "butt-ended" appearance. The interdigitation is a secondary response to imposed biomechanical extrinsic forces [63] and does not follow any special pattern [61], but its widespread presence suggests that the suture is under increased biomechanical stimulation [64]. Some of the interdigitations are united by thin bridges of chondroid tissue which pass through the sutural space, constituting the first microscopic sign of frontal fusion [61]. The location of the fusion point is not invariably endocranial as it is in rats [65], but is sparse and randomly distributed [61].

The MS is the first one to close physiologically as its fusion is a progressive process initiated at the nasion and completed at the anterior fontanelle [62, 66, 67]. The completion of normal fusion occurs between 2 and 14 months in 95% of the normal population with an estimated average age of completion at 8.24 months [68]. After the initiation at an average of 5 months, the process of fusion takes approximately 3–4 months to complete. Furthermore, when the fusion process starts at a younger age, it takes less time to complete [68]. However, the MS has been reported to remain patent up to the seventh year [69].

Premature closure of the MS, metopic craniosynostosis, results in a growth restriction of the frontal bones which leads to a skull deformation known as trigonocephaly [70]. The epidemiology of metopic synostosis has been reported to be 1:5200 newborns, and it is the second most frequently seen type of isolated craniosynostosis after the sagittal one [70]. The etiology of metopic synostosis is multifactorial and has been supposed to be related to intrinsic bone malformation occurred either by genetic, metabolic, or pharmaceutical means [70]. According to Moss [1], the calvaria, dura and cranial base form a single biomechanical entity, and a primary malformation of the cranial base produces abnormal forces within its attached dural fiber tracts, which, in turn, produces premature cranial synostosis. In this sense, the observed neurocranial deformation is the final result. Premature synostosis of the MS, for instance, has been found to be a frequent characteristic of the cleft-palate skull. A cranial base malformation (dysostosis sphenoidalis) was a primary morphological event associated with orofacial clefting. This condition, characterized by a strong basal kyphosis, sets up abnormal tensile condition in the falx cerebri, resulting in the fusion of the overlaying suture [71]. A reported case of trigonocephaly with open MS also suggests that the primary cause is not the MS synostosis, but rather it is a consequence and the underlying cause could be an intrinsic malformation such as hypoplasia of the frontal lobes, which thus require only limited space in the anterior cranial fossa [72]. Furthermore, it has experimentally been established that the normal endocranial fusion of the posterior portion of the MS is well correlated with the structural alterations in the falx cerebri. In rats, normal metopic fusion was inhibited when the underlying dural (falx cerebri) fibre tract was separated from the overlying sutural area. Conversely, periosteal stripping was followed by synostosis of calvarial sutures that normally are patent throughout life [1].

Failed fusion of the MS leads to a condition known as *metopism*. In such cases, the MS runs from *nasion* to *bregma,* the intersection of sagittal and coronal sutures (**Figure 5**). It is

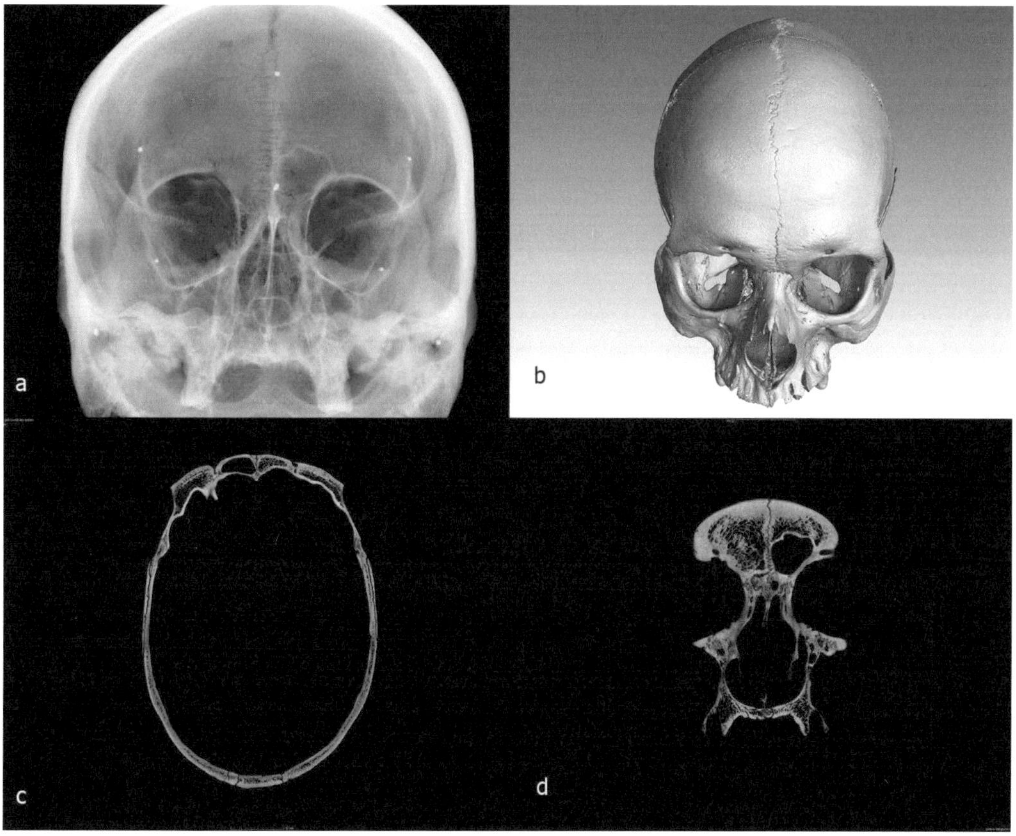

Figure 5. Metopic skull of adult male with aplasia of the right FS: (a) industrial digital radiograph in Caldwell's view; (b) 3D volume representation obtained after scanning with industrial μCT; (c) axial tomogram at the level of FS; and (d) coronal tomogram at the level of FS.

reported that the preserved MS ranges from 0.8 up to 15% in different population groups [14, 73–79]. The persistence of the MS in adults is not reported to cause any abnormalities by itself. However, it has been found as a concomitant finding in numerous disorders [16, 80]. Among the causative factors for *metopism* are considered to be stenocrotaphy, plagiocephaly, brachycephaly, encephalic pressure, diminution of muscular pressure, endocrine dysfunction, atavism, heredity and heredo-specific factors [81], an abnormal growth of the cranial bones, hydrocephaly, growth retardation, sexual influence, scaphocephaly and mechanical causes [82].

It has already been established that metopic skulls possess specific distinctive configuration of the neurocranium characterized by a broad forehead with greater inter-frontal and inter-orbital breadths [4, 81, 83–85], as well as a greater frontal curvature [75]. The metopic skulls attain a given capacity by a greater expansion in the forward direction and a smaller development in the hinder part of the vault. Therefore, the *metopism* could not be explained merely by a supposed expansion of the frontal lobes and namely the prefrontal cortex, but rather as an adjustment of the braincase as a whole to its contents [83]. Furthermore, despite the close developmental interrelation between the neuro- and basicranium, the preservation of the MS along with a specific construction of the neurocranium was not found to be related to an alteration in the cranial base expressed by cranial base angle [86]. All this suggests that the *metopism* is not related to a primary cranial base deformation.

The neurocranial capsule responds secondarily to the primary expansion of the neural mass, consisting of brain, leptomeninges and cerebrospinal fluid, by passive translation of the bones outwards [1]. Hyper- and hypovolumetric growth of the neural mass volume is the primary etiological factor in macro- and microcephaly, respectively. That the volume alone is responsible is well demonstrated by the essentially normal neurocranial sizes and shapes of hydranencephaly [1, 18]. Consequently, the MS persistence is not responsible for the distinctive skull configuration, but rather is an expression of the underlying neural mass specific demands.

5. Metopic suture persistence and frontal sinus development

It has been suggested that the MS preservation suppresses the FS development [27, 40]. A possible explanation has been supposed to be the simultaneous FS development along with the frontal bone growth, most probably with a feedback regulating mechanism. Thus, if the frontal bones fail to fuse, the MS persists and the pneumatization of the frontal sinuses could be retarded or entirely suppressed [32]. Another suggestion is that the MS does not inhibit the FS development itself, but rather the accumulation of both features in nonsyndromic individuals is an expression or an aftereffect of a certain condition during the early development [4]. It is known that the craniosynostosis results in an underdevelopment of the FS due to the increased intracranial pressure (ICP) that hinders pneumatization of the sinuses [87, 88], since the FS development is an inverse ratio to the ICP [89]. However, a surgical enlargement of the neurocranium with an adequate stabilization leads to a decrease in the pressure on the inner frontal cortex; thereafter, the FS pneumatization proceeds normally [88]. Nevertheless, the FS pneumatization seems to depend on the craniosynostosis and on the type of surgery performed [33]. According to McCarthy et al. [87], the fronto-orbital advancement appears to have the detrimental effect on FS development, whereas the strip craniectomy procedures do not. It has been speculated that the path of the ethmoid pneumatization into the FS is interrupted by the saw cut, the gap or defect resulting from the advancement/displacement of the supraorbital bar, as well as residual bone formation. Contrarily, Locher et al. [88] stated that following bilateral fronto-orbital advancement, a nearly regular FS development is possible, with the exception perhaps of the severe cases of Crouzon syndrome. Notwithstanding, if the FS developed after the surgical intervention, it is often located in the roof of the orbits [33].

Besides craniosynostosis, the elevation of the ICP could be a consequence of many other heterogeneous conditions such as haematoma, neoplasm, trauma, seizure, hydrocephalus, meningitis, etc. [90], and most of them are not associated with a distortion of the skull configuration. In newborns and infants, the main signs of acute and chronic elevation of ICP are suture diastasis (mainly coronal and metopic) and bulging of the anterior fontanelle [90]. The excessive head growth is a major feature for an increased ICP until the age of 3 years since the expansion of the skull volume allows partial venting of the increased pressure [91]. Nonetheless, the normal head growth does not preclude the presence of an increased ICP, as the rate of the pressure increase is also important, because the intracranial structures accommodate remarkably well to slowly increasing pressure, while sudden changes are intolerable and result in definite symptoms [91].

The *metopism* has been supposed to be related with the hypofunction of the thymus inducing a condition of prolonged infantilism, which finds expression in the persistence of the MS. Another suggestion is that the hypopituitarism has been concerned in the MS persistence. Both the hypofunction of thymus and pituitary glands independently result in a retardation of bone growth similar to that in rickets, with a marked deficiency in the normal processes of ossification and a tendency for arrested suture obliteration [81]. The iron deficiency anemia (IDA) is a common type of anemia, which has been reported to be associated with an impaired thymus function [92] and a well-known consequence of hypopituitarism [93]. The IDA has been identified as one of the risk factors for vitamin D deficiency in some populations [94]. Patients with IDA have been reported to feature MS preservation [95]. Furthermore, due to the overgrowing red marrow, the severe IDA causes skull thickening, which in turn involves FS underdevelopment [11, 96]. The IDA has also been associated with an increased ICP [97, 98]. The intracranial hypertension has been supposed to be a possible underlying cause for MS persistence along with the FS underdevelopment [4, 59].

The MS preservations, a delayed closure of the anterior fontanelle and wormian bone formation have been found to be common in patients with Down's syndrome [99]. Underdeveloped FS is also typical of the DS [43]. In patients with DS, the thymus function has been significantly impaired [100]; however, it is still unclear whether or not the short stature in DS involves pituitary hypofunction due to the suboptimal production of the growth hormone, or rather involves hypothalamic dysfunction [101, 102]. Interestingly, the IDA is a frequent condition in DS [103].

It could be seen that the persistent MS along with FS underdevelopment and other common symptoms are typical of heterogeneous disorders like DS and IDA, and both conditions involve or are due to an iron deficiency. The iron deficiency is a widespread nutritional disorder in infants, children and women of reproductive age. It has already been suggested that the *metopism* probably is caused by impairment of the ossification process due to a nutritional deficiency and more exactly the lack of calcium. This suggestion has been based on the assumption that the *metopism* has been more prevalent in the medieval than today, in populations with a low life expectancy and among women who have become pregnant and have given birth immaturely [104]. Bearing in mind the symptoms and consequences of IDA, it seems reasonable to suggest that the MS preservation along with the FS underdevelopment could be an expression or aftereffect of nutritional deficiency and more exactly the iron deficiency during early development. This suggestion could be verified through a purposeful monitoring and longitudinal study of patients with confirmed IDA.

6. Conclusion

The peculiar to the metopic skulls frontal bone configuration is rather an expression of the underlying neural mass demands than a consequence of the MS persistence. Moreover, the persistent MS is frequently associated with FS underdevelopment. It is reasonable to suggest that the MS does not inhibit the frontal sinus pneumatization itself, but rather both traits are expression or aftereffect of a certain condition during the early development.

Acknowledgements

This work was supported by the Bulgarian National Science Fund, grants DN01/15-20.12.2016 and DN11/09-15.12.2017.

Conflict of interest

The authors declare no conflict of interest.

Author details

Silviya Nikolova[1*], Diana Toneva[1], Ivan Georgiev[2,3] and Nikolai Lazarov[4,5]

*Address all correspondence to: sil_nikolova@abv.bg

1 Department of Anthropology and Anatomy, Institute of Experimental Morphology, Pathology and Anthropology with Museum, Bulgarian Academy of Sciences, Sofia, Bulgaria

2 Department of Scientific Computations, Institute of Information and Communication Technologies, Bulgarian Academy of Sciences, Sofia, Bulgaria

3 Department of Mathematical Modeling and Numerical Analysis, Institute of Mathematics and Informatics, Bulgarian Academy of Sciences, Sofia, Bulgaria

4 Department of Anatomy and Histology, Medical University of Sofia, Sofia, Bulgaria

5 Department of Synaptic Signaling and Communications, Institute of Neurobiology, Bulgarian Academy of Sciences, Sofia, Bulgaria

References

[1] Moss ML. Functional anatomy of cranial synostosis. Child's Brain. 1975;**1**:22-33. DOI: 10.1159/000119554

[2] Schaeffer J. The Embryology, Development and Anatomy of the Nose, Paranasal Sinuses, Nasolacrimal Passageways and Olfactory Organs in Man. Philadelphia: P Blakiston's Son; 1920

[3] Davis WB. Development and Anatomy of the Nasal Accessory Sinuses in Man. London: WB Saunders Company; 1914

[4] Nikolova S, Toneva D, Georgiev I, Lazarov N. Digital radiomorphometric analysis of the frontal sinus and assessment of the relation between persistent metopic suture and frontal sinus development. American Journal of Physical Anthropology. 2018;**165**:492-506. DOI: 10.1002/ajpa.23375

[5] Marciniak R, Nizankowski C. Metopism and its correlation with the development of the frontal sinuses. Acta Radiologica. 1959;**51**:343-352. DOI: 10.3109/00016925909171105

[6] Hunt DR, Everest K. Frontal sinus size: Sex, population and metopism affinities. American Journal of Physical Anthropology, Abstracts of AAPA poster and podium presentations. 2001;**114**(S32):82-83. DOI: 10.1002/ajpa.1035

[7] Pondé JM, Andrade RN, Via JM, Metzger P, Teles AC. Anatomical variations of the frontal sinus. International Journal of Morphology. 2008;**26**:803-808. DOI: 10.1055/s-2003-37956

[8] Bilgin S, Kantarcı UH, Duymus M, Yildirim CH, Ercakmak B, Orman G, Gunenc Beser C, Kaya M, Gok M, Akbasak A. Association between frontal sinus development and persistent metopic suture. Folia Morphologica. 2013;**72**:306-310. DOI: 10.5603/FM.2013.0051

[9] Rochlin DG, Rubaschewa A. Zum Problem des Metopismus. Zeitschrift für Menschliche Vererbungs- und Konstitutionslehre. 1934;**18**:339-348

[10] Torgersen J. A roentgenological study of the metopic suture. Acta Radiologica. 1950; **33**:1-11

[11] Shapiro R, Schorr SA. A consideration of the systemic factors that influence frontal sinus pneumatization. Investigative Radiology. 1980;**15**:191-202

[12] Baaten PJ, Haddad M, Abi-Nader K, Abi-Ghosn A, Al-Kutoubi A, Jurjus AR. Incidence of metopism in the Lebanese population. Clinical Anatomy. 2003;**16**:148-151. DOI: 10.1002/ca.10050

[13] Guerram A, Le Minor JM, Renger S, Bierry G. Brief communication: The size of the human frontal sinuses in adults presenting complete persistence of the metopic suture. American Journal of Physical Anthropology. 2014;**154**:621-627. DOI: 10.1002/ajpa.22532

[14] Nikolova S, Toneva D, Georgiev I. A persistent metopic suture – Incidence and influence on the frontal sinus development (preliminary data). Acta Morphologica et Anthropologica. 2016a;**23**:83-90

[15] Castriota-Scanderbeg A, Dallapiccola B. Abnormal Skeletal Phenotypes: From Simple Signs to Complex Diagnoses. Berlin Heidelberg: Springer Verlag; 2005

[16] Nikolova S, Toneva D, Yordanov Y, Lazarov N. Multiple Wormian bones and their relation with definite pathological conditions in a case of an adult cranium. Anthropologischer Anzeiger. 2014;**71**:169-190. DOI: 10.1127/0003-5548/2014/0355

[17] Palav S, Vernekar J, Pereira S, Desai A. Hajdu-Cheney syndrome: A case report with review of literature. Journal of Radiology Case Reports. 2014;**8**:1-8. DOI: 10.3941/jrcr.v8i9.1833

[18] Moss ML, Young RW. A functional approach to craniology. American Journal of Physical Anthropology. 1960;**18**:281-292. DOI: 10.1002/ajpa.1330180406

[19] van Schayck R, Niedeggen A. Pneumosinus dilatans after prolonged cerebrospinal fluid shunting in young adults with cerebral hemiatrophy. A report of two cases and review of the literature. Neurosurgical Review. 1992;**15**:217-223. DOI: 10.1007/BF00345938

[20] Washburn SL. The relation of the temporal muscle to the form of the skull. The Anatomical Record. 1947;**99**:239-248. DOI: 10.1002/ar.1090990303

[21] Turner AL. The Accessory Sinuses of the Nose. New York: Longmans, Green & Co; 1901

[22] Yanagisawa E, Smith HM. Radiographic anatomy of the Paranasal sinuses IV. Caldwell view. Archives of Otolaryngology. 1968;**87**:311-322. DOI: 10.1001/archotol.1968.00760060313016

[23] Donald PJ, Gluckmann JL, Rice DH. The Sinuses. New York: Raven Press; 1994

[24] Scheuer L, Black S. Developmental juvenile osteology. San Diego: Academic Press; 2000

[25] Takahashi R. The formation of the human Paranasal sinuses. Acta Oto-Laryngologica. 1984;**97**(408):1-28

[26] Kondrat JW. Frontal Sinus Morphology: An analysis of craniometric and environmental variables on the morphology of modern human frontal sinus patterns [Thesis]. Dekalb (IL): Northern Illinois University; 1995

[27] Samuel E, Lloyd GAS. Clinical Radiology of the Ear, Nose and Throat. 2nd ed. London: Lieut.-Col; 1978

[28] Hanson CL, Owsley DW. Frontal sinus size in Eskimo populations. American Journal of Physical Anthropology. 1980;**53**:251-255. DOI: 10.1002/ajpa.1330530209

[29] Tatlisumak E, Ovali GY, Asirdizer M, Aslan A, Ozyurt B, Bayindir P, Tarhan S. CT study on morphometry of frontal sinus. Clinical Anatomy. 2008;**21**:287-293. DOI: 10.1002/ca.20617

[30] Christensen AM. An empirical examination of frontal sinus outline variability using elliptic Fourier analysis: Implications for identification, standardization, and legal admissibility [Thesis]. University of Tennessee: Knoxville; 2003

[31] Koertvelyessy T. Relationships between the frontal sinus and climatic conditions: A skeletal approach to cold adaptation. American Journal of Physical Anthropology. 1972;**37**:161-172. DOI: 10.1002/ajpa.1330370202

[32] Schuller A. A note on the identification of skull X-ray pictures of the frontal sinus. The Medical Journal of Australia. 1943;**25**:554-556

[33] Arnaud E, Reniet D, Marchac D. Development of the frontal sinus and glabellar morphology after frontocranial remodelling for craniosynostosis in infancy. Journal of Cranio-Maxillo-Facial Surgery. 1994;**5**:81-92. DOI: 10.1097/00001665-199405000-00006

[34] Kim GR. A morphological study of the paranasal sinuses in Koreans. Yonsei Medical Journal. 1962;**3**:11-17

[35] Aydinlioğlu A, Kavakli A, Erdem S. Absence of frontal sinus in Turkish individuals. Yonsei Medical Journal. 2003;**4**:215-218. DOI: 10.3349/ymj.2003.44.2.215

[36] Çakur B, Sumbullu MA, Durna MB. Aplasia and agenesis of the frontal sinus in Turkish individuals: A retrospective study using dental volumetric tomography. International Journal of Medical Sciences. 2011;**8**:278-282. DOI: 10.7150/ijms.8.278

[37] Soman BA, Sujatha GP, Lingappa A. Morphometric evaluation of the frontal sinus in relation to age and gender in subjects residing in Davangere, Karnataka. Journal of Forensic Dental Sciences. 2016;**8**:57. DOI: 10.4103/0975-1475.176945

[38] Danesh-Sani SA, Bavandi R, Esmaili M. Frontal sinus agenesis using computed tomography. The Journal of Craniofacial Surgery. 2011;**22**:e48-e51. DOI: 10.1097/SCS.0b013e318231e26c

[39] Moideen SP, Khizer Hussain Afroze M, Mohan M, Regina M, Sheriff RM, Moideen CP. Incidence of frontal sinus aplasia in Indian population. International Journal of Otolaryngology and Head & Neck Surgery. 2017;**3**:108-111. DOI: 10.18203/issn.2454-5929.ijohns20164811

[40] Hodgson G. In: A Text-Book of x-Ray Diagnosis. 3rd ed. Vol. 1. London: H.K. Lewis; 1939

[41] Ozgursoy OB, Comert A, Yorulmaz I, Tekdemir I, Elhan A, Kucuk B. Hidden unilateral agenesis of the frontal sinus: Human cadaver study of a potential surgical pitfall. American Journal of Otolaryngology. 2010;**31**:231-234. DOI: 10.1016/j.amjoto.2009.02.010

[42] Urken ML, Som PM, Edelstein D, Lawson W, Weber AL, Biller HF. Abnormally large frontal sinus. II. Nomenclature, pathology, and symptoms. The Laryngoscope. 1987;**97**:606-611. DOI: 10.1288/00005537-198705000-00014

[43] Canalis E, Zanotti S. Hajdu-Cheney syndrome: A review. Orphanet Journal of Rare Diseases. 2014;**9**:200. DOI: 10.1186/s13023-014-0200-y

[44] Eggesbø HB, Søvik S, Dølvik S, Eiklid K, Kolmannskog F. CT characterization of developmental variations of the paranasal sinuses in cystic fibrosis. Acta Radiologica. 2001;**42**:482-493. DOI: 10.1080/028418501127347214

[45] Yoshino M, Miyasaka S, Sato H, Seta S. Classification system of frontal sinus patterns by radiography. Its application to identification of unknown skeletal remains. Forensic Science International. 1987;**34**:289-299. DOI: 10.1016/0379-0738(87)90041-7

[46] Christensen AM. Assessing the variation in individual frontal sinus outlines. American Journal of Physical Anthropology. 2005;**127**:291-296. DOI: 10.1002/ajpa.20116

[47] Uthman AT, Al-Rawi NH, Al-Naaimi AS, Tawfeeq AS, Suhail EH. Evaluation of frontal sinus and skull measurements using spiral CT scanning: An aid in unknown person identification. Forensic Science International. 2010;**197**:124.e1-124.e7. DOI: 10.1016/j.forsciint.2009

[48] Quatrehomme G, Fronty P, Sapanet M, Grévin G, Bailet P, Ollier A. Identification by frontal sinus pattern in forensic anthropology. Forensic Science International. 1996;**83**:147-153. DOI: 10.1016/S0379-0738(96)02033-6

[49] Ruder TD, Brun C, Christensen AM, Thali MJ, Gascho D, Schweitzer W, Hatch GM. Comparative radiologic identification with CT images of paranasal sinuses – Development of a standardized approach. Journal of Forensic Radiology and Imaging. 2016;**7**:1-9. DOI: 10.1016/j.jofri.2016.09.001

[50] Cossellu G, De Luca S, Biagi R, Farronato G, et al. Reliability of frontal sinus by cone beam-computed tomography (CBCT) for individual identification. La Radiologia Medica. 2015;**120**:1130-1136. DOI: 10.1007/s11547-015-0552-y

[51] Soares CB, Almeida MS, Lopes Pde M, Beltrão RV, Pontual Ados A, Ramos-Perez FM, Figueroa JN, Pontual ML. Human identification study by means of frontal sinus imaginological aspects. Forensic Science International. 2016;**262**:183-189. DOI: 10.1016/j.forsciint.2016.03.030

[52] Brun CN, Christensen AM, Kravarski M, Gorincour G, Schweitzer W, Thali MJ, Gascho D, Hatch GM, Ruder TD. Comparative radiologic identification with standardized single CT images of the paranasal sinuses-evaluation of inter-rater reliability. Forensic Science International. 2017;**280**:81-86. DOI: 10.1016/j.forsciint.2017.08.029

[53] Belaldavar C, Kotrashetti VS, Hallikerimath SR, Kale AD. Assessment of frontal sinus dimensions to determine sexual dimorphism among Indian adults. Journal of Forensic Dental Sciences. 2014;**6**:25-30. DOI: 10.4103/0975-1475.127766

[54] Tubbs RS, Elton S, Salter G, Blount JP, Grabb PA, Oakes WJ. Superficial surgical landmarks for the frontal sinus. Journal of Neurosurgery. 2002;**96**:320-322. DOI: 10.3171/jns.2002.96.2.0320

[55] Amusa YB, Eziyi JAE, Akinlade O, Famurewa OC, Adewole SA, Nwoha PU, Ameye SA. Volumetric measurements and anatomical variants of paranasal sinuses of Africans (Nigerians) using dry crania. International Journal of Medicine and Medical Sciences. 2011;**3**:299-303

[56] Natsis K, Karabatakis V, Tsikaras P, Chatzibalis T, Stangos N. Frontal sinus anatomical variations with potential consequences for the orbit. Study on cadavers. Morphologie. 2004;**88**:35-38. DOI: 10.1016/S1286-0115(04)97997-0

[57] Pobornikova S. An x-ray investigation of the development of the frontal sinuses in children. Folia Medica (Plovdiv). 1974;**16**:213-220

[58] Nikolova S, Toneva D, Georgiev I, Dandov A, Lazarov N. Morphometric analysis of the frontal sinus: Application of industrial digital radiography and virtual endocast. JOFRI. 2018;**12**:31-39. DOI: 10.1016/j.jofri.2018.02.001

[59] Nikolova S, Toneva D, Georgiev I, Yordanov Y, Lazarov N. Two cases of large bregmatic bone along with a persistent metopic suture from necropoles on the northern Black Sea coast of Bulgaria. Anthropological Science. 2016;**124**:145-153. DOI: 10.1537/ase.160530

[60] Nikolova S, Toneva D, Georgiev I, Harizanov S, Zlatareva D, Hadjidekov V, Lazarov N. A CT-study of the cranial suture morphology and its reorganization during the obliteration. Collegium Antropologicum. 2017;**41**:125-131

[61] Manzanares MC, Goret-Nicaise M, Dhem A. Metopic sutural closure in the human skull. Journal of Anatomy. 1988;**161**:203-215

[62] Faro C, Benoit B, Wegrzyn P, Chaoui R, Nicolaides KH. Three-dimensional sonographic description of the fetal frontal bones and metopic suture. Ultrasound in Obstetrics & Gynecology. 2005;**26**:618-621. DOI: 10.1002/uog.1997

[63] Moss ML. Experimental alteration of sutural area morphology. Anatomical Record. 1957;**127**:569-589. DOI: 10.1002/ar.1091270307

[64] Hinton DR, Becker LE, Muakkassa KF, Hoffman HJ. Lambdoid synostosis. I. The lamboid suture: Normal development and pathology of 'synostosis'. Journal of Neurosurgery. 1984;**61**:333-339. DOI: 10.3171/jns.1984.61.2.0333

[65] Moss ML. Fusion of the frontal suture in the rat. The American Journal of Anatomy. 1958;**102**:141-165. DOI: 10.1002/aja.1001020107

[66] Vu HL, Panchal J, Parker EE, et al. The timing of physiologic closure of the metopic suture: A review of 159 patients using reconstructed 3D CT scans of the craniofacial region. The Journal of Craniofacial Surgery. 2001;**12**:527-532

[67] Weinzweig J, Kirschner RE, Farley A, Reiss P, Hunter J, Whitaker LA, Bartlett SP. Metopic synostosis: Defining the temporal sequence of normal suture fusion and differentiating it from synostosis on the basis of computed tomography images. Plastic and Reconstructive Surgery. 2003;**112**:1211-1218. DOI: 10.1097/01.PRS.0000080729.28749.A3

[68] Bajwa M, Srinivasan D, Nishikawa H, Rodrigues D, Solanki G, White N. Normal fusion of the metopic suture. The Journal of Craniofacial Surgery. 2013;**24**:1201-1205. DOI: 10.1097/SCS.0b013e31829975c6

[69] Skrzat J, Walocha J, Zawiliński J. A note on the morphology of the metopic suture in the human skull. Folia Morphologica. 2004;**63**:481-484

[70] Van der Meulen J. Metopic synostosis. Child's Nervous System. 2012;**28**:1359-1367. DOI: 10.1007/s00381-012-1803-z

[71] Moss ML. Premature synostosis of the frontal suture in the cleft palate patient. Plastic and Reconstructive Surgery. 1957;**20**:199-205

[72] Riemenschneider PA. Trigonocephaly. Radiology. 1957;**68**:863-865. DOI: 10.1148/68.6.863

[73] Bryce TH. Osteology and arthrology. In: Schäfer EA, Symington J, Bryce TH, editors. Quain'S Elements of Anatomy. 11th ed. Vol. IV, Part I;1915. London: Longmans-Green. p. 177

[74] Keith A. Human Embryology and Morphology. 6th ed. London: Edward Arnold; 1948

[75] Woo J-K. Racial and sexual differences in the frontal curvature and its relation to metopism. American Journal of Physical Anthropology. 1949;**7**:215-226. DOI: 10.1002/ajpa.1330070205

[76] Breathnach AS. Frazer'S Anatomy of the Human Skeleton. 5th ed. London: J. & A. Churchill; 1958

[77] Romanes GJ, editor. Cunningham'S Textbook of Anatomy. 11th ed. London: Oxford University Press; 1972

[78] Berry AC. Factors affecting the incidence of non-metrical skeletal variants. Journal of Anatomy. 1975;**120**:519-535

[79] Nikolova S, Toneva D. Frequency of metopic suture in male and female medieval cranial series. Acta Morphologica et Anthropologica. 2012;**19**:250-252

[80] Nikolova S, Toneva D, Georgiev I. A case of skeletal dysplasia in bone remains from a contemporary male individual. Acta Morphologica et Anthropologica. 2015;**22**:97-107

[81] Ashley-Montagu MF. The Medio-frontal suture and the problem of Metopism in the primates. The Journal of the Royal Anthropological Institute of Great Britain and Ireland. 1937;**67**:157-201

[82] Del Sol M, Binvignat O, PDA B, Prates JC. Metopismo no individuo brasileiro. Revista Paulista de Medicina. 1989;**107**:105-107

[83] Bryce TH. Observations on Metopism. Journal of Anatomy. 1917;**51**:153-166

[84] Limson M. Metopism as found in Filipino skulls. American Journal of Physical Anthropology. 1924;**7**:317-324. DOI: 10.1002/ajpa.1330070319

[85] Schultz AH. The metopic Fontanelle, fissure, and suture. Developmental Dynamics. 1929;**44**:475-499. DOI: 10.1002/aja.1000440306

[86] Nikolova S, Toneva D, Georgiev I. Cranial Base angulation in metopic and non-metopic cranial series. Acta Morphologica et Anthropologica. 2017b;**24**:45-49

[87] McCarthy JG, Karp NS, LaTrenta GS, Thorne CH. The effect of early fronto-orbital advancement on frontal sinus development and forehead aesthetics. Plastic and Reconstructive Surgery. 1990;**86**:1078-1084

[88] Locher MC, Sailer HF, Haers PE, Carls FR, Oechslin CK, Grätz KW. Development of frontal sinus following bilateral fronto-orbital osteotomies. Journal of Cranio-Maxillofacial Surgery. 1998;**26**:129-135

[89] Auque J, Bracard S, Roland J, Sakka M. Effects of intracranial pressure on frontal sinus development. Bulletin de l'Association des Anatomistes. 1987;**71**:31-35

[90] Du Boulay GH. Principles of X-Ray Diagnosis of the Skull. London: Butterworths; 1980

[91] Fenichel GM. Increased intracranial pressure. In: Clinical Pediatric Neurology: A Signs and Symptoms Approach. Expert Consult. 6th ed. Philadelphia: Elsevier/Saunders; 2009

[92] Luo C, Chen J, Liao Q, Li Q, Yang X, Li Y. Influence of iron deficiency anemia on development of thymus and spleen and adenosine deaminase activity in rats. Hua Xi Yi Ke Da Xue Xue Bao. 1990;**21**:63-66

[93] Kulaksizoglu M, Ipekci SH, Gonulalan G, Ozturk M, Kaya A, Gonen MS, Cakir M: Do we need to replace GH to correct anemia in hypopituitarism? In: Proceedings of the Endocrine Society's 96th Annual Meeting and Expo; 21-24 June 2014; Chicago; SAT-0729

[94] Katsumata S, Katsumata-Tsuboi R, Uehara M, Suzuki K. Severe iron deficiency decreases both bone formation and bone resorption in rats. The Journal of Nutrition. 2009;**139**:238-243. DOI: 10.3945/jn.108.093757

[95] Reimann FV, Gedikoglu G, Talasli U. Metopism in iron deficiency disease: A roentgenological investigation. Fortschr Roentgenstr. 1978;**129**:246-249. DOI: 10.1055/s-0029-1231005

[96] Reimann FV, Cedikoglu C, Celik E, Ulukurlu L, Kilicözlü I. Deformity of the skull vault due to hypertrophy of red rnarrow in cases of anaemia. RoFo: Fortschritte auf dem Gebiete der Rontgenstrahlen und der Nuklearmedizin. 1981;**135**:20-24. DOI: 10.1055/s-2008-1056822

[97] Capriles FL. Intracranial hypertension and iron-deficiency anemia. Archives of Neurology. 1963;**9**:57-63. DOI: 10.1001/archneur.1963.00460080057008

[98] Mollan SP, Ball AK, Sinclair AJ, Madill SA, Clarke CE, Jacks AS, Burdon MA, Matthews TD. Idiopathic intracranial hypertension associated with iron deficiency anaemia: A lesson for management. European Neurology. 2009;**62**(2):105-108. DOI: 10.1159/000222781

[99] Rivollat M, Castex D, Hauret L, Tillier A. Ancient Down syndrome: An osteological case from saint-Jean-des-Vignes, northeastern France, from the 5-6th century AD. International Journal of Paleopathology. 2014;**7**:8-14. DOI: 10.1016/j.ijpp.2014.05.004

[100] Larocca LM, Lauriola L, Ranelletti FO, Piantelli M, Maggiano N, Ricci R, Capelli A. Morphological and immunohistochemical study of Down syndrome thymus. American Journal of Medical Genetics. Supplement. 1990;**7**:225-230. DOI: 10.1002/ajmg.1320370745

[101] Murdoch JC, Gray CA, McLarty DG, Ratcliffe JG. Pituitary function in Down's syndrome. Journal of Mental Deficiency Research. 1978;**22**:273-275. DOI: 10.1111/j.1365-2788.1978.tb00985.x

[102] Castells S, Beaulieu I, Torrado C, Wisniewski KE, Zarny S, Gelato MC. Hypothalamic versus pituitary dysfunction in Down's syndrome as cause of growth retardation. Journal of Intellectual Disability Research. 1996;**40**:509-517. DOI: 10.1046/j.1365-2788.1996.802802.x

[103] Tenenbaum A, Malkiel S, Wexler ID, Levy-Khademi F, Revel-Vilk S, Stepensky P. Anemia in children with Down syndrome. International Journal of Pediatrics. 2011:5. DOI: 10.1155/2011/813541

[104] Zivanovic S. Ancient Diseases: The Elements of Paleopathology. New York: Pica Press; 1982

Section 2

Challenging Issue on Sinus Augmentation

Chapter 2

Management of the Complications of Maxillary Sinus Augmentation

Alper Sindel, Mehmet Mustafa Özarslan and
Öznur Özalp

Additional information is available at the end of the chapter

http://dx.doi.org/10.5772/intechopen.80603

Abstract

Dental implant rehabilitation of the posterior maxillary region has always been a challenging issue due to both alveolar ridge atrophy and sinus pneumatization. Maxillary sinus augmentation is a well-known and predictable procedure in vertical deficiencies of the posterior maxilla. To date, various techniques have been described based on the physiology of intrasinus bone repair to obtain better outcomes. Nevertheless, these procedures could also be associated with several intra- and postoperative complications such as perforation of the sinus membrane, hemorrhage, infection, graft resorption, and loss of the graft or implants. The aim of this chapter is to review the contemporary methods for maxillary sinus augmentation and to present both recommendations for prevention and management of the associated complications.

Keywords: dental implants, complication, management, sinus augmentation, sinus lift

1. Introduction

Oral rehabilitation with dental implants has been widely practiced with a success rate well over 95% in complete, partial, or single edentulism [1]. However, dental implant placement in the posterior maxillary region is frequently compromised due to certain anatomical and physiological conditions including postextraction alveolar ridge atrophy, pneumatization of the maxillary sinus, and poor quality of residual alveolar bone [2]. Therefore, vertical alveolar ridge augmentation is often mandatory before or in conjunction with the installation of implants [3].

In this regard, maxillary sinus augmentation is a well-known, predictable, and largely required procedure for increasing residual alveolar bone height by elevation of the Schneiderian membrane [4]. Since the introduction of the surgical technique by Tatum [5] in 1976 and Boyne [6] in 1980, various approaches have been extensively studied.

Access to the Schneiderian membrane may generally be achieved directly by lateral approach or indirectly through transcrestal osteotomy. To date, numerous modifications using both approaches have been described, and the vast majority of them have proved their worth and efficacy over the years. Nevertheless, the procedure could also be associated with several intra- and postoperative complications, which may result with a negative impact on the patient's quality of life by additional surgery, hospitalization, and prolonged recovery time. Subsequently, the outcome of the implants and the success of the oral reconstruction procedure may be compromised [4].

Maxillary sinus augmentation procedures are increasingly performed by oral and maxillofacial surgeons, periodontists, dentists, and otorhinolaryngologists worldwide. Prevention and management of the associated complications principally begin with having a thorough knowledge of the sinus augmentation techniques. Thus, the purpose of this chapter is to review the contemporary methods for maxillary sinus augmentation and to present both recommendations for prevention and management of the associated complications.

2. Internal sinus lifting (crestal approach)

The crestal approach involves the elevation of both the Schneiderian membrane and bony floor of the sinus indirectly through the alveolar crest without a preparation on the lateral wall of the sinus. With this technique, the elevation of the sinus floor up to 5 mm without any perforations was shown microscopically [7]. Internal sinus lifting through the transcrestal approach is a well-validated surgical option for situations where there is a minimum of 5–6 mm residual bone height [8]. The technique is considered to be more conservative than the conventional lateral approach and may reduce the operation time and postoperative morbidity [4].

2.1. Surgical technique

Since its introduction in 1986 by Tatum [5], the crestal approach has undergone several modifications in an effort to expand its feasibility and obtain greater success rates with reduced complications [9]. Some of these modifications rely on using medical devices and instruments that are specific to their particular technique. All of these techniques have demonstrated high rates of success; however, there is still insufficient evidence from prospective studies to validate their utility in clinical practice.

2.1.1. Osteotome-mediated sinus floor elevation (OSFE)

OSFE is based on the use of a socket former for the selected implant size for preparing the implant site and hand tapping it in a vertical direction to accomplish a "green-stick fracture" of the sinus floor. Subsequently, implants are placed to support the elevated floor of the maxillary sinus. In 1994, Summers [8] described a modified approach for OSFE by using a set of conical osteotomes with increasing diameters for both implant site preparation and sinus floor elevation (**Figure 1**). This technique allows to increase the bone density, resulting in better primary stability of inserted dental implants.

2.1.2. Bone added osteotome-mediated sinus floor elevation (BAOSFE)

BAOSFE, also referred to as the "Summers technique," is a combination of the OSFE technique with the addition of a bone graft material. The mass of the native bone and the graft material is utilized as a hydraulic plug by the upward push of the osteotome to elevate the sinus floor. Subsequent placement of the implants facilitates the elevation of the sinus membrane by tenting it with their apical end. Various graft materials may be used such as autogenous bone, allografts, xenografts, and alloplastic bone materials [10]. There have been a number of studies claiming the necessity of bone graft material to keep the volume of the sinus membrane [11], whereas others have reported favorable results and reduced risk of infections without the use of any bone graft [12].

2.1.3. Minimally invasive antral membrane balloon elevation (MIAMBE)

MIAMBE is a modification of the BAOSFE method in which sinus lift is performed by the insertion of a specially designed balloon through the osteotomy site on the alveolar crest, insufflating it with saline solution through a catheter in order to detach the sinus membrane. This technique is intended to be applied to alveolar crests measuring 3 mm or less and provide a gain in height up to 10 mm with few intraoperative complications [13].

2.1.4. Hydrostatic sinus lift

Hydrostatic sinus lift technique, first proposed by Chen et al. [14] in 2005, relies on the principle of lifting the Schneiderian membrane using hydraulic pressure. Following the initial drilling, the drill is connected to a pump that produces high hydraulic pressure, which is used to break the sinus floor and to lift the membrane. Along with the recent developments, this technique is supposed to provide reduced risk for sinus membrane perforation, minimal trauma, and postoperative complications for sinus lifting surgery [15].

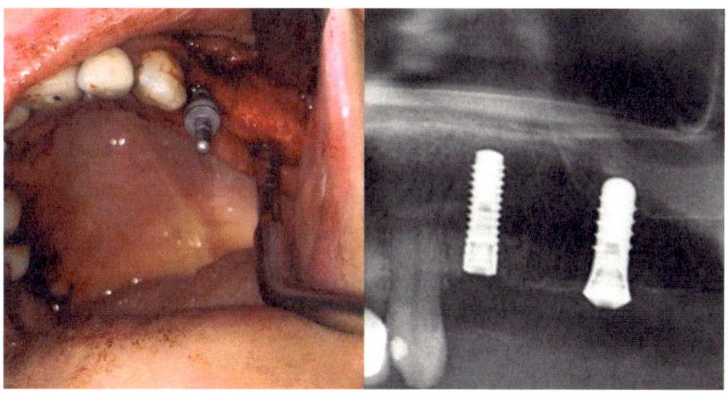

Figure 1. Use of conical osteotomes for both implant site preparation and sinus floor elevation and simultaneous implant installation.

2.2. Internal sinus lift complications: Prevention and management

Internal sinus lifting is associated with several intraoperative and postoperative complications, which may compromise the outcomes of the treatment and health of the patient. An in-depth overview on causes, prevention, and management of these complications is presented later.

2.2.1. *Intraoperative complications*

2.2.1.1. *The Schneiderian membrane perforation*

The main drawback of this procedure is the uncertainty of a possible perforation of the Schneiderian membrane because the sinus lifting procedure is performed blindly due to the impossibility to visualize the sinus floor [5, 6]. The incidence of membrane perforations in osteotome-mediated sinus lift has been reported to range between 4 and 25% [16], while such complication has been described in 25–44% of external sinus lifting cases [17]. It should also be noted that microlacerations are impossible to detect in many cases; thus, the true incidence may be higher than currently reported. Perforation of the sinus membrane may lead to the development of sinusitis, epistaxis, exfoliation of graft particles from the nose, or a patent oral-antral communication. Development of a sinus tear during the internal lifting may not always be determined with the Valsalva maneuver or more accurately by the inspection with an endoscope [18].

Membrane perforation may occur due to several factors related with anatomy, excessive tapping, or overzealous elevation. One possible anatomical challenge may be an oblique sinus floor at the site of preparation, which may lead difficulty in initial in-fracturing and resultant membrane perforation. Likewise, thin sinus mucosa and irregularities of the bony sinus floor such as sharp ridges, antral septa, and spines may pose risks for membrane perforation [19]. Furthermore, elevation of the Schneiderian membrane beyond its capacity may also cause the membrane to tear. To date, a wide range between 2 and 10 mm has been reported for height of sinus elevation using transcrestal techniques [2, 7, 13, 18]. A thorough clinical and radiological examination should be carried out to evaluate the anatomy of the sinus, the presence of sinus pathology, and the residual alveolar bone height. Additionally, intraoperative use of sinuscopy has been suggested to allow for elimination of any sinus pathologies, control of the graft position, and reduction of the risk of sinus membrane perforation and postoperative complications [7].

Although it has been reported that a gain up to 10 mm in alveolar height can be achieved using several modifications of transcrestal approach, it has commonly been assumed that the Schneiderian membrane can be safely elevated for 5 mm through the internal sinus lifting [7, 20]. Therefore, it should be kept in mind that the maximum elevation height obtainable with transcrestal techniques differs interindividually because it highly correlates to the elastic properties of the Schneiderian membrane and the maxillary sinus anatomy as well as the surgical technique of force transmission [21]. The osteotomes should not be tapped or advanced beyond the sinus border. Further attempts for the prevention of membrane perforation may include inserting a collagen membrane into the osteotomy and not to use the particulate graft materials with sharp nature.

Unfortunately, when membrane perforation is detected during the procedure, there is no possibility to repair the torn membrane without changing to a lateral surgical approach because of the limited access [18]. A number of researchers have reported that small perforations show complete recovery in 6 months spontaneously, and it is not required to abort the simultaneous placement of implants or bone grafts [18, 19]. However, if high risk of infection is suspected or the size of perforation is large, postponing the surgery or repairing the perforation through a lateral approach should be considered.

2.2.1.2. *Inadequate primary stability*

Implant stability initially relies on the host bone present at the created osteotomy site, while future additional support is potentially gained by the consolidation and amalgamation of the grafted material with newly formed host bone. Optimal primary stabilization at the time of implant placement is essential for implant success and survival [22]. Lack of primary stabilization may be related to insufficient bone height/width, poor bone quality, or overtreatment with the osteotomes. In cases where poor bone quality is encountered, consideration might be given to greater use of the osteotome versus drilling to increase the bone density and implant stability [22]. Further attempt might include the underpreparation of implant bed with either osteotomes or drills and insert a substantially larger diameter implant to maximize the primary stability. However, it should also be kept in mind that underpreparation may lead to excessive compression during the implant installation and resultant fracture of the bony trabeculae and poor recovery of vital bone. By the same token, the use of tapered implants versus parallel-walled implants has been shown to increase the primary stability in low-density bone as they have higher insertion torque during the placement [23]. Moreover, rough-surface implants are also recommended because they are more prone to adhesion of the bone fragment surfaces resulting in an increased bone formation [24].

2.2.1.3. *Displacement of the implant to the sinus cavity*

Although reportedly uncommon, accidental displacement of the implant into the sinus cavity may occur due to poor bone quality, untreated membrane perforation, and the use of excessive force during the installation [25]. The prevalence is probably underestimated due to the lack of cohort studies and few case reports that have been published [26]. A displaced implant should be removed from maxillary sinus as soon as possible to avoid further complications such as maxillary sinusitis, narrowing of the ostium, or reduced ciliary movements, impaired mucociliary clearance, pseudocyst formation, aspergillosis, migration into the ethmoid sinus, orbital floor, sphenoid sinus, or even the cranial fossa, orbital cellulitis and optic nerve damage, meningitis, or brain abscess [27–31]. Different techniques have been proposed for the removal of a displaced implant from the sinus using a transnasal or transoral approach [32]. The use of transnasal endoscopy has the advantages of a low morbidity, rapid recovery, and treatment of paranasal sinusitis, which, however, has several limitations including the requirement of a specific equipment, specialized surgery rooms, and often general anesthesia [33]. Moreover, the location and size of the implant have to pass through the ostium [25]. Alternatively, a transoral approach with the creation of a bony window in the anterior-lateral wall of the maxillary sinus can be performed. Transoral surgical techniques may remove implants successfully allowing a better visibility combined with the ability to remove even large implants under local anesthesia [32]. On the other hand, since this approach diminishes the integrity of the lateral wall of the maxilla, the access window may not completely reossify [34].

2.2.2. Postoperative complications

Postoperative infection, implant loss, benign paroxysmal positional vertigo, hemorrhage, nasal bleeding, blocked nose, hematomas, and loosening of cover screws are among the reported complications following the OSFE procedure.

2.2.2.1. Infection

Site infection is not only the most common postoperative complication but also among the foremost etiologies of possible complications. Infection may occur due to poor oral hygiene, contamination of the implant surface or graft material, and underlying diseases of the sinus. Particular attention should be paid to minimize the bacterial load during the surgery. The site should be evaluated for the presence of any active periodontal disease or endodontic infection. Moreover, the use of preoperative and postoperative antibiotics and antiseptic mouth rinses is also recommended to decrease potential pathogenic bacteria [35].

2.2.2.2. Benign paroxysmal positional vertigo (BPPV)

BPPV is a common vestibular end organ disorder characterized by short, repeated, brief periods of vertigo that are triggered by certain head movements in the plane of the posterior semicircular canals [36]. Recent evidence suggests that BPPV may occur as an early postoperative complication following OSFE [37]. It has been reported that the percussive forces of the surgical mallet may lead to the detachment of the otoliths from the otoconia layer of the utricular macula and cause them to float around in the endolymph [36, 38]. Moreover, hyperextension of the head during the operation favors the displacement of these free-floating particles into the posterior semicircular canal, creating the position- or motion-induced vertigo [39].

The diagnosis of BPPV is commonly established by the Dix-Hallpike test [40]. The patient experiences vertigo and a characteristic torsional nystagmus when moved quickly into a supine position with the head turned, so that the affected ear is 45° below the horizontal plane [41]. The direction of nystagmus is essential to specify the affected canal as both the vertical and the horizontal semicircular canals may be affected. The posterior canal is by far the most frequently affected canal (80–90%); involvement of the horizontal (lateral) canal is accounting for 5–30%, and the anterior canal is 1–2% of patients [42–44].

The treatment modalities of BPPV include follow-up of the patient, vestibulosuppressant medication, vestibular rehabilitation, repositioning maneuvers, and surgery [45]. Recent evidence supports that the repositioning maneuvers may effectively help in eliminating the vertigo due to BPPV, reducing the risks of falling, and improving the quality of life [44]. To date, several methods with different sequential head movements have been proposed to move otoconial debris from the semicircular canal to the utricle. Among these, the Epley maneuver (canalith repositioning procedure, CRP) and the Semont maneuver (the liberatory maneuver) have been proposed for the treatment of posterior-canal-type BPPV, while the lateral-canal-type BPPV is usually treated with the Lempert maneuver [46–48]. In addition, self-treatment exercises such as the Brandt-Daroff exercise have also been recommended for treatment of any types of BPPV [42, 49].

The incidence of OSFE-induced BPPV has been reported to be less than 3%, and the condition is self-limiting as symptoms subside or disappear within 6 months of onset [39]. However, the symptoms involved may be sufficiently severe to significantly alter the patient's daily life [41]. It is important to be aware of and inform patient about BPPV when performing OSFE. To prevent this complication, gentle hammering with a safe head position should be taken during the procedure. In suspected cases of BPPV, immediate referral to an otorhinolaryngologist is highly recommended.

2.2.2.3. *Implant loss*

Despite the high success rate, implant failures may occur as a consequence of abovementioned complications and patient-related local and systemic factors [50]. It has been reported that implant failures associated with OSFE usually occur before loading [51]. A subantral bone measured 4 mm or less at the time of implant placement has been shown to be associated with an almost 10–20% increase in implant failures [52]. Osteotome technique is usually recommended when more than 6 mm of residual bone height is present, and an increase of about 3–4 mm is expected.

3. External sinus lifting (lateral window technique)

Maxillary sinus floor augmentation using the lateral window technique was originally described by Tatum [5] in 1977 and subsequently published by Boyne [6] in 1980. This technique is still the most frequently used method to increase the amount of bone in the posterior maxilla before or in conjunction with implant placement [53].

3.1. Surgical technique

The technique is mainly based on the sequential steps of a trapdoor osteotomy on the lateral wall of the maxillary sinus and elevation of the Schneiderian membrane to create a confined space for the placement of graft material and dental implant. Over the past 30 years, lateral window technique has undergone numerous modifications including different techniques, graft materials, and implant placement protocols to increase the predictability of the procedure and reduce the rate of complications [53].

3.1.1. *Antrostomy techniques*

An antrostomy is made in the lateral sinus wall to get through to the Schneiderian membrane in order to create a space for the placement of the bone graft material and the implant. The size of the window should be wide enough to achieve sufficient access and vision to perform the membrane elevation and graft placement without complications. On the other hand, redundant expansion of the window should be avoided because it would compromise the blood supply to the graft.

Osteotomy can be made with either the rotary technique or the piezoelectric technique. The rotary technique is performed using a high-speed handpiece or surgical motor and preferably a round diamond or carbide bur. In line with the recent trend toward minimally invasive surgery, the use of piezosurgery has been reported to eliminate the "drag" created by rotary instrumentation and be less associated with the damage to the blood vessels or the Schneiderian membrane [54]. Furthermore, different approaches have also been described regarding the creation technique of the window. One method of creating the access window is abrading away all of the bone in the window area with a lateral cutting motion. As the bone is thinned, the sinus membrane is visualized as a blue shadow, and the thin bony layer is gently removed, creating a complete osteotomy (**Figure 2**). Another method is performing a trapdoor osteotomy in which the superior osteotomy cut is kept partially incomplete, and the lateral wall "window" is rotated (hinged) inward and upward to a horizontal position (**Figure 3**). Alternatively, a complete osteotomy can be performed extending 360° to create a bony island in the center. This can remain pedicled to the membrane and being elevated with it, or it can be removed to be used later for recovering the window (**Figure 4**). In reviewing the literature, there is no evidence that one approach is more favorable than another.

3.1.2. Bone grafting materials

A considerable amount of literature has been published on different types of biomaterials including autograft, allograft, xenograft, alloplast, and growth factors; however, debate continues about the ideal graft material for the maxillary sinus floor augmentation [55].

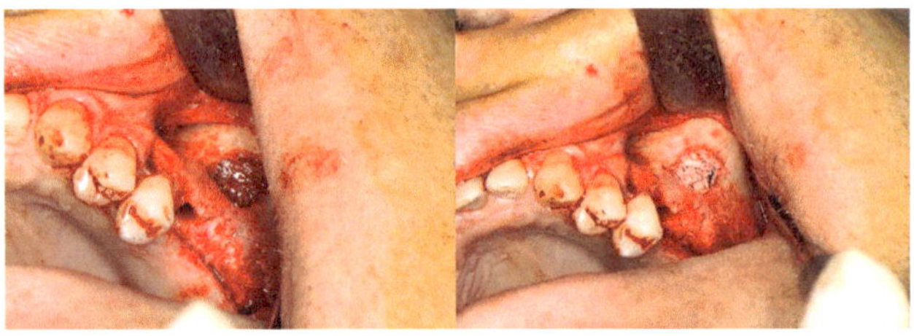

Figure 2. Access to the sinus through the abrasion of the bone and graft placement.

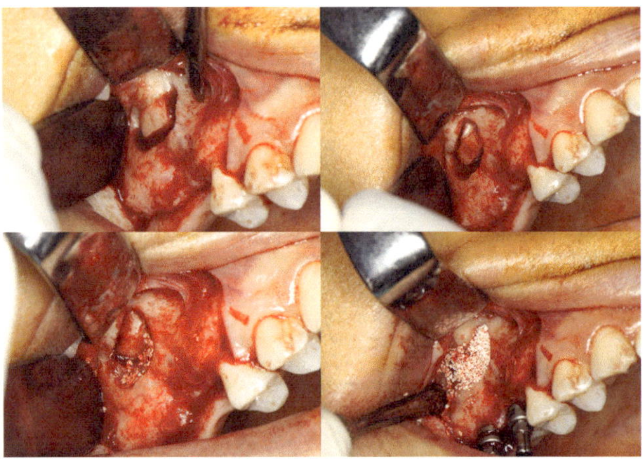

Figure 3. Access to the sinus performing a trapdoor osteotomy and simultaneous implant placement.

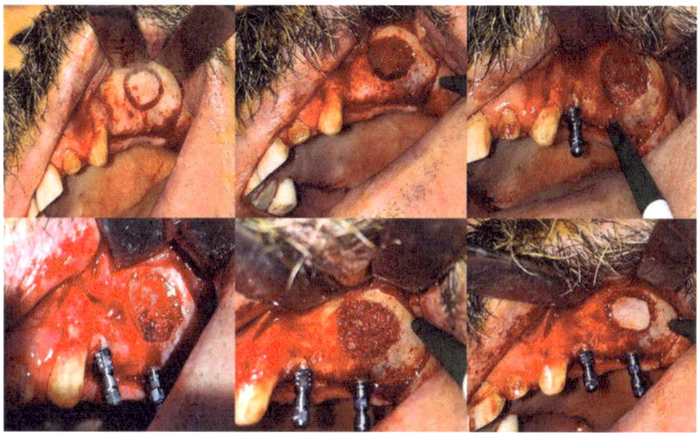

Figure 4. Access to the sinus by creation of a bony island and simultaneous implant placement. The bony island is used to re-cover the window.

Although autogenous bone graft has always been considered the gold standard in augmentation procedures due to its osteoinductive, osteogenic, and osteoconductive characteristics, the procedure is also associated with increased morbidity and significant graft resorption [56]. Therefore, the use of various bone replacement grafts of biologic or synthetic origin has become a major area of interest in order to simplify the surgical procedure by eliminating the need for bone harvesting [57]. Recent evidence suggests that implant survival rates with bone replacement grafts, particularly xenografts as the most rigorously evaluated substitute, are equal to or better than that achieved with autogenous bone [55].

On the other hand, there has also been an alternative concept of lateral window technique, which relies on using the implant to tent the membrane without a bone graft material [58]. Subsequent to the elevation of the Schneiderian membrane similar to the surgical protocol described above, simultaneous implant placement is performed. The blood clot formed around the exposed implant tip or a centrifuged autogenous blood product is used as the sole grafting material. Although several studies have demonstrated favorable results with high survival rates, there is still a lack of long-term clinical and radiographic studies on the amount of bone formation and final treatment outcome with this surgical intervention [58]. Thus, further research is needed to validate the outcomes and predictability of maxillary sinus lift applying the lateral window technique without a graft material and simultaneous implant installation.

3.1.3. Timing of implant placement

A one- or two-stage implant placement approach has been suggested in conjunction with lateral window maxillary sinus lift procedures. In two-stage technique, following the sinus augmentation and a healing period of 6 months or more, implants are placed with a second surgical intervention. Therefore, the one-stage procedure has been proposed in order to shorten the total period of treatment and to eliminate the requirement of a second surgery, thus reducing morbidity and cost [59]. Traditionally, a minimum of 4–5 mm of residual bone height is recommended for simultaneous implant placement with direct sinus lift to ensure initial stability [60]. On the other hand, recent clinical evidence also suggests that the simultaneous placement of implants with direct sinus lift may be a feasible treatment modality as long as adequate primary stability can be ensured, regardless of the recommended minimum residual bone height [61].

3.2. External sinus lift complications: Prevention and management

Although complication rate associated with the direct sinus lift procedure in the literature is quite low, several potential complications have been reported that increase the morbidity and jeopardize the treatment outcome [62].

3.2.1. Intraoperative complications

Surgical difficulties encountered during the course of the procedure may lead to the occurrence of several intraoperative complications. These difficulties may arise from the presence of complex anatomic situations, the choice of less predictable treatment options, inadequate systemic or local diagnosis, or operator error. The most frequent intraoperative complications are the Schneiderian membrane perforation and bleeding, while the others include the obstruction of the antral meatal ostium complex, dislocation of the implant into the sinus cavity, perforations in the buccal flap, and less frequently, injury to the infraorbital nerve [17, 63].

3.2.1.1. The Schneiderian membrane perforation

Sinus membrane perforation, being the most common complication during the sinus lift surgery, has been reported to occur with a range of incidence comprised between 20 and 44% of cases [17]. Membrane perforation may be encountered during different phases of the procedure including preparing the antrostomy, removal or turning over the bony window, raising the membrane, and placing the graft. Moreover, thin membrane, the presence of Underwood's septa, thick or convex lateral walls, a sharp angle between the buccal and palatal walls of the antral cavity, especially when below 30°, irregularities of the sinus floor due to the protrusion of the root profiles, previous interventions of the sinus, and a decreased residual alveolar height less than 3.5 mm are among the anatomical risk factors that prompt the occurrence of membrane perforation [64].

A precise evaluation using computed tomography (CT) may aid to determine the 3D anatomy of the sinus to minimize the rate of perforation. When septa are known to be present, lengthening the window in the anteroposterior direction is recommended in order to allow for a lateral-to-medial elevation of the membrane from both sides of the septum. An alternative to this approach is the creation of two separate windows; however, one should consider that this technique may result in small windows, which can complicate the access and vision [65]. Use of piezoelectric surgery has been proposed to be a valuable adjunct to sinus surgery, which has been shown to result in decreased membrane perforation rates [54]. Other considerations to prevent membrane perforation include using diamond burs and elevation of the membrane from lateral to medial while keeping the instrument in contact with the bone at all times.

Nevertheless, perforation is unavoidable in some cases despite accurate presurgical radiographic evaluation and ideal surgical maneuvers. Perforation of the sinus membrane may result in bacterial contamination and infection of the graft and dispersion of the particulate, leading to impairment of the functional homeostasis of the antral cavity [60]. Once the perforation is confirmed, the exact size of the perforation should be detected by gently raising the surrounding membrane to reduce the tension and to avoid further tearing. Minor perforations of less than 1 mm may self-repair by membrane foldover or clot formation, thus permitting simultaneous implant placement. In perforations smaller than 5 mm, using fibrin glues, collagen tapes, and bioabsorbable membranes or suturing the membrane is usually sufficient for closure that allows simultaneous implant placement. Membrane perforations larger than 5 mm may require bioabsorbable membranes, lamellar bone plates, suturing either alone or in combination with fibrin glue, or abandoning the intervention. Regardless of the size and repair method of the sinus membrane perforation, there should be no doubt about the stability of the perforated area to contain the graft material.

Since large perforations constitute an enormous challenge, several authors have studied and suggested specific repair methods based on the use of collagen membranes, local flaps, and autogenous bone blocks. Among these methods, "the Loma Linda pouch technique," which was introduced by Proussaefs et al. [66] in 2003, involves covering all internal bony walls of the sinus using a slow resorbing collagen membrane simulating the natural membrane and folding the membrane on the lateral wall with external tack fixation. However, pouch formation surrounding the graft material can impair the blood supply coming from the walls of the sinus, thus representing an impediment for the maturation of the graft and the recovery period [67]. More recently, "the intrasinusal locking technique" has been proposed by Sindel et al. [68], which allows for simultaneous implant placement in the presence of a large membrane perforation aiming to decrease the number of surgical interventions and the complications related to surgery. In this technique, autogenous bone ring blocks harvested from mandibular symphysis are placed internal to the floor of the maxillary sinus and stabilized with the simultaneously installed dental implant, using a mechanism similar to that of a screw and nut (**Figure 5**). The authors reported an implant survival rate of 90% without any postoperative complications such as maxillary sinusitis or infection.

3.2.1.2. Excessive bleeding

Intraoperative bleeding is the second most common intraoperative complication of sinus lift procedure [63]. Massive bleeding frequently occurs from damage to the alveolar antral artery (AAA), which is an intraosseous anastomosis between the posterior superior alveolar artery (PSAA) and the infraorbital artery. There is also a possibility of bleeding from extraosseous anastomosis of PSAA and infraorbital artery during the flap elevation and from posterior lateral nasal artery [69].

Although being usually minor, in some cases, bleeding may be difficult to control in a timely manner and induce additional complications such as membrane perforation, impairment of blood supply, and displacement of the graft material [63]. Preoperative evaluation using cone beam–computed tomography (CBCT) may help to create a window respecting the integrity of vascular structures [70]. Further attempts to decrease the risk of bleeding may include preparing the window through the piezosurgery or preferring the diamond burs than carbide burs when rotary instrumentation is used [54]. Management of vascular bleeding during the sinus lift procedure can be carried out by raising the head, applying the direct and firm pressure on the bleeding point, crushing the bone around the vessel, using local vasoconstrictor agents

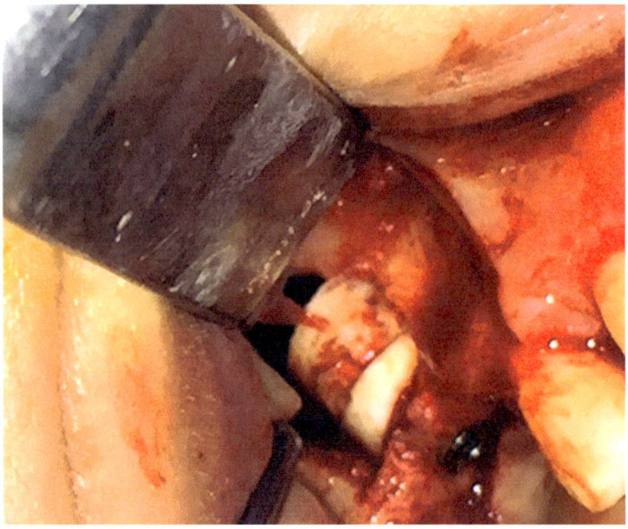

Figure 5. "Intrasinusal locking technique": Autogenous bone ring inside the sinus cavity is locked to the alveolar crest through the dental implant.

or bone wax, and suturing the vessels [17]. In addition, bleeding can be controlled through the use of electrocautery; however, much attention should be paid not to cause membrane perforation [71].

3.2.1.3. Other complications

Improper surgical technique may lead to the tears in the buccal flap while trying to achieve a tension-free closure. Hence, redundant release of the buccal flap should be avoided respecting to the thickness of the flap and convexity of the malar eminence. Likewise, advanced closure methods such as pedicled buccal mucosal flap should be considered in cases where sufficient tension-free closure could not be achieved by buccal flap release. Yet, another complication related to poor surgical technique is the infraorbital nerve damage, which may result from pressure during the flap retraction or dissection for releasing the flap for closure [72]. Care should be taken to identify and protect the nerve while performing surgery near the infraorbital nerve. Additionally, overfilling of the graft material should be avoided because it may lead to the obstruction of the antral meatal ostium complex [63].

3.2.2. Postoperative complications

Infection of the graft, acute sinusitis, flap dehiscence, over-filling necrosis, loss of graft material, formation of oroantral fistula, migration of dental implants into the sinus cavity, implant failure, cyst formation, and BPPV are among the postoperative complications specific to external sinus lift procedure. Furthermore, a number of nonspecific patient responses may also be encountered including edema, hematoma, minor nosebleed, and mild congestion likewise any other surgical procedure.

3.2.2.1. *Graft infection*

Sinus graft infection is a rare but important complication with a reported incidence up to 4.7% [73]. Various factors have been reported to predispose the graft infection such as preexisting sinus infection, membrane perforation, contamination of the graft with saliva, wound dehiscence, and inadequate aseptic technique. The symptoms of the graft infection include tenderness, fistulation, suppuration, severe pain, facial swelling, abscess, elevated body temperature, and loss of graft particles through the fistulous tracts (popcorn sign).

The condition needs to be urgently treated due to the risk of quick spread of the infection to the adjacent structures, which may result in infraorbital abscess, orbital cellulites, and even brain abscess [74]. Several modalities involving irrigation, drainage, administration of systemic antibiotics, and partial or total removal of the graft material have been proposed for the treatment [75]. Superficial infections may be treated with the use of antibiotics alone; however, this modality may result in further progression of the infection requiring the complete removal of the graft. Recently, Mahler et al. [76] have described "the Dome phenomenon," which refers to a dense, solid, hard tissue maintained in the superiormost aspect of the grafted area in case of a graft infection. They reported successful outcomes with partial removal of the infected graft until this dome-shaped area indicating the regenerative potential of the Schneiderian membrane. Generally, the use of a new augmentation material is not recommended to prevent repeated infection because the thorough elimination of infected graft material can enable spontaneous bone fill in majority of the cases.

3.2.2.2. *Acute maxillary sinusitis*

The altered anatomic relation of the antral floor along with a hematoma or a seroma that fills up the maxillary sinus may lead to the obliteration of the osteomeatal unit [77]. Furthermore, the displacement of the graft materials through the sinus membrane or overfilling of the sinus may also result in the impairment of mucociliary clearance. Apart from these, aberrant anatomical factors such as ostium stenosis or preexisting sinus disease may also facilitate the development of acute sinusitis following the sinus lifting procedure [78]. Acute maxillary sinusitis may jeopardize the survival of the implants and the graft. Medical treatment with decongestants and antibiotics should be obtained in patients with a predisposition to sinusitis. In addition, consultation with an otolaryngologist should be considered to confirm whether the management of sinusitis can be carried out conservatively or the sinus patency requires additional surgical intervention.

3.2.2.3. *Other complications*

Increased intrasinus pressure may result in overflow of the graft material through the window and consequent wound dehiscence in the early postoperative period. This rare complication may be avoided by placing and stabilizing a membrane over the window or recovering it with the intact bony window.

As well as being an intraoperative complication, the dental implant migration into the maxillary sinus may also occur after several months or even years of its adequate functioning [79].

Various factors have been suggested to explain the mechanism of late migration including the changes in intrasinusal and nasal pressures, the lack of osseointegration, peri-implant bone destruction due to an autoimmune reaction, and the resorption produced by an incorrect distribution of occlusal force [80]. (See Section 2.2.1 for the management.)

Another unusual complication of direct sinus lift procedure is the formation of an oroantral fistula, which results from the progressive sinus infection and ostium blockage [81]. Following the elimination of the sinus infection, different techniques such as buccal flap, palatal rotation-advancement flap, and buccal fat pad can be used for the treatment of the oroantral communication.

4. Conclusion

Maxillary sinus augmentation, either crestal or lateral window approach, is a well-known, predictable, and often mandatory procedure to increase the alveolar bone height in posterior maxilla for dental implant rehabilitation. However, the procedure is also associated with certain complications that may influence the outcome of the therapy and patients' quality of life. A thorough knowledge of prevention and proper management of these complications is essential to obtain better treatment outcomes.

Author details

Alper Sindel[1]*, Mehmet Mustafa Özarslan[2] and Öznur Özalp[1]

*Address all correspondence to: dtalpersindel@gmail.com

1 Department of Oral and Maxillofacial Surgery, Faculty of Dentistry, Akdeniz University, Antalya, Turkey

2 Department of Prosthodontics, Faculty of Dentistry, Akdeniz University, Antalya, Turkey

References

[1] Buser D, Sennerby L, De Bruyn H. Modern implant dentistry based on osseointegration: 50 years of progress, current trends and open questions. Periodontology 2000. 2017; **73**:7-21

[2] Toffler M. Minimally invasive sinus floor elevation procedures for simultaneous and staged implant placement. New York State Dental Journal. 2004;**70**:38

[3] Raja SV. Management of the posterior maxilla with sinus lift: Review of techniques. Journal of Oral and Maxillofacial Surgery. 2009;**67**:1730-1734

[4] Vazquez JCM, de Rivera ASG, Gil HS, Mifsut RS. Complication rate in 200 consecutive sinus lift procedures: Guidelines for prevention and treatment. Journal of Oral and Maxillofacial Surgery. 2014;**72**:892-901

[5] Tatum JH. Maxillary and sinus implant reconstructions. Dental Clinics of North America. 1986;**30**:207-229

[6] Boyne PJ. Grafting of the maxillary sinus floor with autogenous marrow and bone. Journal of Oral Surgery. 1980;**38**:613-616

[7] Engelke W, Deckwer I. Endoscopically controlled sinus floor augmentation. A preliminary report. Clinical Oral Implants Research. 1997;**8**:527-531

[8] Summers RB. A new concept in maxillary implant surgery: The osteotome technique. Compendium (Newtown, Pa). 1994;**15**(152):154-156. 158 passim; quiz 162

[9] Li T. Sinus floor elevation: A revised osteotome technique and its biological concept. Compendium of Continuing Education in Dentistry (Jamesburg, NJ: 1995). 2005;**26**: 619-620, 622, 624-616 passim; quiz 630, 669

[10] Del Fabbro M, Corbella S, Weinstein T, Ceresoli V, Taschieri S. Implant survival rates after osteotome-mediated maxillary sinus augmentation: A systematic review. Clinical Implant Dentistry and Related Research. 2012;**14**:e159-e168

[11] Pjetursson BE, Ignjatovic D, Matuliene G, Brägger U, Schmidlin K, Lang NP. Transalveolar maxillary sinus floor elevation using osteotomes with or without grafting material. Part ii: Radiographic tissue remodeling. Clinical Oral Implants Research. 2009;**20**:677-683

[12] Pérez-Martínez S, Martorell-Calatayud L, Peñarrocha-Oltra D, García-Mira B, Peñarrocha-Diago M. Indirect sinus lift without bone graft material: Systematic review and meta-analysis. Journal of Clinical and Experimental Dentistry. 2015;**7**:e316

[13] Peñarrocha-Diago M, Galán-Gil S, Carrillo-García C, Peñarrocha-Diago D, Peñarrocha-Diago M. Transcrestal sinus lift and implant placement using the sinus balloon technique. Medicina Oral, Patología Oral y Cirugía Bucal. 2012;**17**:e122

[14] Chen L, Cha J. An 8 year retrospective study: 1100 patients receiving 1557 implants using the minimally invasive hydraulic sinus condensing technique. Journal of Periodontology. 2005;**76**:482-491

[15] Kao DW, DeHaven HA Jr. Controlled hydrostatic sinus elevation: A novel method of elevating the sinus membrane. Implant Dentistry. 2011;**20**:425-429

[16] Reiser GM, Rabinovitz Z, Bruno J, Damoulis PD, Griffin TJ. Evaluation of maxillary sinus membrane response following elevation with the crestal osteotome technique in human cadavers. The International Journal of Oral & Maxillofacial Implants. 2001;**16**:833-840

[17] Zijderveld SA, van den Bergh JP, Schulten EA, Christiaan M. Anatomical and surgical findings and complications in 100 consecutive maxillary sinus floor elevation procedures. Journal of Oral and Maxillofacial Surgery. 2008;**66**:1426-1438

[18] Nkenke E, Schlegel A, Schultze-Mosgau S, Neukam FW, Wiltfang J. The endoscopically controlled osteotome sinus floor elevation: A preliminary prospective study. The International Journal of Oral & Maxillofacial Implants. 2002;**17**:557-566

[19] Berengo M, Sivolella S, Majzoub Z, Cordioli G. Endoscopic evaluation of the bone-added osteotome sinus floor elevation procedure. International Journal of Oral and Maxillofacial Surgery. 2004;**33**:189-194

[20] Nedir R, Bischof M, Vazquez L, Szmukler-Moncler S, Bernard JP. Osteotome sinus floor elevation without grafting material: A 1 year prospective pilot study with ITI implants. Clinical Oral Implants Research. 2006;**17**:679-686

[21] Pommer B, Unger E, Sütö D, Hack N, Watzek G. Mechanical properties of the schneiderian membrane in vitro. Clinical Oral Implants Research. 2009;**20**:633-637

[22] Aparicio C, Lang NP, Rangert B. Validity and clinical significance of biomechanical testing of implant/bone interface. Clinical Oral Implants Research. 2006;**17**:2-7

[23] Wilson T Jr, Miller R, Trushkowsky R, Dard M. Tapered implants in dentistry: Revitalizing concepts with technology: A review. Advances in Dental Research. 2016;**28**:4-9

[24] Javed F, Ahmed HB, Crespi R, Romanos GE. Role of primary stability for successful osseointegration of dental implants: Factors of influence and evaluation. Interventional Medicine and Applied Science. 2013;**5**:162-167

[25] Chiapasco M, Felisati G, Maccari A, Borloni R, Gatti F, Di Leo F. The management of complications following displacement of oral implants in the paranasal sinuses: A multicenter clinical report and proposed treatment protocols. International Journal of Oral and Maxillofacial Surgery. 2009;**38**:1273-1278

[26] Ridaura-Ruiz L, Figueiredo R, Guinot-Moya R, Piñera-Penalva M, Sanchez-Garcés MA, Valmaseda-Castellón E, Gay-Escoda C. Accidental displacement of dental implants into the maxillary sinus: A report of nine cases. Clinical implant dentistry and related research. 2009;**11**:e38-e45

[27] Cascone P, Ungari C, Filiaci F, Gabriele G, Ramieri V. A dental implant in the anterior cranial fossae. International Journal of Oral and Maxillofacial Surgery. 2010;**39**:92-93

[28] Kastner J, Taudy M, Lisy J, Grabec P, Betka J. Orbital and intracranial complications after acute rhinosinusitis. Rhinology. 2010;**48**:457-461

[29] De Foer C, Fossion E, Vaillant J-M. Sinus aspergillosis. Journal of Cranio-Maxillofacial Surgery. 1990;**18**:33-40

[30] Haben CM, Balys R, Frenkiel S. Dental implant migration into the ethmoid sinus. The Journal of Otolaryngology. 2003;**32**:342

[31] Felisati G, Lozza P, Chiapasco M, Borloni R. Endoscopic removal of an unusual foreign body in the sphenoid sinus: An oral implant. Clinical Oral Implants Research. 2007; **18**:776-780

[32] Jeong K-I, Kim S-G, Oh J-S, You J-S. Implants displaced into the maxillary sinus: A systematic review. Implant Dentistry. 2016;**25**:547-551

[33] González-García A, González-García J, Diniz-Freitas M, García-García A, Bullón P. Accidental displacement and migration of endosseous implants into adjacent craniofacial structures: A review and update. Medicina Oral, Patología Oral y Cirugía Bucal. 2012;**17**:e769

[34] Bassi MA, Andrisani C, Lico S, Ormanier Z, Arcuri C. Endoscopic retrieval of a dental implant into the maxillary sinus: A case report. ORAL & Implantology. 2016;**9**:69

[35] Testori T, Drago L, Wallace SS, Capelli M, Galli F, Zuffetti F, Parenti A, Deflorian M, Fumagalli L, Weinstein RL. Prevention and treatment of postoperative infections after sinus elevation surgery: Clinical consensus and recommendations. International journal of dentistry. 2012;**2012**:365809

[36] Penarrocha-Diago M, Rambla-Ferrer J, Perez V, Perez-Garrigues H. Benign paroxysmal vertigo secondary to placement of maxillary implants using the alveolar expansion technique with osteotomes: A study of 4 cases. The International Journal of Oral & Maxillofacial Implants. 2008;**23**:129-132

[37] Giannini S, Signorini L, Bonanome L, Severino M, Corpaci F, Cielo A. Benign paroxysmal positional vertigo (bppv): It may occur after dental implantology. A mini topical review. European Review for Medical and Pharmacological Sciences. 2015;**19**:3543-3547

[38] Saker M, Ogle O. Benign paroxysmal positional vertigo subsequent to sinus lift via closed technique. Journal of Oral and Maxillofacial Surgery. 2005;**63**:1385-1387

[39] Sammartino G, Mariniello M, Scaravilli MS. Benign paroxysmal positional vertigo following closed sinus floor elevation procedure: Mallet osteotomes vs. Screwable osteotomes. A triple blind randomized controlled trial. Clinical Oral Implants Research. 2011;**22**:669-672

[40] Dix M, Hallpike C. The pathology, symptomatology and diagnosis of certain common disorders of the vestibular system. In: Proceedings of the Royal Society of Medicine. SAGE Publications; 1952;**45**:341-354

[41] Su GN-C, Tai P-W, Su P-T, Chien H-H. Protracted benign paroxysmal positional vertigo following osteotome sinus floor elevation: A case report. The International Journal of Oral & Maxillofacial Implants. 2008;**23**:955-959

[42] Bhattacharyya N, Baugh RF, Orvidas L, Barrs D, Bronston LJ, Cass S, et al. Clinical practice guideline: Benign paroxysmal positional vertigo. Otolaryngology–Head and Neck Surgery. 2008;**139**:47-81

[43] Çakir BÖ, Ercan İ, Çakir ZA, Civelek Ş, Sayin İ, Turgut S. What is the true incidence of horizontal semicircular canal benign paroxysmal positional vertigo? Otolaryngology–Head and Neck Surgery. 2006;**134**:451-454

[44] Imai T, Takeda N, Ikezono T, Shigeno K, Asai M, Watanabe Y, et al. Classification, diagnostic criteria and management of benign paroxysmal positional vertigo. Auris, Nasus, Larynx. 2017;**44**:1-6

[45] Tang H, Li W. Advances in the diagnosis and treatment of benign paroxysmal positional vertigo. Experimental and Therapeutic Medicine. 2017;**14**:2424-2430

[46] Epley JM. The canalith repositioning procedure: For treatment of benign paroxysmal positional vertigo. Otolaryngology–Head and Neck Surgery. 1992;**107**:399-404

[47] Semont A, Freyss G, Vitte E. Curing the bppv with a liberatory maneuver. Advanced Otorhinolaryngology. 1988;**42**:290-293

[48] Lempert T, Tiel-Wilck K. A positional maneuver for treatment of horizontal-canal benign positional vertigo. The Laryngoscope. 1996;**106**:476-478

[49] Brandt T, Daroff RB. Physical therapy for benign paroxysmal positional vertigo. Archives of Otolaryngology. 1980;**106**:484-485

[50] Sakka S, Coulthard P. Implant failure: Etiology and complications. Medicina Oral, Patología Oral y Cirugía Bucal. 2011;**16**:e42-e44

[51] Shi J-Y, Gu Y-X, Zhuang L-F, Lai H-C. Survival of implants using the osteotome technique with or without grafting in the posterior maxilla: A systematic review. The International Journal of Oral & Maxillofacial Implants. 2016;**31**:1077-1088

[52] Toffler M, Rosen PS. Complications with transcrestal sinus floor elevation: Etiology, prevention, and treatment. In: Dental Implant Complications: Etiology, Prevention, and Treatment. Hoboken, New Jersey, United States: Wiley-Blackwell; 2015;**2**:427-456

[53] Starch-Jensen T, Aludden H, Hallman M, Dahlin C, Christensen A-E, Mordenfeld A. A systematic review and meta-analysis of long-term studies (five or more years) assessing maxillary sinus floor augmentation. International Journal of Oral and Maxillofacial Surgery. 2018;**47**:103-116

[54] Blus C, Szmukler-Moncler S, Salama M, Salama H, Garber D. Sinus bone grafting procedures using ultrasonic bone surgery: 5 year experience. The International Journal of Periodontics & Restorative Dentistry. 2008;**28**:221-229

[55] Wallace SS, Tarnow DP, Froum SJ, Cho S-C, Zadeh HH, Stoupel J, et al. Maxillary sinus elevation by lateral window approach: Evolution of technology and technique. The Journal of Evidence-Based Dental Practice. 2012;**12**:161-171

[56] Shanbhag S, Shanbhag V, Stavropoulos A. Volume changes of maxillary sinus augmentations over time: A systematic review. The International Journal of Oral & Maxillofacial Implants. 2014;**29**:881-892

[57] Danesh-Sani SA, Loomer PM, Wallace SS. A comprehensive clinical review of maxillary sinus floor elevation: Anatomy, techniques, biomaterials and complications. British Journal of Oral and Maxillofacial Surgery. 2016;**54**:724-730

[58] Borges FL, Dias RO, Piattelli A, Onuma T, Gouveia Cardoso LA, Salomão M, et al. Simultaneous sinus membrane elevation and dental implant placement without bone graft: A 6 month follow-up study. Journal of Periodontology. 2011;**82**:403-412

[59] Lambert F, Lecloux G, Rompen E. One-step approach for implant placement and subantral bone regeneration using bovine hydroxyapatite: A 2-6 year follow-up study. The International Journal of Oral & Maxillofacial Implants. 2010;**25**:598-606

[60] Jensen OT, Shulman LB, Block MS, Iacono VJ. Report of the sinus consensus conference of 1996. The International Journal of Oral & Maxillofacial Implants. 1998;**13**:11-45

[61] Cha HS, Kim A, Nowzari H, Chang HS, Ahn KM. Simultaneous sinus lift and implant installation: Prospective study of consecutive two hundred seventeen sinus lift and four hundred sixty-two implants. Clinical Implant Dentistry and Related Research. 2014;**16**:337-347

[62] Lee H-W, Lin W-S, Morton D. A retrospective study of complications associated with 100 consecutive maxillary sinus augmentations via the lateral window approach. The International Journal of Oral & Maxillofacial Implants. 2013;**28**:860-868

[63] Maridati P, Stoffella E, Speroni S, Cicciu M, Maiorana C. Alveolar antral artery isolation during sinus lift procedure with the double window technique. The Open Dentistry Journal. 2014;**8**:95

[64] Al-Dajani M. Incidence, risk factors, and complications of schneiderian membrane perforation in sinus lift surgery: A meta-analysis. Implant Dentistry. 2016;**25**:409-415

[65] Betts NJ, Miloro M. Modification of the sinus lift procedure for septa in the maxillary antrum. Journal of Oral and Maxillofacial Surgery. 1994;**52**:332-333

[66] Proussaefs P, Lozada J. The "Loma linda pouch": A technique for repairing the perforated sinus membrane. The International Journal of Periodontics & Restorative Dentistry. 2003;**23**:593-597

[67] Meleo D, Mangione F, Corbi S, Pacifici L. Management of the schneiderian membrane perforation during the maxillary sinus elevation procedure: A case report. Annali di Stomatologia. 2012;**3**:24

[68] Sindel A, Özarslan M, Özalp Ö. Intrasinusal locking technique: A novel use of the ring block technique at sinus perforations for simultaneous implant placement. International Journal of Oral and Maxillofacial Surgery. 2018;**47**:499-504

[69] Flanagan D. Arterial supply of maxillary sinus and potential for bleeding complication during lateral approach sinus elevation. Implant Dentistry. 2005;**14**:336-339

[70] Rosano G, Taschieri S, Gaudy JF, Weinstein T, Del Fabbro M. Maxillary sinus vascular anatomy and its relation to sinus lift surgery. Clinical Oral Implants Research. 2011; **22**:711-715

[71] Katranji A, Fotek P, Wang H-L. Sinus augmentation complications: Etiology and treatment. Implant Dentistry. 2008;**17**:339-349

[72] Tourbah B, Maarek H. Complications of maxillary sinus bone augmentation: Prevention and management. In: Sinus Grafting Techniques. Cham, Switzerland: Springer; 2015. pp. 195-233

[73] Jensen SS, Terheyden H. Bone augmentation procedures in localized defects in the alveolar ridge: Clinical results with different bone grafts and bone-substitute materials. The International Journal of Oral & Maxillofacial Implants. 2009;**24**:218-236

[74] Hong S-B, Kim J-S, Shin S-I, Han J-Y, Herr Y, Chung J-H. Clinical treatment of postoperative infection following sinus augmentation. Journal of Periodontal & Implant Science. 2010;**40**:144-149

[75] Urban IA, Nagursky H, Church C, Lozada JL. Incidence, diagnosis, and treatment of sinus graft infection after sinus floor elevation: A clinical study. The International Journal of Oral & Maxillofacial Implants. 2012;**27**:449-457

[76] Mahler D, Levin L, Zigdon H, Machtei EE. The "dome phenomenon" associated with maxillary sinus augmentation. Clinical Implant Dentistry and Related Research. 2009;**11**:e46-e51

[77] Timmenga NM, Raghoebar GM, Liem RS, Van Weissenbruch R, Manson WL, Vissink A. Effects of maxillary sinus floor elevation surgery on maxillary sinus physiology. European Journal of Oral Sciences. 2003;**111**:189-197

[78] Melen I, Friberg B, Andreasson L, Ivarsson A, Jannert M, Lindahl L. Ostial and nasal patency in chronic maxillary sinusitis: A long-term post-treatment study. Acta Oto-Laryngologica. 1986;**102**:500-508

[79] Laureti M, Ferrigno N, Rosella D, Papi P, Mencio F, De Angelis F, Pompa G, Di Carlo S. Unusual case of osseointegrated dental implant migration into maxillary sinus removed 12 years after insertion. Case Reports in Dentistry. 2017;**2017**:9634672

[80] Galindo P, Sánchez-Fernández E, Avila G, Cutando A, Fernandez JE. Migration of implants into the maxillary sinus: Two clinical cases. The International Journal of Oral & Maxillofacial Implants. 2005;**20**:291-295

[81] Fugazzotto P, Melnick PR, Al-Sabbagh M. Complications when augmenting the posterior maxilla. Dental Clinics. 2015;**59**:97-130

Chapter 3

Sinus Lifting and Leucocyte- and Platelet-Rich Fibrin

Berkem Atalay

Additional information is available at the end of the chapter

http://dx.doi.org/10.5772/intechopen.81163

Abstract

The insufficient alveolar bone height due to the maxillary sinus in the posterior maxilla and postextraction bone resorption may limit implant placement. The sinus lifting procedure creates space between the maxillary alveolar bone and the Schneiderian membrane, which is filled with graft materials to maintain adequate space for new bone formation. Leucocyte- and platelet-rich fibrin (L-PRF)-mixed bone substitute or L-PRF has been used solely as a graft material for sinus lifting. The clinical and radiological findings of the application of PRF for sinus augmentation have been shown to have good results regarding new bone formation. The L-PRF can be an efficient biomaterial for graft particles in maxillary sinus lifting.

Keywords: sinus lifting, leucocyte- and platelet-rich fibrin, bone graft, L-PRF block, Schneiderian membrane

1. Introduction

Alveolar bone resorption in the edentulous ridge can cause insufficient bone volume for placing dental implants and consequently cannot be rehabilitated by prosthetics. Sinus lifting is a surgical approach with the elevation of the Schneiderian membrane to place the bone grafts for treatment of atrophic posterior maxilla [1]. This surgical technique is a successful treatment for augmentation of the atrophic posterior maxilla and to gain bone volume for dental implant procedure [2].

Sinus lifting shows complexity due to anatomical variations and Schneiderian membrane. The lateral bone's thickness changes the risk of membrane perforation. Evaluation of the thickness of the lateral wall before surgical treatment may affect the integrity of the Schneiderian membrane during the surgery [3].

Sinus lifting is a predictable technique, but various complications can occur during surgery or postoperative period [3]. These complications can be listed as edema, perforation of Schneiderian membrane, sinusitis development, bleeding, wound dehiscence, postoperative wound and bone graft material infection, implant failure if it is placed simultaneously, and disruption of normal sinus physiologic function. These complications can delay the healing process and may require additional surgeries [4–6]. Cone-beam computed tomography (CBCT) provides an accurate evaluation of the sinus and related anatomical structures. Danesh-Sani et al. recommend using CBCT before surgery to minimize the risk of Schneiderian membrane perforation [7].

Presurgical evaluation with CBCT has become an essential tool for diagnosis and surgical planning, including sinus lifting. Before performing a sinus lift, the clinician's attention should not be only directed to the patency of the ostium through CBCT, because many anatomical features could influence the surgical approach of sinus lifting.

Postoperative swelling of the Schneiderian membrane mostly occurs with maxillary sinus lifting procedure. The mucosa of the Schneiderian membrane heals rapidly and recovers its homeostasis. If the ostiomeatal complex is unfavorable due to anatomic variations, its healing can be delayed, and risk of sinusitis is increased. The ostiomeatal complex plays an essential role in the development of maxillary sinusitis by dysfunction of the mucociliary system. If the patency of the ostiomeatal complex is interrupted, clearance of the maxillary sinus can be delayed and can increase the risk for development of sinusitis [8].

Surgeons must consider the risk of infectious sequelae after sinus lifting. The inflammatory reaction after any surgical procedure is unavoidable. Because of the interference of ciliary activity caused by the elevation of the Schneiderian membrane, altered mucous composition and bacterial infection can occur [9]. After sinus lifting, the maxillary sinus may be filled with hematoma or seroma. However, a mild inflammatory reaction can occur as a regular physiological activity of the nasal airway, and swelling of the mucosa can cause obstruction of the patency of the ostiomeatal complex. As a result, sinus lifting might compound the physiological drainage of the maxillary sinus into the middle meatus by inflammatory swelling on the mucosa of the ostium can predispose the patient to acute maxillary sinusitis [10]. Persisting effect on the ciliated mucosa can be expected because of raising the mucosa of the maxillary sinus [11]. The maxillary sinus mucosa can adapt adequately to the alteration following sinus lifting [12]. It is generally assumed that altered maxillary sinus, such as elevation of the Schneiderian membrane with curving outward or injured sinus mucosa, might change the physiological activity of the maxillary sinus.

Anatomic variations of the maxillary sinus are commonly detected, with an estimated prevalence of 68% [13]. Some anatomic variations on the lateral nasal wall, such as the deviated nasal septum, concha bullosa or paradoxical middle turbinate, and bending of the uncinate process are significant because of their help to the blockage of ostiomeatal complexes. These variants can interfere with drainage and ventilation of the maxillary sinus, and can affect the risk of sinusitis [14]. Compromised maxillary sinus drainage is closely associated with a reduction of the maxillary ostium. Reduced size of the ostium diameter can cause sinusitis [15].

The risk of Schneiderian membrane perforation during sinus lifting, in the presence of antral septa, can be increased [1]. Antral septa divide the sinus into compartments and smaller accessory sinuses [16, 17]. The presence of septa may constitute a risk factor by causing the Schneiderian membrane to become perforated during surgery. The development of sinusitis is one of the possible complications associated with perforation of the Schneiderian membrane [9]. For the repair of such perforations, there are a variety of techniques, including a buccal fat flap, fibro-mucosal grafts, connective tissue, resorbable collagen membranes, amnion-chorion barriers, and the leucocyte- and platelet-rich fibrin (L-PRF) [18]. Obtaining L-PRF consists of a very simple and inexpensive protocol that produces a strong membrane after compression [19].

L-PRF acts as a bioactive bridge and releases growth factors. The release increases day by day and reaches its highest level on the 14th day and continues until the 28th day [20–22]. L-PRF has certain effects on wound healing [19]. The leukocytes and cytokines have a significant role in controlling infectious and inflammatory processes. While the fibrin matrix is resorbed, cytokines are released to accelerate neovascularization and protect from infection. So, when L-PRF is used in membrane form, it stabilizes the graft material, covers the perforation since it has an inherent attachment to the Schneiderian membrane [23], and protects the wound [18, 24] (https://youtu.be/vuHPSpBVCl8).

The limited quantity of autogenous bone graft in sinus lifting with high morbidity rates is important for the clinicians using bone substitutes rather than the autogenous grafts. So, the investigation of optimal biomaterial combinations to enhance bone regeneration properties is in progress [25, 26]. L-PRF with bone graft for sinus lifting is accelerating bone regeneration. Choukroun et al. reported that healing time between sinus lifting and implant placement could be reduced by using L-PRF [27].

The use of L-PRF with a high concentration of platelets, growth factors, and leucocytes may increase the development of new bone. The liquid L-PRF (i-PRF) has been proposed to agglutinate the bone substitute [28]. Mixing i-PRF with bone substitute creates the L-PRF block.

2. L-PRF block

Prior to sinus lifting surgery, 8–16 tubes of venous blood needed to be collected from the patients. Two tubes should be separated as a white cap, plastic coating, and placed in the centrifuge at 2700 rpm for 3 minutes. The remaining tubes as a red cap, glass coating should be placed in the centrifuge at 2700 rpm for 12 minutes.

The liquid fibrinogen in the white cap tubes has to be aspirated with a sterile syringe. When the centrifugation of the red cap tubes finishes, the L-PRF clots can be removed from the tubes and compressed using a sterile metal box to mold membranes (**Figure 1**).

For the preparation of the L-PRF block as described by Cortellini et al., L-PRF membranes are cut and mixed with a bone substitute at a ratio of two membranes with 0.5 g bone substitute. The liquid fibrinogen needed to be added to the homogenous mix and stirred for at least 10 seconds for the ideal form. By the chopped membranes, fibrinogen is polymerizing into platelets and leucocyte, forming the L-PRF block (**Figure 2**).

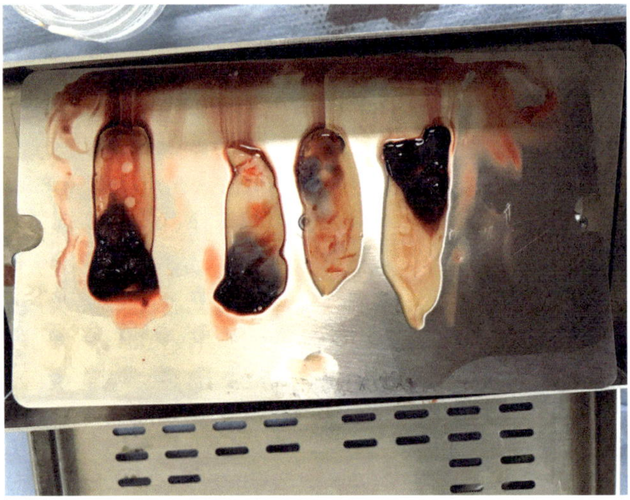

Figure 1. The ready-to-use L-PRF membranes in preparation kit.

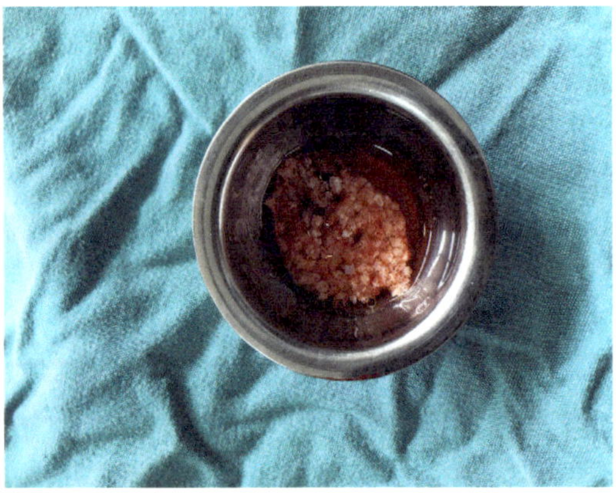

Figure 2. The L-PRF block.

3. Conclusion

The L-PRF block is secreting bioactive molecules like; a platelet-derived growth factor, bone morphogenetic proteins, insulin-like growth factor, vascular endothelial growth factor, transforming growth factor-β1, and transforming growth factor-β2 [29].

L-PRF can have a positive effect on bone regeneration and osseointegration. Easy preparation of L-PRF, biological properties, and low cost could be considered as reliable support in sinus lifting surgery. The use of sufficient L-PRF clots and membranes, avoiding to close the patency of ostium, is crucial to gain a covetable bone volume [30] (**Figure 3**).

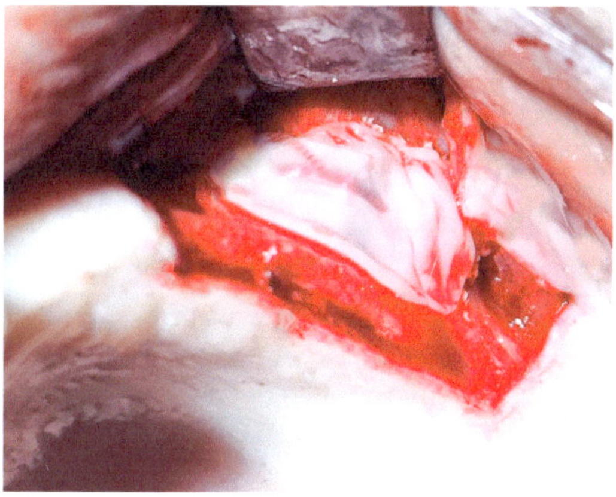

Figure 3. The use of the L-PRF membrane to cover the lateral window.

The L-PRF block maintains the volumetric stability of the biomaterial during healing and by this way, it can prevent the shrinkage of the scaffold. The effects of L-PRF on tissue healing by the release of growth factors and increasing angiogenesis and osteogenesis can lead to the higher volume of newly formed bone with the L-PRF block [31]. The L-PRF block can be a successful new procedure for sinus lifting after further investigations with histological analysis and randomized controlled clinical trials.

Author details

Berkem Atalay

Address all correspondence to: berkematalay@istanbul.edu.tr

Faculty of Dentistry, Department of Oral and Maxillofacial Surgery, İstanbul University, Turkey

References

[1] Tatum H. Maxillary and sinus implant reconstructions. Dental Clinics of North America. 1986;**30**:207-229

[2] Pjetursson BE, Tan WC, Zwahlen M, Lang NP. A systematic review of the success of sinus floor elevation and survival of implants inserted in combination with sinus floor elevation. Journal of Clinical Periodontology. 2008;**35**:216-240

[3] Zijderveld SA, Van den Bergh JP, Schulten EA, Bruggenkate CM. Anatomical and surgical findings and complications in 100 consecutive maxillary sinus floor elevation procedures. Journal of Oral and Maxillofacial Surgery. 2008;**66**:1426-1438

[4] Moreno Vazquez JC, Gonzalez de Rivera AS, Gil HS, Mifsut RS. Complication rate in 200 consecutive sinus lift procedures: Guidelines for prevention and treatment. Journal of Oral and Maxillofacial Surgery. 2014;**72**:892-901

[5] Schwartz-Arad D, Herzberg R, Dolev E. The prevalence of surgical complications of the sinus graft procedure and their impact on implant survival. Journal of Periodontology. 2004;**75**:511-516

[6] Nkenke E, Schlegel A, Schultze-Morgau S, Neukam FW, Wiltfang J. The endoscopically controlled osteotome sinus floor elevation: A preliminary prospective study. The International Journal of Oral & Maxillofacial Implants. 2002;**17**:577-566

[7] Danesh-Sani SA, Movahed A, ElChaar ES, Chong Chan K, Amintavakoli N. Radiographic evaluation of maxillary sinus lateral wall and posterior superior alveolar artery anatomy: A cone-beam computed tomographic study. Clinical Implant Dentistry and Related Research. 2017;**19**:151-160

[8] Bertrand B, Eloy P. Relationship of chronic ethmoidal sinusitis, maxillary sinusitis, and ostial permeability controlled by sinusomanometry: A statistical study. Laryngoscope. 1992;**102**:1281-1284

[9] Zimbler MS, Lebowitz RA, Glickman R, Brecht LE, Jacobs JB. Antral augmentation, osseointegration, and sinusitis: The otolaryngologist's perspective. American Journal of Rhinology. 1998;**12**:311-316

[10] Timmenga NM, Raghoebar GM, van Weissenbruch R, Vissink A. Maxillary sinusitis after augmentation of the maxillary sinus floor: A report of 2 cases. Journal of Oral and Maxillofacial Surgery. 2001;**59**:200-204

[11] Timmenga NM, Raghoebar GM, Liem RS, van Weissenbruch R, Manson WL, Vissink A. Effects of maxillary sinus floor elevation surgery on maxillary sinus physiology. European Journal of Oral Sciences. 2003;**111**:189-197

[12] Stammberger H. Endoscopic endonasal surgery concepts in the treatment of recurring rhinosinusitis. Part II. Surgical technique. Otolaryngology and Head and Neck Surgery. 1986;**94**:147-156

[13] Bolger WE, Butzin CA, Parsons DS. Paranasal sinus bony anatomic variations and mucosal abnormalities: CT analysis for endoscopic sinus surgery. Laryngoscope. 1991;**101**:56-64

[14] Bayram M, Sirikci A, Bayazit YA. Important anatomic variations of the sinonasal anatomy in light of endoscopic surgery: A pictorial review. European Radiology. 2001;**11**:1991-1997

[15] Laine FJ, Smoker WR. The ostiomeatal unit and endoscopic surgery: Anatomy, variations, and imaging findings in inflammatory diseases. AJR. American Journal of Roentgenology. 1992;**159**:849-857

[16] van den Bergh JP, ten Bruggenkate CM, Disch FJ, Tuinzing DB. Anatomical aspects of sinus floor elevations. Clinical Oral Implants Research. 2000;**11**:256-265

[17] Tidwell JK, Blijdorp PA, Stoelinga PJ, Brouns JB, Hinderks F. Composite grafting of the maxillary sinus for placement of endosteal implants. A preliminary report of 48 patients. International Journal of Oral and Maxillofacial Surgery. 1992;**21**:204-209

[18] Aricioglu C, Dolanmaz D, Esen A, et al. Histological evaluation of the effectiveness of platelet-rich fibrin on the healing of sinus membrane perforations: A preclinical animal study. Journal of Cranio-Maxillo-Facial Surgery. 2017;**45**:1150-1157

[19] Dohan Ehrenfest DM, Del Corso M, Diss A, et al. Three-dimensional architecture and cell composition of a Choukroun's platelet-rich fibrin clot and membrane. Journal of Periodontology. 2010;**81**:546-555

[20] Dohan DM, Choukroun J, Diss A, et al. Platelet-rich fibrin (PRF): A second-generation platelet concentrate. Part I: Technological concepts and evolution. Oral Surgery, Oral Medicine, Oral Pathology, Oral Radiology, and Endodontics. 2006;**101**:37-44

[21] Choukroun J, Diss A, Simonpieri A, et al. Platelet-rich fibrin (PRF): A second-generation platelet concentrate. Part V: Histologic evaluations of PRF effects on bone allograft maturation in sinus lift. Oral Surgery, Oral Medicine, Oral Pathology, Oral Radiology, and Endodontics. 2006;**101**:299-303

[22] Sohn DS, Heo JU, Kwak DH, Kim DE, Kim JM, Moon JW, et al. Bone regeneration in the maxillary sinus using an autologous fibrin-rich block with concentrated growth factors alone. Implant Dentistry. 2011;**20**:389-395

[23] Simonpieri A, Choukroun J, Del, Corso M, Sammartino G, Dohan DM. Simultaneous sinus-lift and implantation using micro-threaded implants and leukocyte- and platelet-rich fibrin as sole grafting material: A six-year experience. Implant Dentistry. 2011;**20**:2-12

[24] Öncü E, Kaymaz E. Assessment of the effectiveness of platelet-rich fibrin in the treatment of Schneiderian membrane perforation. Clinical Implant Dentistry and Related Research. 2017;**19**:1009-1014

[25] Corbella S, Taschieri S, Weinstein R, Del Fabbro M. Histomorphometric outcomes after lateral sinus floor elevation procedure: A systematic review of the literature and meta-analysis. Clinical Oral Implants Research. 2016;**27**:1106-1122

[26] Shanbhag S, Shanbhag V, Stavropoulos A. Volume changes of maxillary sinus augmentations over time: A systematic review. The International Journal of Oral & Maxillofacial Implants. 2014;**29**:881-892

[27] Choukroun J, Diss A, Simonpieri A, et al. Platelet-rich fibrin (PRF): A second-generation platelet concentrate. Part IV: Clinical effects on tissue healing. Oral Surgery, Oral Medicine, Oral Pathology, Oral Radiology, and Endodontics. 2006;**101**:56-60

[28] de Almeida Barros MCF, Helder V, Rodrigues ME, Freitas MNBM, Diuana-Calasans MM. Obtenção da fibrina rica em plaquetas injetável (i-PRF) e sua polimerização com enxerto ósseo: Nota técnica. Revista do Colégio Brasileiro de Cirurgiões. 2015;**42**:421-423

[29] Cortellini S, Castro AB, Temmerman A, et al. Leucocyte- and platelet-rich fibrin block for bone augmentation procedure: A proof of concept study. Journal of Clinical Periodontology. 2018;**45**:624-634

[30] Castro AB, Meschi N, Temmerman A, Pinto N, Lambrechts P, Teughels W, et al. Regenerative potential of leucocyte- and platelet-rich fibrin. Part B: Sinus floor elevation, alveolar ridge preservation and implant therapy. A systematic review. Journal of Clinical Periodontology. 2017;**44**:225-234

[31] Pichotano EC. The İnfluence of Leukocyte and Platelet-Rich Fibrin on Bone Formation after Maxillary Sinus Floor Elevation with a Deproteinized Bovine Bone: A Randomized Clinical Trial [thesis]. UNESP Institutional Repository; 2018

Section 3

Challenging Issue on Rhinosinusitis and Sinonasal Neoplasms

Chapter 4

Medical Management of the Paranasal Sinus Infections

Mehmet Şentürk

Additional information is available at the end of the chapter

http://dx.doi.org/10.5772/intechopen.81040

Abstract

Rhinosinusitis is a common disease among all the sinus diseases, and unsuccessful attempts to these infections may result not only in economic burdens but also in increasing the numbers of untreated patients in the community. Medical management of the rhinosinusitis includes antibiotics, antihistamines, nasal decongestants, corticosteroids, mucolytics, leukotriene antagonists, and nasal irrigations. Each treatment option must be selected for appropriate patient and prescriptions must be tailored according to the patient's need. These needs must depend on the endoscopic examination, symptoms, and sinus cultures and computed tomography. It is also a matter of debate whether these investigations lead to treatment or not, but it would be wrong to expect that a single examination method and physical examination alone should direct treatment in the first place. As a result, managing the process with the most appropriate examination methods for the patient's complaints will be the most beneficial approach.

Keywords: acute rhinosinusitis, chronic rhinosinusitis, pediatric, adult, nasal polyp, antibiotic

1. Introduction

Rhinosinusitis is the major public health problem among the upper respiratory tract infections that produce enormous consequences that source the negative effect on the quality of life of the patient and cause significant morbidity and mortality. Rhinosinusitis also has a significant effect on the health economics. In the United States, the predicted yearly amount of the burden has been estimated at $3.5–5.8 billion, especially $1.8 billion for first 12 years of age [1]. It seems that rhinosinusitis affect the quality of life of the children and cause economic loss. It is imperative to obtain up-to-date and accurate information for each physician who is involved in the treatment of this disease group and related ones. In this chapter, updated information has been given about the medical treatments on pediatric acute rhinosinusitis, pediatric chronic sinusitis, adult acute rhinosinusitis, adult chronic rhinosinusitis without nasal polyp (CRSsNP), and adult chronic rhinosinusitis with nasal polyp (CRSwNP). This information has been compiled from very important guidelines and articles by authors. In this way, the reader will be able to acquire much more detailed and accurate information as well as the source of the information to be obtained.

2. Medical management of pediatric acute rhinosinusitis

2.1. Oral antibiotics

Oral antibiotic treatment is not necessitating the majority of the acute rhinosinusitis (ARS) patients. Viral infections that resolve without therapy are the main cause of rhinosinusitis [2]. A minor proportion of these patients develop a subsequent bacterial inflammation that will heal with antimicrobial treatment. *Streptococcus pneumoniae, Haemophilus influenzae, Moraxella catarrhalis,* Group A beta-hemolytic *streptococci,* and *Staphylococcus aureus* are the most common cause of the development of rhinosinusitis. Therefore, the patient who has taken oral antibiotic therapy is the most important concern in clinical practice. However, acute rhinosinusitis with viral etiology may be resolved without any treatment but bacterial rhinosinusitis is treated by antibiotics. The diagnosis of bacterial ARS may be considered when symptoms prolonged over 10 days or there is deterioration after drug-free follow-up period [3]. The guideline from the American Academy of Pediatrics [4] suggested that physicians must use antibiotic treatment for ARS in children with intense beginning or deteriorating progression. As well, reporters also advised that physicians should either use antibiotic therapy or offer further outpatient observation for 3 days to children with persistent disorder. This report also confirmed that if there is no improving in symptoms or if there is a failure to recover, clinicians should modify antibiotics or initiate antibiotics in child treated with observation [4]. The recommendation of using antibiotics for severe or worsening acute bacterial sinusitis in consequence of the benefits showed a theoretically higher risk of suppurative complications than for children who existed lasting symptoms.

It is recommended that when the clinical diagnosis of acute bacterial rhinosinusitis (ABRS) is established, empirical antimicrobial therapy should be initiated directly [5]. Amoxicillin-clavulanate (45 mg/kg/day, divided into two doses) instead of amoxicillin alone is recommended as the initial therapy of ABRS in children. The cephalosporins such as cefuroxime, cefdinir or cefpodoxime, clindamycin (or linezolid) + cefixime, and levofloxacin may be preferred in the condition of a penicilin allergy. Cephalosporins are usually used as the suitable treatment for ARS. Cephalexin and cefadroxil, which are the first-generation agents, are not the first choice for *H. influenzae* infection. Beta-lactamase-producing *M. catarrhalis* and some *H. influenzae* strains has reduce the response to cefaclor (50 mg/kg/day in two doses), and early second-generation cephalosporins. On the other hand, beta-lactamase-producing bacteria have a good response to second-generation cephalosporins (cefuroxime axetil, 30 mg/kg/day and cefprozil, in two doses as oral suspension). Third-generation cephalosporins such as cefixime, ceftibuten, cefpodoxime axetil (10 mg/kg once daily), and cefdinir (14 mg/kg/day in one or two doses) seem to be an alternative option for the therapy. Macrolides (clarithromycin and azithromycin) are not recommended for empirical treatment due to elevated resistance rates of *S. pneumoniae*. Because of high resistance rates between *S. pneumoniae* and *Haemophilus influenzae*, trimethoprim-sulfamethoxazole is not recommended for empirical treatment. Ampicillin-sulbactam (100 mg/kg/day for three times a day) or ceftriaxone (100 mg/kg/day at single or double dose) given intravenously or intramusculary can be used in patients who do not endure oral antibiotics due to vomiting or in patients who do not recover after 24–48 hours of treatment with a second antibiotic therapy. If there is a suspicion of an aerobic pathogen as a cause of ARS, clindamycin or metronidazole may be added to a wide spectrum antibiotics. In patients with acute bacterial RS, the appropriate treatment duration is not definitively defined, but 10–14 days of treatment appear to be adequate for mild acute forms, but 14–21 days of treatment appear to be appropriate for severe acute forms and subacute forms [5].

2.2. Intranasal saline irrigation

Nasal saline irrigation has been shown to be effective and well tolerated in children with rhinosinusitis [6]. Management of sinus disease often involves the use of saline irrigations. Saline irrigation helps patients with rhinosinusitis by improving mucociliary clearance, slenderizing mucus, and providing anti-inflammatory effects [7]. Decreasing in symptoms after nasal irrigations is associated with an increase in quality of life in patients with acute rhinosinusitis [3, 8, 9].

2.3. Intranasal corticosteroids

It has been also shown that the use of intranasal corticosteroids significantly improved the symptoms of ARS [3]. Intranasal corticosteroids are recommended for both moderate (monotherapy) and severe (oral antibiotics) types of acute rhinosinusitis [10]. A double-blind, placebo-controlled trial revealed the efficacy of topical corticosteroid therapy in comparison with both monotherapy and antibiotics [11]. In this study, mometasone furoate (MF) was compared with amoxicillin and placebo in patients with ARS. MF 200 μg twice a day was significantly better than placebo and amoxicillin for correction of symptom score. MF was used once a day and was superior to placebo but not to amoxicillin. This study is the first study to show that topical corticosteroids are effective when given twice daily in the treatment of ARS and are more effective than amoxicillin. The results of this study were also supported by two other studies with a similar design. However, in another study, the use of antibiotics and topical steroids alone and in combination has not been effective in changing the severity of symptoms or duration of bacterial ARS. However, in this study, the patients with 4 days of symptoms and only those with colds and not ARS have been included. It is supported by the use of intranasal corticosteroids alone or as adjuvant therapy to antibiotics. High doses of intranasal corticosteroids (mometasone furoate 400 versus 200 μg) have a stronger effect on the reduction or complete improvement of symptoms. There was no significant adverse effect for both treatment groups, and there was no significant difference in the reduction in symptoms and recurrence rates with higher doses of intranasal corticosteroids. Further randomized clinical trials are needed to examine the effectiveness and proper use of antibiotics and intranasal corticosteroids as a single or combined therapy for the treatment of different severe ARS. There are some studies comparing the effectiveness of mometasone furoate nasal spray and amoxicillin and placebo in patients with acute, uncomplicated RS. It is concluded that the use of mometasone furoate twice daily as 200 μg in acute, uncomplicated RS patients significantly reduced symptoms when compared with amoxicillin and placebo without predisposing factors or bacterial infection [12]. Rahmati et al. [13] revealed that the use of fluticasone in children has been associated with reducing the severity of acute sinusitis symptoms. Foden et al. [7] stated that intranasal corticosteroids (INCS) are the basis for the treatment of rhinosinusitis. As a monotherapy in ARS, INCS had a significant improvement in symptoms compared to placebo and amoxicillin [12]. On regarding the use of INCS, either as monotherapy or adjuvant to antibiotics, these studies have also been designed based on the approval of diagnosis. Intranasal corticosteroids (INCSs) are recommended in patients with a history of allergic rhinitis, especially as an adjunct to antibiotics for the empirical treatment of ABRS [5].

2.4. Other treatment modalities

It was accepted as a symptomatic treatment of viral upper respiratory tract infections with analgesic, antipyretic, and decongestant drugs (topical or systemic) [6]. Decongestants should be used with caution in pediatric patients because there is a small number of studies on the efficacy and side effects of decongestants. Concurrent use of decongestant and antihistamine in the treatment of pediatric upper respiratory tract infection and inflammation is still debated. In patients with ABRS, topical or oral decongestants and/or antihistamines are not recommended as adjuvant therapy (strong, low to moderate). Oral corticosteroids may be added to the treatment of cases with nasal polyposis or marked mucosal edema when the initial treatment is not received [14]. Antihistamines are useful in the case of accompanying acute bacterial RS and allergic RS because they reduce the inflammatory component and respond positively to antibiotics. Except the current allergic rhinitis, there is no indication for the use of antihistamines (both intranasal and oral) in the treatment of postviral ARS [10].

2.5. Nonresponsive patients

The patients who have worsened clinically during the first 72 hours or who have not recovered after 3–5 days of empirical antimicrobial therapy with a first-step agent should be evaluated for resistance pathogens, nontoxic etiology, structural abnormality, or other reasons for treatment failure (strong, low). In patients with suspected sinus infection who cannot respond to empirical antimicrobial therapy, cultures are recommended to be obtained with direct sinus aspiration rather than nasopharyngeal swab (strong, moderate). Endoscopic-guided cultures of medium meatus may be considered as an alternative in adults, but their reliability was not determined in children (weak, moderate). Nasopharynx cultures are not considered reliable and are not recommended for microbiological diagnosis of ABRS [5].

3. Medical management of pediatric chronic rhinosinusitis

3.1. Intranasal saline irrigation

Nasal saline irrigation should be considered as the primary therapeutic tool in CRS, even in the child age group, which is a long-term CRS [15–17]. Nasal saline lavage can significantly reduce chronic sinusitis symptoms, improve disease-specific quality of life, and be well tolerated in children with chronic rhinosinusitis symptoms [6, 18]. Nasal saline solutions make it easier to mechanically remove the mucus and increase the ciliary rhythm [19]. Nasal saline sprays or irrigations when tolerated are also used in the treatment of CRS, and primarily, sinonasal secretion, pathogens and debris removal are thought to help. Although Cochrane collection does not support any advice on nasal saline irritation, some studies have shown some degree of efficacy in CRS [16].

3.2. Intranasal corticosteroids

Topical steroids, although the absolute resolution of the CRS does not improve, may accelerate the solution of CRS symptoms when evaluated in the short term. In the management of CRS, it may be affected by suspected or proven allergic disease, including steroids. In particular, nasal steroids should be maintained when an allergic patient is treated for CRS. Topical nasal steroids suppress mucosal inflammation [9]. Examples include fluticasone propionate, commonly found in generic form, and mometasone furoate, which is indicated for use in nasal congestion due to allergic rhinitis in children aged 2 years and older. Topical nasal steroids are usually preferred for children with CRS due to low systemic bioavailability. Therefore, systemic side effects are rare in children with CRS and the most common complication is epistaxis. Although long-term prophylactic use often seems to be safe, it helps to suppress chronic symptoms and recurrent diseases, and typically conflicts with long-term antibiotic medicines used in CRS every 3–6 weeks [16].

3.3. Antibiotic treatment in the management of pediatric chronic rhinosinusitis

3.3.1. Oral antibiotics

Long-term and broad-spectrum antibiotics have been the basis for treating pediatric chronic rhinosinusitis. Amoxicillin/clavulanate is a good choice for first-line treatment, but antibiotics to be selected must also be effective against possible pathogens in CRS, including *S aureus*, Pseudomonas and anaerobes. Encompassing for MRSA may be indicated. Long-period treatment with macrolides for up to 12 weeks may also benefit patients with CRS. A culture should be obtained, preferably directly from the sinus cavity or endoscopic, in patients who do not recover or develop worsening despite treatment. For the last 20 years, antimicrobial resistance has been increasing. These contain the creation of beta lactamases and cephalosporins. Clindamycin can be administered in the event of penicillin allergy or who suspect MRSA. Other oral agents covering MRSA include trimethoprim-sulfamethoxazole and linezolid. The dose of amoxicillin-clavulanate recommended for children is 45 mg/kg. Another recommended antibiotic management procedure is high-dose amoxicillin or amoxicillin/clavulanate (90 mg/kg/day orally twice daily) for children from environmental areas with high endemic degrees (>10%) of aggressive penicillin-nonsusceptible (PNS) *S. pneumoniae*. In addition, high-dose amoxicillin or amoxicillin/clavulanate therapy is recommended for the children with severe infection, attendance at nursery, age<2, latest hospitalization, antibiotic usage within the past month, and immunocompromisation [6, 16, 20]. Metronidazole can be administered in addition to one of the following antibiotics: cefazolin, cefuroxime, cefixime proksetil, clarithromycin, azithromycin, or trimethoprim-sulfamethoxazole and is administered as three times a day for 30–50 mg/kg/day and maximum daily dose for 2.250 mg/day. Antimicrobial therapy is given for a three-week period and can be extended up to 10 weeks in patients with antibiotic resistance [19].

3.3.2. *Parenteral antibiotics*

Parenteral treatment is applied to children who are extremely ill, who undergo surgery or who have a problem of adaptation to the oral regimen. Among the parenteral antimicrobials such as ampicillin-sulbactam, piperacillin-tazobactam, clindamycin, moxifloxacin, carbapenems (imipenem, meropenem, doripenem), and second-generation cephalosporins, cefoxitin effective against both anaerobes and aerobes are included. Vancomycin, linezolid, and daptomycin and ceftaroline are among the parenteral antimicrobials effective against MRSA. Metronidazole may be given as parenteral against anaerobes in combination with an agent with aerobic activity [9, 20].

3.3.3. *Intranasal antibiotics*

Although topical antibiotic treatment is not recommended in the best part of CRS cases, further studies should be required according to the initial findings. Demands about the combination potential with dose, treatment time, optimal treatment method, and other therapies carry on to be responded [9].

3.4. Systemic corticosteroids

Oral methylprednisolone has a good tolerance and offers additional benefit to treatment with antibiotics for children with CRS [21]. Combination treatment with systemic corticosteroids and antibiotics was established to be favorable in children (age between 6 and 17 years) with CRS whose management with at least three 10–14–day sequences of wide-spectrum antibiotics was unsuccessful. Minimal side effects may be seen. It was observed that children treated with corticosteroids plus antibiotics had meaningfully better declines in entire symptom and sinus CT scores compared with those given placebo plus antibiotics. Complete clinical healing observed more frequently and reverts within 6 months less commonly in the active management group. Moreover, Ozturk et al. [21] conducted a randomized trial comparing amoxicillin-clavulanate with and without methylprednisolone, and examined the advantage of addition of systemic corticosteroids to oral antibiotics for the management of CRS. Both management arms revealed progress compared with baseline with the steroid management being meaningfully more effective regarding dropping CT scores and total rhinosinusitis symptoms, such as nasal obstruction, cough, and postnasal drainage [22].

3.5. Adjuvant medical treatments

Adjuvant medical treatment involving antihistamines and decongestants for pediatric CRS has been used widely with unconfirmed benefits. Oral antihistamines and decongestants may offer symptomatic advance; but the general period of the disease may not be affected. Moreover, the effects of antihistamines and decongestants on secretions and mucosa may undesirably affect the innate physiologic mechanisms of the sinuses and nose to cope with infection and inflammation [9, 16, 19].

3.6. Treatment for gastroesophageal reflux

It is not proved to use proton pump inhibitors (PPI) for pediatric CRS. The International Consensus Statement on Allergy and Rhinology: rhinosinusitis [23] summaries the facts about CRS and laryngopharyngeal reflux. It has set grade B evidence to prove the relationship between these situations but expresses that treatment guidelines or mechanistic trials are requiring. This statement further endorses to establish accurately diagnosing laryngopharyngeal reflux before starting PPI management in patients with difficult to treat CRS [24].

4. Medical management of adult acute rhinosinusitis

4.1. Nasal saline spray/saline irrigation

In the treatment of adult ABRS, there has been a recommendation of topical nasal saline irrigation with either isotonic or hypertonic form as a combined treatment. Saline sprays have an effect on reducing rhinitis symptoms. Also, it revealed a better sinus-related quality of life, decreased symptoms, and drug use with routine hypertonic nasal saline irrigation. No serious side effect has been determined with saline irrigation. When compared to isotonic saline, hypertonic saline treatment may have a better anti-inflammatory result and ability to subtilize mucous and rapidly recover mucociliary clearance [5, 25].

4.2. Intranasal corticosteroids

In the routine treatment of acute bacterial rhinosinusitis, intranasal corticosteroids (INCSs) are recommended as a supplement to antibiotics, especially in patients with allergic rhinitis [5, 12, 26]. Intranasal corticosteroids improved the symptoms and had only minor side events, consisting of headache, nasal itching, and epistaxis [25].

4.3. Antibiotic treatment

In acute bacterial rhinosinusitis, the most common determined pathogens are *S. pneumoniae or H. influenzae,* so the use of amoxicillin (with or without clavulanate) is commonly recommended for empirical treatment in adult patients [25, 27]. On the other hand, Chow et al. [5] recommends amoxicillin-clavulanate rather than amoxicillin as empirical antimicrobial therapy for ABRS in adults. Also, it is recommended to use penicillin or amoxicillin for 7–14 days [10]. Macrolides (azithromycin and clarithromycin) are not recommended for initial therapy because of high rates of resistance to *S. pneumoniae*. By the way, trimethoprim-sulfamethoxazole is also not recommended for initial therapy due to high rates of resistance to both *S. pneumoniae* and *Haemophilus influenzae*. As an alternative treatment to amoxicillin-clavulanate for empirical therapy of adult ABRS, doxycycline may be chosen for being highly effective against airway pathogens and having superb pharmacokinetic/pharmacodynamics features [5].

Because of the inconstant proportions of resistance among *S. pneumoniae*, there is no recommendation for second- and third-generation oral cephalosporin antibiotics in the initial monotherapy of ABRS. Combined treatment with a third-generation oral cephalosporin (cefpodoxime or cefixime) plus clindamycin may be used as a second-line treatment for children from geographic regions with high endemic rates of penicillin nonsusceptible *Streptococcus pneumoniae* or for children with non-type I penicillin allergy. İt is strongly recommended that the use of doxycycline, levofloxacin, or moxifloxacin may be an alternative treatment for initial antimicrobial therapy in adults who are sensitive to penicillin. According to the up-to-date data, it is not a recommended routine antimicrobial coverage for *S. aureus* or MRSA for the initial treatment of ABRS, even though *S. aureus* (including methicillin-resistant *S. aureus* [MRSA]) is a possible agent in ABRS, and 5–7 days' therapy is recommended for uncomplicated ABRS in adults [5].

*H. influenza*e can be highly resistant to amoxicillin and ampicillin [28]. Fluoroquinolones remain highly effective against both *H. influenzae* and *S. pneumoniae* [29]. Though the role of the fluoroquinolones is growing, these drugs are commonly recommended as second-line treatment, or as first-line treatment in patients with moderate illness who have had recent antimicrobial treatment, or for clinically moderate to severe disease patients [30, 31]. In these cases, another treatment option may be using high-dose amoxicillin/clavulanate (4 g/250 mg per day). High-dose amoxicillin with clavulanate treatment (2 g orally twice daily or 90 mg/kg/d orally twice daily) is recommended for adult patients with ABRS who have high risk of being infected with an amoxicillin-resistant organism. High-dose amoxicillin/clavulanate (4 g/250 mg per day) is recommended for severe infection, findings such as evidence of temperature of 39°C [102°F] or higher and trend of suppurative complications, age over 65 years, necessity of hospitalization, antibiotic usage within the last month, immunocompromisation and living in geographic regions with high endemic rates (>10%) of invasive PNS S *pneumoniae*. Alternative treatment choice of acute rhinosinusitis comprises of cephalosporins. Third-generation cephalosporins, such as cefdinir or ceftriaxone, are enough effective against *H. influenzae* but have much lower effectiveness against *S. pneumoniae* [27].

4.3.1. Penicillin-allergic patients

Though resistance rates of macrolide antibiotics to *H. influenzae* and *S. pneumoniae* are rising throughout the world, as first-line agents in patients with β-lactam allergies, they are still preferred [31]. For these patients, either a fluoroquinolone (levofloxacin or moxifloxacin) or doxycycline is recommended as another agent for initial antimicrobial treatment. For patients who do not have penicillin allergy, fluoroquinolones are not considered as the first-line treatment of ABRS, because results are similar to amoxicillin-clavulanate, and side effects are seen higher [27].

4.4. Additional treatments

Clinicians may recommend analgesics, nasal saline, and/or topical intranasal steroids, for symptomatic relief of ABRS. Nonsteroidal anti-inflammatory agents or acetaminophen are generally adequate for facial pain related to ABRS [25].

4.4.1. Decongestants

4.4.1.1. Topical decongestants

There are no recommendation about topical and oral decongestants as combined therapy. Decongestants may offer short-term relief for nasal congestion. Xylometazoline or oxymetazoline is the frequently existing topical decongestants. They can be found in the form of drops or spray and act by contracting the sinusoids in the nasal tissues. After applying these agents intranasally, within 10 minutes, local vasoconstriction occurs. Their effects last up to 12 hours. Decreased nasal mucosal blood flow and mucosal clearance may cause this long effect: the topical nasal decongestants. Topical nasal decongestants have important side effects such as nasal mucosal irritation, dryness, or ulceration. Long-term use (>10 days) of topical nasal decongestants may cause tachyphylaxis and rhinitis medicamentosa (rebound swelling of the nasal mucosa). Therefore, the use of topical nasal decongestants must be limited to 10 days [5].

4.4.1.2. Oral decongestants

Phenylephrine, pseudoephedrine, and ephedrine are frequently used as oral decongestants. As they offer rapid relief on a short term, they are preferred commonly. When compared to topical nasal decongestants, oral decongestants have a lower effect on the nasal obstruction. Because they have no effect of rebound phenomenon, they may be preferred for a long term. After oral intake, nasal decongestion starts within 30 minutes and continues for up to 6 hours. Phenylephrine is the least effective agent among the oral decongestants. There are some side effects related to the oral decongestants such as nervousness, drowsiness, agitation, and arrhythmias. There are some risks that should be avoided to use oral decongestants in combinations with alcohol or some medications such as sedatives and monoamine oxidase inhibitors. For patients with stable hypertension, commonly, there is no noteworthy rise in blood pressure. However, careful use is recommended in patients with prostatic hypertrophy, glaucoma, or ischemic heart disease [27].

4.4.2. Topical anticholinergics

Topical intranasal anticholinergics, such as ipratropium bromide, are mainly preferred to stop symptom of rhinorrhea. On nasal congestion, sneezing and itching has no significant effect. Nasal irritation, burning, and dryness are the most common adverse effects followed by a headache, dry mouth and stuffy nose, etc. On mucociliary clearance, nasal mucosal alteration, and olfaction, they have no effect with long-term usage [25].

4.4.3. Antihistamines

For management of acute rhinosinusitis, no clinical trials recommend the use of antihistamines. First-generation antihistamines have the anticholinergic effects, and thus, mucociliary clearance may be impaired. On the other hand, second-generation antihistamines have no anticholinergic effect and are not recommended for acute rhinosinusitis [25].

4.4.4. Mucolytics

As a mucolytic agent, guaiphenesin is a frequently used for mucolysis. It is commonly preferred together with a decongestant drug. While it is used to thin the nasal secretions and increase drainage, trials evaluate the effects of placebo and guaiphenesin on ciliary beat frequency and nasal mucociliary clearance, and could not reveal any assessable impact [25].

4.4.5. Oral corticosteroids

When oral corticosteroid steroids are used as monotherapy for ABRS, there is no recommendation to use of systemic steroids for ABRS and they have no advantage over placebo. Among their adverse events, in mild condition, gastrointestinal complaints, nausea, and vomiting may also be seen. But the effects of these agents must take into account on the systems of glucose metabolism, bone turnover, and cardiovascular circulation [25].

5. Medical management of adult chronic rhinosinusitis without nasal polyp (CRSsNP)

5.1. Saline treatment

Nasal saline irrigations have beneficial effects and are accepted treatment modality as strong recommendation for chronic rhinosinusitis. Among the advantageous effects of saline are healing of symptoms and improving quality of life, increase in mucous clearance, improved ciliary activity, interruption and elimination of inflammatory mediators, biofilms and antigens, and protection of the sinonasal mucosa [25]. Nasal saline treatment has beneficial safety profile, no risk of systemic absorption, and well patient tolerance make it a potent long-term topical nasal therapy approach. Irrigation solutions may be either isotonic or hypertonic saline. High-volume (>200 mL) nasal saline irrigations in addition to other medical treatments is strongly recommended for CRS. Hypertonic nasal saline irrigations notably enhanced CRS-specific quality of life, symptom scores, and diminished drug usage. For establishing the hygiene, microwave decontamination of the irrigation bottles may be considered as a useful disinfecting method. It has been established that saline irrigation is superior to saline spray in throwing out secretions and enhancing the quality of life [23, 25].

5.2. Intranasal corticosteroids

It has been shown that the patients with CRSsNP benefited significantly from topical nasal steroids. The direct transmission of INCS to the sinuses has a greater impact. Patients with previous sinus surgery have a favorable impact of INCS in comparison with nonsurgical patients. INCS have only slight side effects. Modern INCS have no additional clinical effectiveness than the first-generation INCS [23, 32].

5.2.1. Standard delivery (sprays)

The standard measured dose of INCS should be used in the treatment of CRSsNP. There is a significant improvement in the endoscopic and symptom scores. Dominance of benefit outweighs harm. Aggregated degree of evidence is A. Epistaxis and headache may be seen as side effects [23].

5.2.2. Nonstandard delivery (sprays)

Penetration of topical nasal sprays behind the nasal cavities into the paranasal sinuses, especially in preoperative patients, is expected to be limited. This situation caused a need to use of new delivery devices to offer improving corticosteroid deposition in the sinus tissues and for possible clinic healing. There are four prominent nonstandard delivery methods: (i) intranasal irrigation, (ii) maxillary antrostomy sinusotomy tubes (MAST), (iii) mucosal atomization devices (MAD), (iv) YAMIK sinus catheter. As a consequence, intranasal corticosteroid irrigations are the option in CRSsNP. They may be mostly beneficial for postoperative patients. The utilization of MAST or MAD is an option. Use of the YAMIK device is not recommended based on up-to-date data [23].

5.3. Oral corticosteroids

There is no clear evidence on the benefits of oral corticosteroids in CRSsNP. Oral steroid usage in CRSsNP is optional, due to inadequate strong evidence. Oral steroid use in perioperative period with CRSsNP is not recommended. The risks of oral steroids are uncommon, but significant side effects should be taken into consideration [10, 23, 33].

5.4. Antibiotics

5.4.1. Oral antibiotics

Sabino et al. [34] stated that 14 days of amoxicillin-clavulanate usage did not change any clinical course of acute exacerbations of chronic rhinosinusitis (AECRS) compared to placebo. Interestingly, combination of an oral antibiotic with a topical intranasal steroid spray may not offer further benefits for managing AECRS. When intranasal corticosteroids and saline irrigations have failed to reduce symptoms, long-term antibiotic treatment should be considered. Macrolide antibiotics have been used in the majority of trials. These antibiotics have revealed a response proportion of 60–80%. Roxithromycin has acceptable effects in patients without polyp. In a placebo-controlled azithromycin study, [35] suggests that the population with high serum IgE are less likely to respond to macrolide treatment. Long-term treatment with doxycycline or trimethoprim-sulfamethoxazole could reveal hopeful options. Level of evidence for macrolides in patients with CRSsNP is Ib, and strength of recommendation C, but in CRSsNP patients with normal IgE, the recommendation level is A [10].

5.4.2. Oral out of macrolide antibiotics for <3 weeks

When considering the use of antibiotic treatment less than 3 weeks in the management of CRS, current data are related to the treatment of AECRS. In addition, there is a shortage of suitable prospective trial at present. Because there is no sufficient clinical study and data, the ability to make recommendations regarding the use of nonmacrolide antibiotic for less than 3 weeks in CRSsNP is not applicable [10].

5.4.3. Oral out of macrolide antibiotics for >3 weeks

Although there are significant data on the role of long-term treatment with macrolide antibiotics for CRSsNP, there are little data in the literature concerning similar management with nonmacrolide agents. Dubin et al. [36] conducted an observational study with long-term oral antibiotics in patients with CRSsNP. Thirty five patients with CT scan and culture-approved CRSsNP were prescribed antibiotics for 6 weeks. At the end of the study, there was no considerable improvement between third and sixth weeks and only 38% of the patients reported improvement in CT scan scores. For the treatment of CRSsNP, the recommendation of nonmacrolide oral antibiotics for longer than 3 weeks has inadequate evidence. So, there is no applicable degree of evidence for the use of oral nonmacrolide antibiotics in CRSsNP [23].

5.4.4. Macrolide antibiotics

Macrolide antibiotics have both anti-inflammatory and antimicrobial functions, and for this reason, they may be considered to be effective in the treatment of CRS. Previous studies on lower respiratory diseases have led to be used macrolide antibiotics in the treatment of CRS. In those studies, erythromycin had been used in panbronchiolitis to improve clinical symptoms. Aggregated grade of evidence of these therapeutic agents is B. They offer, especially for patients without elevated IgE, a decline in endoscopy scores and some symptoms in patients with CRSsNP. Their effects are comparable to INCS. The effect of the agents may not sustain for long term after termination of treatment. They have important risks of drug interactions, in frequent mild undesirable events, and severe cardiovascular complications. Their benefits seem to outweigh harms. The convenient drug, dosage, and length of therapy are not recognized. Macrolides have an optional effect for patients with CRSsNP and were judged for the evidence of moderate quality [37].

5.4.5. Intravenous antibiotics

Intravenous antibiotics have a weak evidence in the treatment of CRSsNP. Their aggregated grade of evidence is C. There has been possible healing with patient-reported symptoms in case-controlled and cohort trials. Among their side effects, bleeding, deep vein thrombosis, drug adverse events, elevated liver enzymes, neutropenia, rash, thrombophlebitis, and sepsis may be determined. Their cost is high. The harm during the use of these agents outweighs the benefits. There is no recommendation for the use of intravenous antibiotics and should not be prescribed routinely in CRSsNP [23].

5.4.6. Topical antibiotics

The aim of topical antibiotic treatment for CRS is to transport high amounts of antibiotics into the sinonasal tissues, hence enhancing efficiency, diminishing systemic absorption and related side effects. It has been demonstrated that endoscopic sinus surgery increases the penetration of topical antibiotic agents from 2 to more than 95%. There is an aggregated grade of evidence of B for this management strategy, but randomized controlled trials have been unsuccessful to demonstrate any benefit from the application of topical antibiotic agents. Among their side effects, epistaxis, irritation, and nasal congestion may be seen. There is no recommendation regarding the topical antibiotic treatment in the management of CRSsNP at present [10].

5.5. Antifungal treatment in the management of adult chronic rhinosinusitis without nasal polyp (CRSsNP)

5.5.1. Topical antifungals

Physicians should avoid prescribing any topical antifungal therapy for routine patients with CRSsNP due to the systemic review of randomized controlled trials. Also, clinicians must avoid cost of ineffective therapy, unnecessary side effects, and shift of sinonasal flora [10].

5.5.2. Oral antifungals

For a significant subgroup of patients, fungi are considered as a causative agent of CRS with eosinophilic inflammation. Hence, it has been thought that antifungals have a possible effect in this subgroup of CRS patients. So, in the standard management of CRSsNP, there has been no confirmation about the use of oral antifungal treatment and aggregated grade of evidence is not applicable [10].

5.6. Combination treatment with nasal irrigation treatment in the management of adult chronic rhinosinusitis without nasal polyp (CRSsNP)

The antimicrobial effects of the sodium hypochlorite (NaOCl), particularly against *S. aureus* and *P. aeruginosa*, have been well established. Topical nasal irrigation with 0.05% NaOCl in saline solution has been found to be more effective than saline alone after 3 months usage [10, 38]. For nasal irrigation, xylitol in water is a well-tolerated substance. Xylitol irrigations lead to a further healing in chronic rhinosinusitis symptoms compared to saline irrigation [10]. It is considered that biofilms have the pathophysiological role in CRS. Surfactants have reductive effects on water surface tension and may facilitate dissolving of the biofilms. The use of sodium hypochlorite or xylitol nasal irrigations is supported by up-to-date with grade of recommendations B, but baby shampoo irrigations are not supported [10].

5.7. Proton pump inhibitors

There is no satisfactory evidence of the use for proton pump inhibitor therapy for CRSsNP in adults. Hence, there is also no support for the use of proton pump inhibitors, H2-receptor antagonists, antacids, or prokinetic therapy for chronic rhinosinusitis [39].

5.8. Topical alternative therapies

5.8.1. *Surfactants*

The benefits of surfactants are clearance of thick secretions and interruption of biofilm formation. Surfactants have the effects of clearance of secretions and blockage of biofilm development. Their side effects comprise ciliary dysfunction and nasal irritation. Although they have balanced effects regarding benefit and harm and limited clinical information, it is not possible to recommend for the use of surfactants in CRSsNP [23].

5.8.2. *Manuka honey*

Manuka honey and chief component methylglyoxal have in vitro effects against both the biofilm and planktonic formations of *Pseudomonas aeruginosa* and *Staphylococcus aureus*. But, regarding the routine use of Manuka honey in CRSsNP, no clinical study exists. Possible respiratory epithelial damage, nasal irritation, and burning may also be seen. As of the lack of evidence, it is not possible to recommend to use Manuka honey in CRSsNP [23].

5.8.3. *Xylitol*

Xylitol is composed of five-carbon sugar and has the property of improving the innate immune system. The main effect of xylitol is to increase the activity of natural antimicrobial factors in respiratory secretions [23].

6. Medical management of adult chronic rhinosinusitis with nasal polyp (CRSwNP)

6.1. Saline (spray and irrigation) treatment

In the management of CRSwNP, saline is strongly recommended as grade A evidence. Both isotonic and hypertonic saline irrigations seem to offer similar subjective results and are well tolerated. There is a dominance of benefit rather than harm. It is important to use nasal saline irrigation in addition to other topical treatment approaches. There is a superiority of higher volume (>200 mL) irrigations over low-volume topical nasal sprays [10, 23, 40, 41]. Regarding the patients with difficult to treat sphenoid sinus disease, it has been suggested that the irrigation position of nose-to-ceiling head position is more effective than the nose-to-floor position in delivering a 120-mL irrigation to the sphenoid sinuses [42].

6.2. Intranasal corticosteroids: standard delivery (drops and sprays)

In the management of CRSwNP, the use of topical corticosteroids have keystone role. Intranasal corticosteroids (sprays or drops) are recommended before or after the surgery for CRSwNP. The use of INCS as sprays or drops have noteworthy benefits. Its advantages include improved symptoms, endoscopic views, size of polyp, quality of life, objective tests of smell, airway, and polyp relaps. Headache, epistaxis, and nasal mucosal damage may be seen as side effects [23, 40, 41, 43].

http://dx.doi.org/10.5772/intechopen.81040

6.3. Intranasal corticosteroids: nonstandard delivery (irrigation and nebulizers)

Nonstandard topical corticosteroid delivery system, especially after sinus surgery, is an option in CRSwNP. General benefits are not available to statistically approve therapeutic recovery on existing evidence. Although evidence of adrenal suppression has not been seen, this cannot be ruled out by nonstandard delivery and dosing regimens. They have off-label use and possible minor side effects in comparison with oral corticosteroids [23].

6.4. Oral corticosteroids

The short-term oral corticosteroids usage in treatment of CRSwNP is strongly recommended. Both in subjective and objective measurements, this treatment provides a considerable short-term healing in the patients with CRSwNP. Patients must be prescribed systemic corticosteroids in acute aggravations of CRSwNP. The recovery time may take 8–12 weeks with the use of INCS. Further gastrointestinal complications may also be seen. There may be temporary adrenal inhibition, insomnia, and elevated bone turnover. With long-term management, the entire well-known corticosteroid complications may be seen. Corticosteroid agents have significant benefits over harm in short-term usage. The use of corticosteroids in long term or frequently is not encouraged by the literature and has further risk of damage to the patients [10, 33, 37, 40, 43].

6.5. Antibiotics

6.5.1. Oral out of macrolide antibiotics for <3 weeks

In general, there is no recommendation to prescribe nonmacrolide antibiotics less than 3 weeks course for the patients with nonacute clinic conditions of CrSWNP. Oral doxycycline therapy for 3 weeks decreases the polyp size and postnasal discharge, but this therapy cannot decrease the other complaints in patients with CRSwNP compared to the placebo. Because there is no placebo in the erdosteine study, it is impractical to establish a benefit. There may have gastrointestinal discomfort and risk of resistance and anaphylaxis. There may be more harm than benefits [10, 23, 40].

6.5.2. Oral out of macrolide antibiotics for >3 weeks

Long-term oral nonmacrolide antibiotics for more than 3 weeks course in the management of adult chronic rhinosinusitis with nasal polyp (CRSwNP) is not currently recommended [10, 23].

6.5.3. Macrolide antibiotics

Macrolides may have advantageous effects after endoscopic sinus surgery to reduce polyp recurrence and recover symptoms of CRSwNP. Benefits have shown outweigh harm. They may have considerable drug interactions. Also, they may cause infrequent but serious cardiovascular complications [10, 23].

6.5.4. Topical antibiotics

Topical antibiotic agents have efficiency in just lower stage studies and have unidentified systemic absorption and side-effect scale. So, they should be prescribed only if conventional management modalities (oral antibiotics, steroid sprays, saline) are unsuccessful [10, 23].

6.6. Antifungals

6.6.1. Oral antifungals

For the treatment of CRSwNP, there is no recommendation for prescribing oral antifungal agents. Liver function tests may be deteriorated during systemic usage. Because there is a lack of evidence for the use of oral antifungal therapy, there is a greater risk of adverse effects than potential advantages. For the usual management of CRSwNP, clinicians should not prescribe the oral antifungal drugs [10, 23].

6.6.2. Intranasal antifungals

For the usual CRSwNP treatment, topical antifungal medications should not be utilized. In the management of typical CRSWNP, there is no benefit of topical antifungals, but there may be some benefits in some CRSwNP subdivisions, such as allergic fungal sinusitis. Because they have unconfirmed systemic absorption and side-effect scale, topical antifungal agents should only be considered if routine treatment modalities failed [10, 23, 41].

6.7. Anti-LT therapy

For patients with CRSwNP, montelukast may be useful and an option to substitute or supplement to INCS. Symptoms can be improved when compared to the INCS and may have limited benefits in addition to the INCS. Montelukast is in association with infrequent neuropsychiatric side effects in post-sale records. In addition, there has been also in association with high liver enzymes and Zileuton and other medications [23]. On the contrary, anti-leukotriene treatment is not supported for the patients with CRSwNP and this treatment modality is not recommended [10, 23].

6.8. Aspirin desensitization

This therapy must be considered and recommended in patients with aspirin exacerbated rhinitis disease to impede postoperative nasal polyp renewal. The aggregated grade of evidence is B. Benefits include decreased polyp reformation after surgery, decreased CRS symptoms in increased QoL and AERD, reduced the need for systemic corticosteroids, and decreased number of reoperations. It is necessary to be vigilant for gastrointestinal bleeding. It should be noted that this treatment has the potential to increase morbidity in patients with kidney disease and blood clotting problems with the increasing doses. There has been lower than 3% gastrointestinal complaints throughout the low-dose treatments. Absolute benefit is present rather than harm. Aspirin desensitization is a unique treatment modality for aspirin-sensitive patients with CRSwNP [10, 23].

6.9. Immunotherapy

For postoperative period of AFRS patients, this treatment modality offers an option with balanced benefit and harm. There is a limited data and the grade of evidence is C. If a patient represents enhanced sensitivity to the certain antigens, immunotherapy may be used to diminish the inflammatory load [23, 40].

6.10. Anti-IL 4 and anti-IL13 treatment

An anti-IL-4/13α subunit receptor antibody, dupilumab, has been approved for atopic dermatitis [44]. Add-on therapy of dupilumab may have a role in nasal symptom relief for patients with uncontrolled persistent asthma and comorbid persistent allergic rhinitis [45]. It has been observed that for the patient with nasal polyp, addition of subcutaneous dupilumab to mometasone furoate nasal spray reduced endoscopic nasal polyp scores after treatment. More sophisticated studies are needed to evaluate for longer treatment duration and larger patient samples [46].

6.11. Anti-IL5

Reslizumab is an anti-IL5 mAb derived from human tissues and acts diminishing the amount of eosinophils both in tissue and blood. Anti-IL5 antibodies may have benefit in the management of CRSwNP patients [10].

Mepolizumab, FDA approved for severe eosinophilic asthma, is another anti-IL-5 human derived antibody that has been studied in patients with CRS. For the patients with recurrent nasal polyposis, who receiving topical corticosteroids and required surgery, mepolizumab treatment showed a huge reduction in the need for surgery and a huge improvement in symptoms than placebo [44, 47]. Also, there is a continued clinical trial of mepolizumab in the patients with CRSwNP refractory to medical and surgical therapy [48].

Benralizumab is another anti-IL5 molecule that could potentially have some benefits for inhibiting the IL-5 pathway in CRS [44].

6.12. Anti-IL13

Lebrikizumab did not substantially heal FEV1 in mild-to-moderate asthma patients by inhibiting IL-13 pathway. Inhibiting IL-13 in this patient population was not satisfactory to improve lung function [49].

Tralokinumab, an agent of anti-IL13, in severe asthma exacerbations, has not been considered as a key role for interleukin 13, and it was stated that Tralokinumab is unsuccessful for management of severe, uncontrolled asthma [50–52].

Anrukinzumab is a humanized anti-IL-13 monoclonal antibody, which acts to block the cytokine and prevent the activation of IL-13Rα1 and IL-13Rα2 [53, 54].

So far, there is no approved anti-IL13 treatment modality for the patients with CRwNP.

6.13. Anti IgE

Omalizumab is a human-derived anti-IgE monoclonal antibody that prevents binding of IgE to receptors on mast cells and basophils. Omalizumab has been approved for severe allergic asthma [44]. Anti-IgE therapy also reduces nasal polyp score in patients with severe comorbid asthma [55].

6.14. Intranasal triamcinolone acetonide/carboxymethylcellulose foam

For acute exacerbations of postoperative CRSwNP patients, it has been observed that topical triamcinolone acetonide/carboxymethylcellulose foam reduced systemic steroid need, is well tolerant, and a good treatment option [56].

Author details

Mehmet Şentürk

Address all correspondence to: drmehmetsenturk@gmail.com

Department of Otorhinolaryngology, Head and Neck Surgery, Ozel Konya Hospital, Karatay, Konya, Turkey

References

[1] Abzug MJ. Acute sinusitis in children: Do antibiotics have any role? Journal of Infection. 2014;**68**(Suppl 1):S33-S37. DOI: 10.1016/j.jinf.2013.09.012

[2] Brook I. Acute sinusitis in children. Pediatric Clinics of North America. 2013;**60**:409-424. DOI: 10.1016/j.pcl.2012.12.002

[3] Victores AJ, Takashima M. Management of acute rhinosinusitis. In: Yen MT, Johnson TE, editors. Orbital Cellulitis and Periorbital Infections. 1st ed. Cham: Springer; 2018. pp. 75-87. DOI: 10.1007/978-3-319-62606-2

[4] Wald ER, Applegate KE, Bordley C, Darrow DH, Glode MP, Marcy SM, et al. Clinical practice guideline for the diagnosis and management of acute bacterial sinusitis in children aged 1 to 18 years. Pediatrics. 2013;**132**:e262-e280. DOI: 10.1542/peds.2013-1071

[5] Chow AW, Benninger MS, Brook I, Brozek JL, Goldstein EJ, Hicks LA, et al. IDSA clinical practice guideline for acute bacterial rhinosinusitis in children and adults. Clinical Infectious Diseases. 2012;**54**:e72-e112. DOI: 10.1093/cid/cir1043

[6] Chandran SK, Higgins TS. Chapter 5: Pediatric rhinosinusitis: Definitions, diagnosis and management—An overview. American Journal of Rhinology & Allergy. 2013;**27**(Suppl 1):S16-S19. DOI: 10.2500/ajra.2013.27.3896

[7] Foden N, Burgess C, Shepherd K, Almeyda R. A guide to the management of acute rhinosinusitis in primary care: Management strategy based on best evidence and recent European guidelines. British Journal of General Practice. 2013;**63**:611-613. DOI: 10.3399/bjgp13X674620

[8] Para AJ, Clayton E, Peters AT. Management of rhinosinusitis: An evidence based approach. Current Opinion in Allergy and Clinical Immunology. 2016;**16**:383-389. DOI: 10.1097/ACI.0000000000000276

[9] Magit A. Pediatric rhinosinusitis. Otolaryngologic Clinics of North America. 2014;**47**:733-746. DOI: 10.1016/j.otc.2014.06.003

[10] Fokkens WJ, Lund VJ, Mullol J, Bachert C, Alobid I, Baroody F, et al. European position paper on rhinosinusitis and nasal polyps 2012. Rhinology Supplement. 2012;**23**:1-298

[11] Meltzer EO, Bachert C, Staudinger H. Treating acute rhinosinusitis: Comparing efficacy and safety of mometasonefuroate nasal spray, amoxicillin, and placebo. The Journal of Allergy and Clinical Immunology. 2005;**116**:1289-1295. DOI: 10.1016/j.jaci.2005.08.044

[12] Meltzer EO, Hamilos DL. Rhinosinusitis diagnosis and management for the clinician: A synopsis of recent consensus guidelines. Mayo Clinic Proceedings. 2011;**86**:427-443. DOI: 10.4065/mcp.2010.0392

[13] Rahmati MB, Mohebi S, Shahmohammadi S, Rezai MS. Fluticasone nasal spray as an adjunct to amoxicillin for acute sinusitis in children: A randomized controlled trial. Europen Review for Medical and Pharmacological Sciences. 2013;**17**:3068-3072

[14] Mori F, Fiocchi A, Barni S, Beghi G, Caddeo A, Calcinai E, et al. Management of acute rhinosinusitis. Pediatric Allergy and Immunology. 2012;**23**(Suppl 22):27-31. DOI: 10.1111/j. 1399-3038.2012.01321.x

[15] Wei JL, Sykes KJ, Johnson P, He J, Mayo MS. Safety and efficacy of once-daily nasal irrigation for the treatment of pediatric chronicrhinosinusitis. The Laryngoscope. 2011; **121**:1989-2000. DOI: 10.1002/lary.21923

[16] Rose AS, Thorp BD, Zanation AM, Ebert CS Jr. Chronic rhinosinusitis in children. Pediatric Clinics of North America. 2013;**60**:979-991. DOI: 10.1016/j.pcl.2013.04.001

[17] Hong SD, Kim JH, Kim HY, Jang MS, Dhong HJ, Chung SK. Compliance and efficacy of saline irrigation in pediatric chronic rhinosinusitis. Auris, Nasus, Larynx. 2014;**41**:46-49. DOI: 10.1016/j.anl.2013.07.008

[18] Lin SY, Baugher KM, Brown DJ, Ishman SL. Effects of nasal saline lavage on pediatric sinusitis symptoms and disease-specific quality of life: A case series of 10 patients. Ear Nose Throat Journal. 2015;**94**:E13-E18

[19] Cazzavillan A, Castelnuovo P, Berlucchi M, Baiardini I, Franzetti A, Nicolai P, et al. Management of chronic rhinosinusitis. Pediatric Allergy and Immunology. 2012;**23**(Suppl 22):32-44. DOI: 10.1111/j.1399-3038.2012.01322.x

[20] Brook I. The role of antibiotics in pediatric chronic rhinosinusitis. Laryngoscope Investigative Otolaryngology. 2017;**2**:104-108. DOI: 10.1002/lio2.67

[21] Ozturk F, Bakirtas A, Ileri F, Turktas I. Efficacy and tolerability of systemic methylprednisolone in children and adolescents with chronic rhinosinusitis: A double-blind, placebo-controlled randomized trial. Journal of Allergy and Clinical Immunology. 2011; **128**:348-352. DOI: 10.1016/j.jaci.2011.04.045

[22] Hamilos DL. Pediatric chronic rhinosinusitis. American Journal of Rhinology and Allergy. 2015;**29**:414-420. DOI: 10.2500/ajra.2015.29.4238

[23] Orlandi RR, Kingdom TT, Hwang PH, Smith TL, Alt JA, Baroody FM, et al. International consensus statement on allergy and rhinology: Rhinosinusitis. International Forum of Allergy & Rhinology. 2016;**6**(Suppl 1):S22-S209. DOI: 10.1002/alr.21695

[24] Bock JM, Poetker DM. Reflux and chronic rhinosinusitis. JAMA Otolaryngology Head and Neck Surgery. 2016;**142**:633-634. DOI: 10.1001/jamaoto.2016.1050

[25] Rosenfeld RM, Piccirillo JF, Chandrasekhar SS, Brook I, Ashok Kumar K. Clinical practice guideline (update): Adult sinusitis. Otolaryngology Head and Neck Surgery. 2015;**152**(Suppl 2):S1-S39. DOI: 10.1177/0194599815572097

[26] Demoly P. Safety of intranasal corticosteroids in acute rhinosinusitis. American Journal of Otolaryngology. 2008;**29**:403-413. DOI: 10.1016/j.amjoto.2007.11.004

[27] Masood A, Moumoulidis I, Panesar J. Acute rhinosinusitis in adults: An update on current management. Postgraduate Medical Journal. 2007;**83**:402-408. DOI: 10.1136/pgmj.2006.054767

[28] Karlowsky JA, Draghi DC, Thornsberry C, Jones ME, Critchley IA, Sahm DF. Antimicrobial susceptibilities of *Streptococcus pneumoniae, Haemophilus influenzae* and *Moraxella catarrhalis* isolated in two successive respiratory seasons in the US. International Journal of Antimicrobial Agents. 2002;**20**:76-85

[29] Hoban D, Felmingham D. The PROTEKT surveillance study: Antimicrobial susceptibility of *Haemophilus influenzae* and *Moraxella catarrhalis* from community-acquired respiratory tract infections. Journal of Antimicrobial Chemotherapy. 2002;**50**(Suppl S1):49-59. DOI: 10.1093/jac/dkf810

[30] MD1 P, Portugal LG. Treatment of rhinosinusitis in the outpatient setting. American Journal of Medicine. 2005;**118**(Suppl 7A):45S-50S. DOI: 10.1016/j.amjmed.2005.05.013

[31] Anon JB. Current management of acute bacterial rhinosinusitis and the role of moxifloxacin. Clinical Infectious Diseases. 2005;**41**(Suppl 2):167-176. DOI: 10.1086/428057

[32] Chong LY, Head K, Hopkins C, Philpot C, Burton MJ, Schilder AG. Different types of intranasal steroids for chronic rhinosinusitis. Cochrane Database of Systematic Reviews 2016;**4**:1-82. DOI: 10.1002/14651858.CD011993.pub2

[33] Poetker DM, Jakubowski LA, Lal D, Hwang PH, Wright ED, Smith TL. Oral corticosteroids in the management of adult chronic rhinosinusitis with and without nasal polyps: An evidence-based review with recommendations. International Forum of Allergy & Rhinology. 2013;**3**:104-120. DOI: 10.1002/alr.21072 (Epub Aug 7, 2012)

[34] Sabino HA, Valera FC, Aragon DC, Fantucci MZ, Titoneli CC, Martinez R, et al. Amoxicillin-clavulanate for patients with acute exacerbation of chronic rhinosinusitis: A prospective, double-blinded, placebo-controlled trial. International Forum of Allergy & Rhinology. 2017;**7**:135-142. DOI: 10.1002/alr.21846

[35] Haruna S, Shimada C, Ozawa M, Fukami S, Moriyama H. A study of poor responders for long-term, low-dose macrolide administration for chronic sinusitis. Rhinology. 2009;**47**:66-71

[36] Dubin MG, Kuhn FA, Melroy CT. Radiographic resolution of chronic rhinosinusitis without polyposis after 6 weeks vs 3 weeks of oral antibiotics. Annals of Allergy, Asthma & Immunology. 2007;**98**:32-35. DOI: 10.1016/S1081-1206(10)60856-3

[37] Head K, Chong LY, Piromchai P, Hopkins C, Philpott C, Schilder AG, et al. Systemic and topical antibiotics for chronic rhinosinusitis. Cochrane Database Systematic Reviews. 2016;**26**(4):CD011994. DOI: 10.1002/14651858.CD011994.pub2

[38] Raza T, Elsherif HS, Zulianello L, Plouin-Gaudon I, Landis BN, Lacroix JS. Nasal lavage with sodium hypochlorite solution in *Staphylococcus aureus* persistent rhinosinusitis. Rhinology. 2008;**46**:15-22

[39] Gilani S, Pynnonen MA, Shin JJ. National practice patterns of antireflux medication for chronic rhinosinusitis. JAMA Otolaryngology Head and Neck Surgery. 2016;**142**:627-633. DOI: 10.1001/jamaoto.2016.0937

[40] McCoul ED, Tabaee A. A practical approach to refractory chronic rhinosinusitis. Otolaryngologic Clinics of North America. 2017;**50**:183-198. DOI: 10.1016/j.otc.2016.08.014

[41] Huang A, Govindaraj S. Topical therapy in the management of chronic rhinosinusitis. Current Opinion in Otolaryngology Head and Neck Surgery. 2013;**21**:31-38. DOI: 10.1097/MOO.0b013e32835bc4ab

[42] Craig JR, Palmer JN, Zhao K. Computational fluid dynamic modeling of nose-to-ceiling head positioning for sphenoid sinus irrigation. International Forum of Allergy & Rhinology. 2017;**7**:474-479. DOI: 10.1002/alr.21908

[43] Ocampo CJ, Peters AT. Medical therapy as the primary modality for the management of chronic rhinosinusitis. Allergy and Asthma Proceedings. 2013;**34**:132-137. DOI: 10.2500/aap.2013.34.3636

[44] Ghadersohi S, Tan BK. Contemporary pharmacotherapy for allergic rhinitis and chronic rhinosinusitis. Otolaryngologic Clinics of North America. 2017;**50**:1135-1151. DOI: 10.1016/j.otc.2017.08.009

[45] Weinstein SF, Katial R, Jayawardena S, Pirozzi G, Staudinger H, Eckert L, et al. Efficacy and safety of dupilumab in perennial allergic rhinitis and comorbid asthma. Journal of Allergy and Clinical Immunology. 2018;**142**:171-177.e1. DOI: 10.1016/j.jaci.2017.11.051

[46] Bachert C, Mannent L, Naclerio RM, Mullol J, Ferguson BJ, Gevaert P, et al. Effect of subcutaneous dupilumab on nasal polyp burden in patients with chronic sinusitis and nasal polyposis: A randomized clinical trial. Journal of the American Medical Association. 2016;**315**:469-479. DOI: 10.1001/jama.2015.19330

[47] Bachert C, Sousa AR, Lund VJ, Scadding GK, Gevaert P, Nasser S, et al. Reduced need for surgery in severe nasal polyposis with mepolizumab: Randomized trial. Journal of Allergy and Clinical Immunology. 2017;**140**:1024-1031.e14. DOI: 10.1016/j.jaci.2017.05.044

[48] GlaxoSmithKline. Mepolizumab in Nasal Polyposis. 2009. Available from: https://ClinicalTrials.gov/show/NCT01362244 [Accessed: August 20, 2018]

[49] Korenblat P, Kerwin E, Leshchenko I, Yen K, Holweg CTJ, Anzures-Cabrera J, et al. Efficacy and safety of lebrikizumab in adult patients with mild-to-moderate asthma not receiving inhaled corticosteroids. Respiratory Medicine. 2018;**134**:143-149. DOI: 10.1016/j.rmed.2017.12.006

[50] Chung KF. Tralokinumab unsuccessful for management of severe, uncontrolled asthma. Lancet Respiratory Medicine. 2018;**6**:480-481. DOI: 10.1016/S2213-2600(18)30194-2

[51] Russell RJ, Chachi L, FitzGerald JM, Backer V, Olivenstein R, Titlestad IL, et al. Effect of tralokinumab, an interleukin-13 neutralising monoclonal antibody, on eosinophilic airway inflammation in uncontrolled moderate-to-severe asthma (MESOS): A multicentre, double-blind, randomised, placebo-controlled. Lancet Respiratory Medicine. 2018;**6**: 499-510. DOI: 10.1016/S2213-2600(18)30201-7

[52] Panettieri RA Jr, Sjöbring U, Péterffy A, Wessman P, Bowen K, Piper E, et al. Tralokinumab for severe, uncontrolled asthma (STRATOS 1 and STRATOS 2): Two randomised, double-blind, placebo-controlled, phase 3 clinical trials. Lancet Respiratory Medicine. 2018 Jul;**6**(7):511-525. DOI: 10.1016/S2213-2600(18)30184-X

[53] F H, J R, W R, F C, S M. A pharmacokinetic comparison of anrukinzumab, an anti- IL-13 monoclonal antibody, among healthy volunteers, asthma and ulcerative colitis patients. British Journal of Clinical Pharmacology. 2015;**80**:101-109. DOI: 10.1111/bcp.12589

[54] D1 B, Ferrando M, Varricchi G, Passalacqua G, Canonica GW. A critical evaluation of anti-IL-13 and anti-IL-4 strategies in severe asthma. International Archieves of Allergy and Immunology. 2016;**170**(2):122-131. DOI: 10.1159/000447692

[55] Rivero A, Liang J. Anti-IgE and anti-IL5 biologic therapy in the treatment of nasal polyposis: A systematic review and meta-analysis. Annals of Otology Rhinology and Laryngology. 2017;**126**:739-747. DOI: 10.1177/0003489417731782

[56] Chaudhry AL, Chaaban MR, Ranganath NK, Woodworth BA. Topical triamcinolone acetonide/carboxymethylcellulose foam for acute exacerbations of chronic rhinosinusitis/nasal polyposis. American Journal of Rhinology and Allergy. 2014;**28**:341-344. DOI: 10.2500/ajra.2014.28.4053

Chapter 5

Orbital Cellulitis

Lizette Mowatt

Additional information is available at the end of the chapter

http://dx.doi.org/10.5772/intechopen.79983

Abstract

Infection in the soft tissues of the orbit, posterior to the orbital septum results in orbital cellulitis. This is a very serious condition, which may occur as a complication of sinusitis by contiguous spread or may result from haematogenous spread or from trauma. Orbital cellulitis presents with periorbital swelling, proptosis, conjunctival chemosis and injection, extraocular motility deficits and visual loss. It requires comanagement by the ophthalmologist and otorhinolaryngologist when secondary to sinusitis. It is important that this condition is recognized early, and immediate management is done to prevent impending visual loss and further complications of periosteal abscesses, meningitis, cavernous sinus thrombosis and death. This chapter reviews the epidemiology of orbital cellulitis, pathogenesis, causative organisms, investigations (including imaging of the sinuses) and treatment. Prognostic factors and conditions that complicate this such as diabetes will also be discussed.

Keywords: orbital, sinusitis, periorbital swelling, proptosis, brain abscess, meningitis

1. Introduction

Orbital cellulitis is the involvement of the orbital tissues behind the orbital septum with inflammation or infection. The orbital septum is an important dividing landmark, as infection and inflammation occurring anterior to it is called preseptal cellulitis, which is managed differently than that occurring posterior to it, orbital cellulitis.

Orbital cellulitis is an inflammatory process and is generally used to describe infectious inflammation [1]. The sinuses are closely associated with the orbit and are commonly the source of infection from direct contiguous spread. It is important that orbital cellulitis is diagnosed, investigated with imaging to determine if the source is from the sinuses and treatment (medical and/or surgical) commenced early to prevent serious complications, including cerebral abscess and meningitis. Sinus surgery may be required for the treatment of orbital cellulitis secondary to sinusitis or pansinusitis. The management of this condition may, therefore, require a multidisciplinary team of the ophthalmologist, otolaryngologist, infection specialist and neurosurgeon.

2. Orbital anatomy

The bony orbit is a pear-shaped cavity which houses the eyeball with its adnexae (lacrimal gland) and orbital fat. The volume of the orbit is ~30 ml of which the eyeball takes up 6 ml (20%). The orbit is related superiorly to the frontal sinus, inferiorly to the maxillary sinus, medially the ethmoid sinus and anterior aspect of the sphenoid sinus.

The anterior border of the orbit is the **orbital septum**, which separates the lid from the orbit. The orbital septum, a fibrous tissue arises from the periosteum of the superior and inferior orbital rims, divides the plane of the inflammation or infection into preseptal or postseptal (orbital cellulitis) (**Figure 1**). Infection anterior to the orbital septum is called preseptal cellulitis and can be managed by oral antibiotics. However, when the infection is posterior to the orbital septum, it results in orbital cellulitis which is an ophthalmic emergency requiring in hospital treatment.

The orbit is bounded superiorly by the **roof** (the lesser wing of the sphenoid bone and orbital plate of the frontal bone), which is below the anterior cranial fossa and frontal sinus. The greater wing of the sphenoid and the zygomatic bone make up the **lateral wall** (**Figure 2**).

Three bones make the **floor of the orbit,** the zygomatic, maxillary and palatine. Blow out fractures commonly occur in the posterior medial aspect of the maxilla. The orbital floor is also the superior boundary of the maxillary sinus.

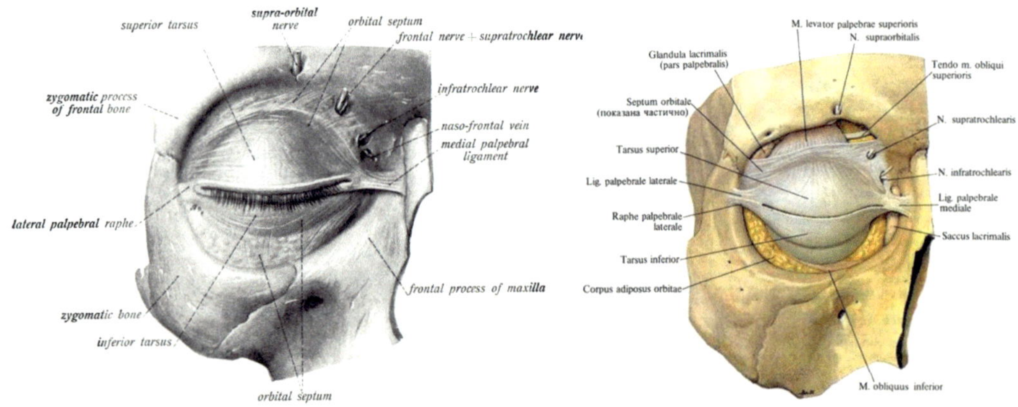

Figure 1. An anatomical illustration from the 1909 edition of Sobotta's Anatomy. https://commons.wikimedia.org/wiki/File:Sobo_1909_770.png#/media/File:Sobo_1909_770.png. Source: Riordan-Eva and Cunningham [2].

Four bones make up the **medial wall**; maxillary (frontal process), lacrimal, ethmoid and sphenoid bone (**Figure 3**). The lamina papyracea, which forms part of the medial wall, is paper-thin and perforated by numerous foramina for nerves and blood vessels, which makes easy contiguous spread from the ethmoid sinuses to the orbit in the spread of orbital cellulitis.

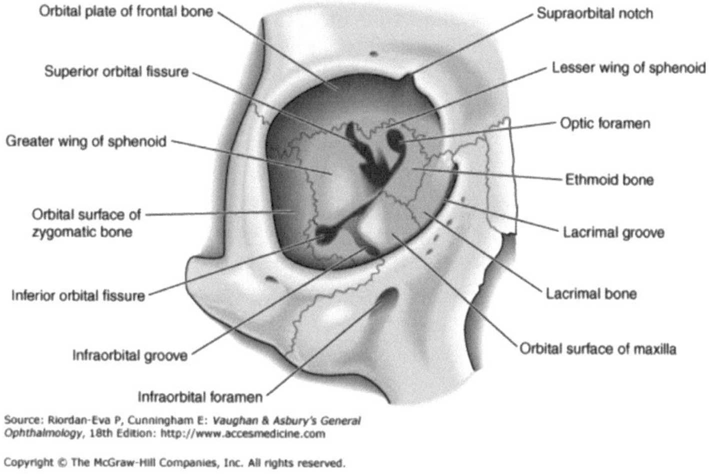

Figure 2. Anterior view of bones of right orbit. Source: Riordan-Eva and Cunningham [2]. Copyright © 2018 McGraw-Hill Education. All rights reserved.

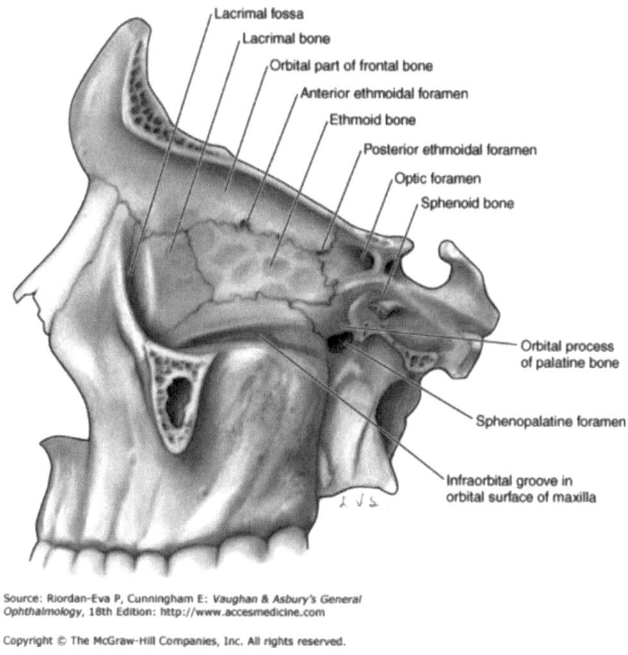

Figure 3. Medial wall of the orbit. Source: Riordan-Eva and Cunningham [2]. Copyright © 2018 McGraw-Hill Education. All rights reserved.

The **superior orbital fissure** is between the greater and lesser wings of the sphenoid and allows communication between the cranium and the orbit (**Figure 2**). This fissure is divided into the superior and inferior portion. The superior portion transmits the superior ophthalmic vein, lacrimal, frontal and trochlear nerves. The inferior portion transmits the abducens nerve, superior and inferior divisions of the oculomotor nerve and the sympathetic fibres from the cavernous plexus. Inflammation of the superior orbital fissure and orbital apex is called Tolosa-Hunt syndrome.

The **inferior orbital fissure** is located between the greater wing of the sphenoid and the maxillary bone, which divides the lateral orbital wall from the orbital floor (**Figure 2**). It connects the pterygopalatine and infratemporal fossae with the orbit and transmits the maxillary and zygomatic nerves in addition to the branches of the inferior ophthalmic vein.

The lesser wing of the sphenoid has the **optic foramen** through which the optic nerve and ophthalmic artery is transmitted from the middle cranial fossa to the orbit.

2.1. Epidemiology of orbital cellulitis

Orbital cellulitis may occur at all age groups but is more commonly seen in children. The incidence in children is 1.6 per 100,000 compared to adults 0.1 per 100,000 [3]. Gender distribution is usually equal; however, the males predominate in some countries because of work-related injuries as in India and Nigeria [1]. Orbital cellulitis has its peak incidence in winter and early spring [1, 4] and is least frequent (19.4%) in the summer months [5].

In the western countries, patients have an average duration of symptoms for 4.4 days and an average hospital stay of 5.8–6.2 days compared with developing countries, where the average symptom duration is 5.2–10.6 days, prior to presentation and have a longer average hospital stay of 9–13.7 days [1]. In developing countries, late presentation results in poor prognosis [6].

2.2. Pathogenesis of orbital cellulitis

Orbital cellulitis may result from direct contiguous spread (e.g. sinuses or dental), exogenous (e.g. trauma or surgery) and endogenous (haematogenous). Orbital cellulitis is unilateral in greater than 90% of cases [7]. Most cases of orbital cellulitis result from the extension of infection from the paranasal sinuses [1, 6]. Approximately, 1.3–5.6% of sinusitis results in orbital cellulitis and 80% of all complications of acute rhinosinusitis are orbital (**Table 1**) [4, 10–12].

The ethmoid sinuses are the most frequent source of infection in 43–100% of cases [1]. This may be due to the thin medial orbital wall. Other predisposing factors for the orbital spread include lack of lymphatics and valveless veins of the orbit and foramina of the orbital bones. Childhood orbital cellulitis may involve more than one sinus in 15.7–38% of cases, whereas in adults the multiple sinus involvement was <11%.

Upper respiratory tract infections are a major cause of orbital cellulitis and can reflect the seasonal distribution of the disease [1, 4]. Contiguous spread may also occur from endophthalmitis, pan ophthalmitis, dental abscesses and extension from preseptal cellulitis. Dental infections can result

http://dx.doi.org/10.5772/intechopen.79983

Group	Chandler et al.	Moloney et al.
I	Preseptal cellulitis	Preseptal cellulitis
II	Orbital cellulitis	Subperiosteal abscess
III	Subperiosteal abscess	Orbital cellulitis
IV	Orbital abscess	Orbital abscess
V	Cavernous sinus thrombosis	Cavernous sinus thrombosis

Table 1. Classification of the complications of sinusitis by Chandler et al. [8] and modification by Moloney [9].

in odontogenic orbital cellulitis with spread through the maxillary sinus. Haematogenous spread from a bacteraemia may occur and a bilateral orbital cellulitis has been reported in a case of infective endocarditis [13].

Trauma is a predisposing factor, which may be a direct penetrating injury or orbital fractures. Orbital cellulitis may occur from direct spread from the sinuses as seen in trauma resulting in a blow-out fracture of the orbit. Orbital foreign bodies can be metallic or organic, with the latter (e.g. wood) containing significant bacteria [14]. Less commonly it has been reported after surgery usually with the use of an explant such as aqueous drainage device (glaucoma surgery) or silicone scleral sponges (retinal detachment repair) [15, 16].

2.2.1. *Microorganisms*

Staphylococcus aureus and *Streptococcus* species are the most common causative organisms [1]. There are increasing cases of methicillin resistant *Staphylococcus aureus* (MRSA). *Streptococcus pneumoniae* is seen more commonly in younger children and *Group A Streptococcus* in older children. In one study from Scotland, *Streptococcus* (66%) and *Haemophilus* (46%) were the most common pathogens in children [3]. Less commonly coagulase-negative *Staphylococcus, Haemophilus influenza, Klebsiella pneumoniae, Moraxella catarrhalis* and other respiratory tract anaerobes were implicated [17]. *H. Influenzae* used to be a common pathogen; however, this has significantly reduced after the introduction of the *H. influenzae* vaccine [17–19].

Post traumatic cases are usually due to *S. aureus* and *S. pyogenes. Streptococcus* infections can lead to a necrotizing lid disease and necrotizing fasciitis [1]. Trauma with penetration of organic foreign body may have *Staphylococcus epidermidis, Staphylococcus aureus, Enterobacter agglomerans and Clostridium perfringens* as the offending organisms [14]. Odontogenic infections resulting in orbital cellulitis usually have mixed aerobic and anaerobic bacteria.

Fungal infections are usually seen in high risk patients such as diabetes mellitus, immunocompromised patients, patients on chronic steroids or antibiotic treatment. Mucormycosis and aspergillosis are the most common types. Fungi can invade blood vessel walls causing a thrombosing vasculitis. This can cause significant severe complications of ophthalmic vascular thrombosis, cavernous sinus thrombosis, meningoencephalitis, brain abscess and ultimately a high mortality rate [1].

2.3. Clinical features

Orbital cellulitis presents with periorbital oedema and cellulitis of the eyelids, ptosis, red eye with conjunctival chemosis and pain on eye movements. As it worsens proptosis, reduced vision and double vision occur due to limitation of extraocular movements with the orbital swelling (**Figure 4**). Most common symptoms are reduction in vision (66.6%), proptosis and ptosis (33.3%) [12]. Patients may also experience pain on eye movements due to inflammation of the extraocular muscles. Patients may give a history of sinusitis or an upper respiratory tract infection.

Constitutional signs such as fever, malaise, loss of appetite are usually present. Headache may occur in 10% of patients. Children are more likely to have a fever and a higher leukocytosis [7]. Children less than a year may present with fever, periorbital edema and erythema with reduced appetite and lethargy [1]. Patients between 1 and 7 years old are less likely to have proptosis and ophthalmoplegia compared to older children and adults.

Clinical signs include proptosis, limitation of extraocular movements, reduced vision, a relative afferent pupillary defect (RAPD) and impaired colour vision. Compression of the central retinal artery can compromise vision from optic nerve ischemia with resulting infarction of the sclera, choroid and retina [7]. Secondary inflammation can result in iridocyclitis, vitritis and septic pan ophthalmitis. Increase in the intraocular pressure, glaucoma, due to the increased congestion of the episcleral vessels can further reduce the vision.

This patient requires urgent ophthalmic admission, imaging, commencement of intravenous (IV) antibiotics and monitoring. Colour vision and pupillary reactions should be monitored every 4–6 h, in addition to the proptosis with the Hertel exophthalmometer.

Increased inflammation and congestion in the orbit can result in an orbital apex syndrome. The pupillary reactions should be monitored for a RAPD which suggests an optic neuropathy secondary to an orbital apex syndrome. Patients with a RAPD, elevated intraocular pressures and complete ophthalmoplegia can develop permanent loss of vision in that eye if orbital pressure is not relieved urgently.

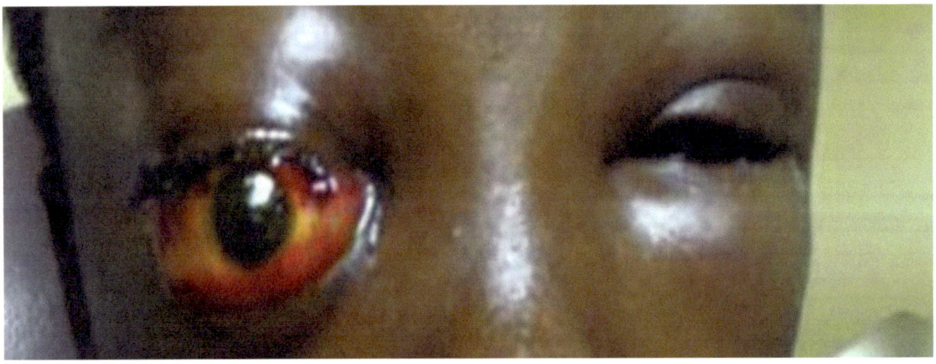

Figure 4. Right orbital cellulitis with periorbital swelling and proptosis.

Odontogenic orbital cellulitis can rapidly progress and cause blindness from a severe tense orbit, with resulting central retinal artery occlusion and ischemic optic neuropathy [20]. With increasing proptosis, corneal ulceration from exposure keratopathy may occur.

2.3.1. *Special clinical scenarios*

2.3.1.1. *Fungal orbital cellulitis*

This condition can be caused by the fungus of the order *Mucorales*, usually found in the soil among decaying organic matter [21]. *Rhizopus, Rhizomucor and Mucor* species are most common and are related to pathogenesis of vascular invasion with resulting thrombosis and necrosis of tissues. Elevated levels of iron and glucose in the serum are a predisposing factor [21]. Aspergillosis, caused by the fungus *Eurotiales*, genus *Aspergillus* can be non-invasive or invasive and is associated with vascular involvement and bony erosion, initially affecting the sinuses then spreading to the orbit.

Diagnosis is usually done by biopsy or culture and requires aggressive treatment with intravenous antifungals and may require orbital exenteration. Cases of non-invasive aspergillosis do not require orbital exenteration. Invasive aspergillosis has been reported to masquerade as giant cell arteritis, with symptoms of jaw claudication, scalp tenderness and weight loss [21]. The initial onset of fungal orbital cellulitis can be insidious then rapidly progressive, so a high index of suspicion must be present.

2.3.1.2. *Rhino-orbital mucormycosis*

This is a rare opportunistic infection caused by the fungi "Mucoraceae." This usually occurs in patients with immunosuppression and diabetic ketoacidosis but has been seen in patients with myelodysplastic syndrome, chronic hepatitis C infection, polysubstance abuse, alcoholic liver cirrhosis and Crohn's disease with systemic immunosuppression [21]. Uncontrolled diabetic ketoacidosis is the most commonly associated condition in orbital mucormycosis.

Patients may present with gradual onset of facial and periorbital swelling, double vision and loss of vision. Septic necrosis can cause black eschar from ischemic infarction on the palate, turbinates, skin and eye lids. Complications can result in retinal vascular occlusion, cranial palsies and cerebrovascular occlusion. The onset may be insidious in immunosuppressed patients and a high index of suspicion must be present to prevent the delay in diagnosis and treatment.

Fungal infections can be acquired from inhalation of spores with resulting upper respiratory tract infection then sinus involvement, orbital cellulitis with contiguous spread to the brain. Mucormycosis initially involves the maxillary and ethmoid sinus, thereafter spreading to the orbit and brain. The severity of the hyphae invasion of blood vessels results in an occlusive vasculitis with ischemia and infarction of orbital tissues, which can eventually become fatal.

Fungal orbital cellulitis from aspergillosis has been reported in a patient with myelodysplastic syndrome and portal hypertension, with the initial presentation mimicking giant cell arteritis [21]. Gradual onset of periorbital and facial swelling, diplopia and visual loss may occur. Black eschar results from ischemic infarction and septic necrosis of the palates, turbinates, nasal septum and eyelids and may present with ophthalmoplegia. The progression is slower than bacterial orbital cellulitis.

High risk of mortality is associated with bilateral orbital involvement, diabetes, renal transplantation with immunosuppression, leukaemia and hemiparesis [21]. A rare case of spread from a fungal nasal septal abscess *Scedosporium apiospermum* resulting in an orbital apex syndrome has been reported in a diabetic patient, which resulted in blindness [22]. Mucormycosis in immunocompetent patients is rare, and there has only been one reported case of zygomycetes infection in an immunocompetent child [23].

2.3.1.3. Allergic aspergillosis sinusitis

Allergic aspergillosis sinusitis occurs in immunocompetent patients who have nasal polyposis and chronic sinusitis. About 17% of allergic fungal sinusitis will present as orbital cellulitis. Patients will have an eosinophilia, with thick mucin in the sinuses on CT scans. Sinus biopsy reveals peanut butter like mucus with eosinophils and extra-mucosal fungal hyphae. Endoscopic debridement of the sinuses, treatment with corticosteroids is recommended [24].

2.3.2. Investigations (bloods and swabs)

Patients with orbital cellulitis require in hospital management. Blood investigations include full blood count. The leukocytosis is usually over 15,000 cells/microliter. Erythrocyte sedimentation rate (ESR) and blood cultures should also be done. Blood cultures are infrequently positive.

Conjunctival swabs and blood cultures usually have a low yield and may not be representative of organisms causing an orbital abscess. If meningeal or cerebral signs develop a lumbar puncture may be indicated to rule out intracranial complications in additional to imaging.

When fungal orbital cellulitis is suspected, intranasal biopsies sent for frozen section looking for hyphae elements can be helpful [21]. Diagnosis is confirmed by biopsy by the necrotic tissues in the nasopharynx or involved sinus. Zygomycosis has non-septate large branching hyphae that stain with hematoxylin-eosin stain. Aspergillus species stain with the Grocott-Gomori methenamine-silver nitrate showing septate branching hyphae of uniform width.

2.3.3. Investigations (imaging)

The most commonly affected sinus is the ethmoid (91.6%) (**Figure 5**) [12]. X-rays of the sinuses can show fluid-filled cavities in the sinus and may show thickened mucous membranes. However, CT scan imaging of the orbit and sinuses is the usual modality of choice for diagnosis and monitoring as it shows more definition. It is indicated in inflammation with proptosis, external ophthalmoplegia and reduced vision. Other indications include no improvement or deterioration of the patient's condition within 24 h or non-resolving pyrexia over 36 h.

The CT scan demonstrates the sinuses involved and size and location of possible orbital abscesses (**Figures 5** and **6a**, **b**). Sinus X-ray can show an air-fluid level, for orbital abscesses with gas [25]. Ultrasound can detect abscesses of the anterior orbit with 90% accuracy [6].

CT scans have additional benefits as it also determines the inflammatory changes in the orbit and identifies potential sources of infection including a foreign body. It defines size and location of an orbital abscess and subperiosteal abscesses (**Figure 7**). Early abscesses may appear as increased soft tissue density and when enlarged, a fluid collection with rim enhancement may be present. Identification of orbital abscesses can be challenging on CT and a third of abscesses may be missed if the coronal sections are not done [26]. Contrast media can enhance

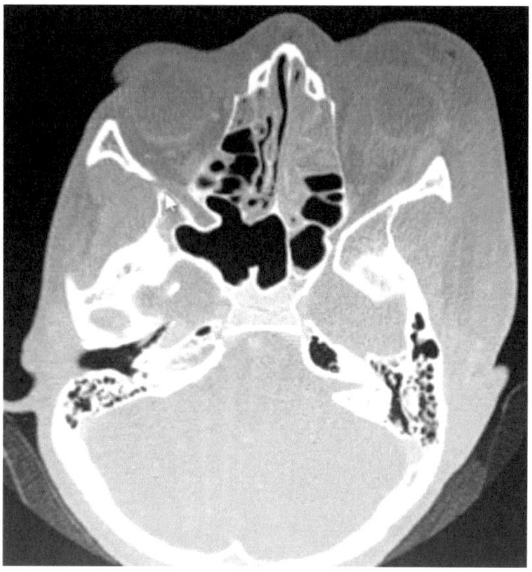

Figure 5. Left orbital cellulitis secondary to a left ethmoiditis with left periorbital oedema and associated mucosal thickening in the right ethmoid sinus (axial CT scan).

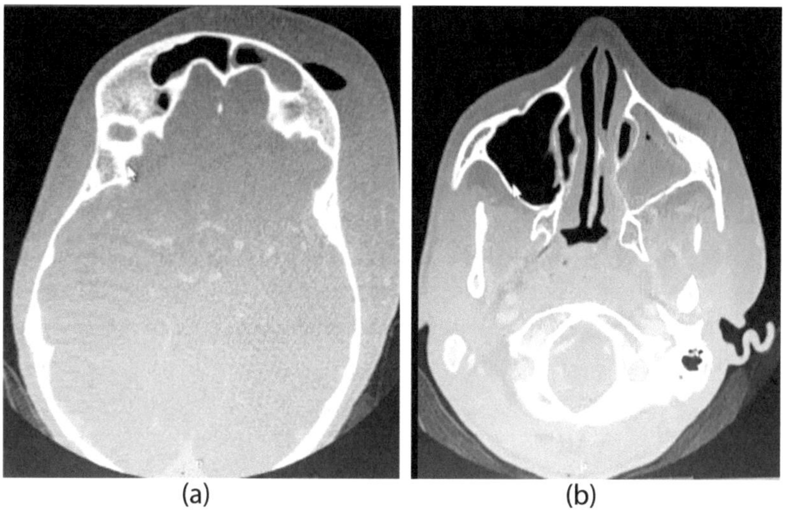

Figure 6. (a) Axial CT scan showing left frontal sinusitis associated with swelling of the left side of the face and air in the soft tissues. There is associated mild mucosal thickening in the right frontal sinus. (b) Axial CT scan showing left maxillary sinusitis.

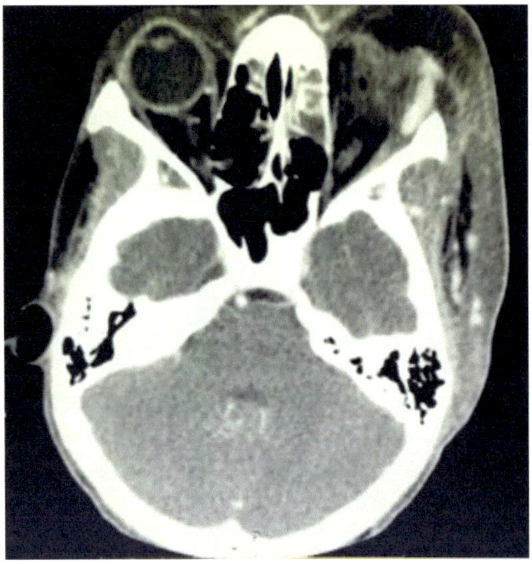

Figure 7. CT scan of the orbits showing air present in a localized loculated collection in the superior orbit.

the surrounding wall of the abscess on CT scanning and can differentiate between an abscess and orbital inflammation. The orbital abscess size may increase during the first few days of intravenous antibiotics [26].

The presence of neurological signs requires imaging for intracranial extension. MRI imaging can supplement CT scans with better resolution of orbital soft tissues. Fat saturated T2weighted MRI and diffusion weighted imaging are helpful. MRI is superior to CT for imaging orbital and subperiosteal abscesses and intracranial involvement and reduces the exposure to radiation [6]. In cases with possible complications, a MRI or CT venogram can help elucidate the presence of a cavernous sinus thrombosis.

2.4. Treatment

Orbital cellulitis requires in hospital management with intravenous broad-spectrum antibiotics. This should cover most Gram-positive and Gram-negative bacteria. Treatment of the predisposing factor, for example sinusitis, should be implemented early. Treatment is initially with 1–2 weeks of intravenous antibiotics followed by 4 weeks of oral antibiotics [4]. Management of these cases is multidisciplinary with involvement of the ophthalmologist, otolaryngologist, infectious disease and neurosurgical specialists.

Nasal decongestants help to promote spontaneous drainage of the infected sinus and early intervention to drain the involved sinus.

2.4.1. Antibiotics

Broad spectrum intravenous antibiotics are used empirically. In a Canadian study on orbital cellulitis in children, the commonest combination was IV cefuroxime (24%), IV clindamycin +

IV cephalosporin (21%) and IV cloxacillin + IV cefotaxime (18%) [17]. Subperiosteal abscess were noted in 31.5% of patients but only 21% of patients required surgical intervention [17]. In adults, high dose IV {Augmentin (amoxil and claviolonic), ceftriaxone and sulbactum} and metronidazole have been found to be effective [12].

Children have simpler infections than adults with one aerobic pathogen [7]. Children, 9 years and older and adults may have multiple aerobic and anaerobic organisms which may require medical and surgical treatment. There is a sliding scale of risk and older patients should undergo sinus surgery early before the development of orbital or intracranial abscesses.

CT scans are not predictive of clinical course for orbital abscesses [7]. Expansion of an abscess on CT scan in the first few days is not indicative of failure of antibiotics [26]. However, if visual function is compromised, drainage of the abscess is warranted. Drainage within 24 h is recommended if the orbital abscess is large (superior or inferior), dental involvement (children >9 years), evidence of intracranial extension, involvement of the frontal sinuses [7]. Children <9 years can be monitored with an expectant approach if they have a medial subperiosteal abscess (modest size), no visual loss, nor intracranial or frontal sinus involvement [7]. The patient must undergo continual monitoring of their optic nerve function (Snellen vision, RAPD, colour vision, pupillary reactions) and level of consciousness.

Fungal cellulitis requires aggressive antifungal treatment and may require orbital exenteration and yet still have a high mortality rate [21]. The treatment regime for fungal orbital cellulitis involves:

- Intravenous (IV) amphotericin and irrigation of amphotericin
- Aggressive surgical debridement -Wide excision of devitalized and necrotic tissues
- Adjunctive hyperbaric oxygen
- Correction of metabolic defect
- Exenteration in severe unresponsive cases.

Orbital fungal cellulitis is treated with intravenous anti-fungal. Intravenous amphotericin B can be used initially then posaconazole orally when discharged. Voriconazole or amphotericin B can be used for invasive aspergillosis. In mucormycosis, intravenous amphotericin B may be used or IV micafungin as an adjunctive treatment. In some cases, a suture tarsorrhaphy (closure of the eye lids) can be done and an irrigation cannula placed to deliver intraorbital amphotericin B [21].

Intra orbital catheter delivery of amphotericin B can be used as an adjunctive therapy with early aggressive surgical debridement when required. For invasive aspergillosis, voriconazole or amphotericin B may be used. The onset of fungal orbital cellulitis can initially be insidious then progress rapidly, so a high index of suspicion is important.

2.4.2. *Surgical treatment*

Approximately, 12–15% of patients require surgical management [5, 27]. Children 10–19 years old were more likely to require surgical intervention and much older patients with leukocytosis

[5]. The presence of acute and chronic sinusitis, proptosis, diplopia, conjunctival chemosis increases the odds ratio of surgical intervention.

Surgical treatment is used for treatment of the source of infections (pan sinusitis) and complication of orbital cellulitis (intraorbital or intracranial) with good result (**Figure 8a** and **b**). Drainage of a subperiosteal abscess requires an incision to the periosteum. Insertion of a drain for several days may be used. Functional endoscopic sinus surgery (FESS) can be done for some periosteal abscesses, eliminating the need for an external ethmoidectomy and facial scar [4]. In fungal orbital cellulitis, early diagnosis and initiation of treatment may also require limited debridement. However, severe invasive fungal orbital cellulitis may require exenteration.

2.4.3. Role of corticosteroids

Oral steroids may be used with caution as an adjunct to intravenous antibiotic therapy, as it can hasten the resolution of the inflammation, reducing the duration of the intravenous antibiotics and length of the hospital stay. It also has a low risk of exacerbating infection [28]. Steroids are started after a positive response to intravenous antibiotics has occurred [28]. Children with orbital cellulitis treated concurrently with intravenous steroids (IV dexamethasone 0.3 mg/kg/d Q6H for 3 days) had significantly shorter hospital stays than those without (3.8 vs. 6.7 days, $p < 0.001$) [29]. A short course of systemic steroids concurrent with IV antibiotics appears to be safe and efficacious [29]. The hospital stay was shorter for the children who had IV steroids, whether they had surgical intervention.

2.5. Complications

Complications from orbital cellulitis can result from mechanical factors in the orbit or haematogenous and contiguous spread. There are valveless veins around the orbit which predispose to this spread.

Ocular complications result from proptosis and increased pressure in the orbit. It includes exposure keratopathy, glaucoma, central retinal artery or vein occlusion, optic neuropathy from an orbital apex syndrome.

The other complications of orbital cellulitis include subperiosteal abscess, intracranial complications (cavernous sinus thrombosis, meningitis and brain abscess) [12]. Approximately, 0.3–5.1% develop orbital or subperiosteal abscess [10, 11]. Development of orbital abscess does not correlate specifically with the patient's vision, proptosis or any other sign [25].

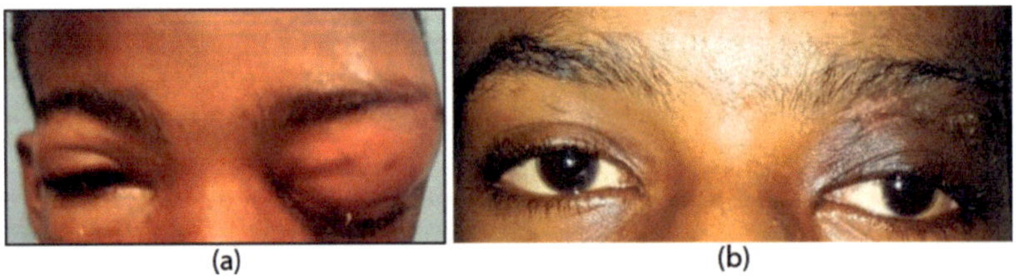

Figure 8. (a) Left orbital cellulitis. (b) Six weeks post-surgical intervention and intravenous antibiotics.

Orbital or periosteal abscesses should be suspected in patients with progressive proptosis with globe displacement, swinging pyrexia and failure to improve despite intravenous antibiotics. They are usually localized adjacent to the affected sinus in the subperiosteal space, usually the medial orbital wall. Serial imaging may be required.

In younger children <9 years, they may develop isolated medial or inferior subperiosteal orbital abscesses with good vision and mild to moderate proptosis, however, may settle with medical treatment.

Indications for surgical intervention for subperiosteal abscess [30] are:

- Patients ≥9 year old
- Non-medial location of subperiosteal abscess
- Involvement of frontal sinusitis
- Large subperiosteal abscess
- Suspicion of anaerobic infection
- Chronic sinusitis
- Acute optic nerve compromise
- Infection of dental origin

Orbital abscess is more likely in post-traumatic or post-operative cases. Before antibiotics, death from **meningitis** occurred in 17% of cases and blindness in 20% [8]. Present day, ~ 1.9% of patients will develop meningitis and 7–23% can result in blindness, from ocular complications such as corneal ulcer, central retinal artery occlusion or optic atrophy. Delay in required surgical intervention also results in a poor prognosis [8].

Orbitocranial complication of acute sinusitis in children, though uncommon can be life threatening causing high morbidity if diagnosed late. They may require additional procedures such as endoscopic sinus surgery, orbital decompression or subdural empyema drainage [31].

Intracranial complications are uncommon but can be very serious. Meningitis, brain abscess and cavernous sinus thrombosis can occur. Brain abscesses must be considered in patients who have the classic triad of headache, fever and neurological deficit, but may be present in <50% of cases, however, a headache may be present in 70% of cases [30, 32]. The neurosurgical team must be involved as neurosurgical drainage may be required. Cavernous sinus thrombosis must be considered in patients with rapid progression of proptosis, ipsilateral ophthalmoplegia. These patients may also have clinical signs of severe headache, nausea and vomiting. Orbital cellulitis is an inflammatory and infective disease of the orbit which can have visual threatening and life-threatening complications. It is important to diagnose, investigated and treat early to reduce complication and morbidity.

Conflict of interest

The author has no conflict of interest.

Author details

Lizette Mowatt

Address all correspondence to: lizettemowatt@yahoo.com

University of the West Indies, Kingston, Jamaica

References

[1] Tsirouki T, Dastiridou AI, Ibánez Flores N, Cerpa JC, Moschos MM, Brazitikos P, Androudi S. Orbital cellulitis. Survey of Ophthalmology. Jul–Aug 2018;**63**(4):534-553

[2] Riordan-Eva P, Cunningham Jr ET. Chapter 1. Anatomy & embryology of the eye. In: Vaughan & Asbury's General Ophthalmology. 18th ed. The McGraw-Hill Companies. 2011. Available from: http://accessmedicine.mhmedical.com/content.aspx?bookid=387&sectionid=40229318 [Accessed: March 26, 2018]

[3] Murphy C, Livingstone I, Foot B, Murgatroyd H, MacEwen CJ. Orbital cellulitis in Scotland: current incidence, aetiology, management and outcomes. The British Journal of Ophthalmology. Nov 2014;**98**(11):1575-1578

[4] Wan Y, Shi G, Wang H. Treatment of orbital complications following acute rhinosinusitis in children. Balkan Medical Journal. Jul 2016;**33**(4):401-406. DOI: 10.5152/balkanmedj.2016.141065. [Epub Jul 1, 2016]

[5] Segal N, Nissani R, Kordeluk S, Holcberg M, Hertz S, Kassem F, et al. Orbital complications associated with paranasal sinus infections-A 10-year experience in Israel. International Journal of Pediatric Otorhinolaryngology. Jul 2016;**86**:60-62

[6] Uhumwangho OM, Kayoma DH. Current trends in treatment outcomes of orbital cellulitis in a tertiary hospital in Southern Nigeria. Nigerian Journal of Surgery. Jul–Dec 2016; **22**(2):107-110

[7] Chaudhry IA, Al-Rashed W, Arat YO. The hot orbit: Orbital cellulitis. Middle East African Journal of Ophthalmology. Jan 2012;**19**(1):34-42

[8] Chandler JR, Langenbrunner DJ, Stevens ER. The pathogenesis of orbital complications in acute sinusitis. The Laryngoscope. Sep 1970;**80**(9):1414-1428

[9] Moloney JR, Badham NJ, McRae A. The acute orbit preseptal (periorbital) cellulitis, subperiosteal abscess and orbital cellulitis due to sinusitis. The Journal of Laryngology and Otology. 1987;**101**(Suppl. 12):1-14

[10] Radovani P, Vasili D, Xhelili M, Dervishi J. Orbital complications of sinusitis. Balkan Medical Journal. 2013;**30**(2):e59-e61

[11] Al-Madani MV, Khatatbeh AE, Rawashdeh RZ, Al-Khtoum NF, Shawagfeh NR. The prevalence of orbital complications among children and adults with acute rhinosinusitis. Brazilian Journal of Otorhinolaryngology. Nov–Dec 2013;**79**(6):716-719

[12] Gupta S, Goyal R, Gupta RK. Clinical presentation and outcome of the orbital complications due to acute infective rhino sinusitis. Indian Journal of Otolaryngology and Head & Neck Surgery. Aug 2013;**65**(Suppl 2):431-434

[13] Asif T, Hasan B, Ukani R, Pauly RR. Infective endocarditis presenting as bilateral orbital cellulitis: An unusual case. Cureus. Jun 14, 2017;**9**(6):e1350

[14] Taş S, Top H. Intraorbital wooden foreign body: clinical analysis of 32 cases, a 10-year experience. Ulusal Travma ve Acil Cerrahi Dergisi. Jan 2014;**20**(1):51-55

[15] Beck DE, El-Assal KS, Doherty MD, Wride NK. Orbital cellulitis following uncomplicated aqueous shunt surgery. Journal of Glaucoma. Feb 2017;**26**(2):e101-e102

[16] Nemet AY, Ferencz JR, Segal O, Meshi A. Orbital cellulitis following silicone-sponge scleral buckles. Clinical Ophthalmology. 2013;**7**:2147-2152

[17] Fanella S, Singer A, Embree J. Presentation and management of pediatric orbital cellulitis. Canadian Journal of Infectious Diseases and Medical Microbiology. Fall 2011;**22**(3):97-100

[18] Donahue SP, Schwartz G. Preseptal and orbital cellulitis in childhood. A changing microbiologic spectrum. Ophthalmology. Oct 1998;**105**(10):1902-1905

[19] Sharma A, Liu ES, Le TD, Adatia FA, Buncic JR, Blaser S, Richardson S. Pediatric orbital cellulitis in the *Haemophilus influenzae* vaccine era. Journal of AAPOS. Jun 2015;**19**(3): 206-210

[20] Park CH, Jee DH, La TY. A case of odontogenic orbital cellulitis causing blindness by severe tension orbit. Journal of Korean Medical Science. Feb 2013;**28**(2):340-343

[21] Farooq AV, Patel RM, Lin AY, Setabutr P, Sartori J, Aakalu VK. Fungal orbital cellulitis: Presenting features, management and outcomes at a referral center. Orbit. Jun 2015;**34**(3): 152-159

[22] Kishimoto I, Shinohara S, Ueda T, Tani S, Yoshimura H, Imai Y. Orbital apex syndrome secondary to a fungal nasal septal abscess caused by *Scedosporium apiospermum* in a patient with uncontrolled diabetes: A case report. BMC Infectious Diseases. Sep 26, 2017;**17**(1): 649. DOI: 10.1186/s12879-017-2753-6

[23] Badiee P, Jafarpour Z, Alborzi A, Haddadi P, Rasuli M, Kalani M. Orbital mucormycosis in an immunocompetent individual. Iranian Journal of Microbiology. Dec 2012;**4**(4):210-214

[24] Klapper SR, Lee AG, Patrinely JR, Stewart M, Alford EL. Orbital involvement in allergic fungal sinusitis. Ophthalmology. Dec 1997;**104**(12):2094-2100

[25] Hornblass A, Herschorn BJ, Stern K, Grimes C. Orbital abscess. Survey of Ophthalmology. Nov–Dec 1984;**29**(3):169-178

[26] Harris GJ. Subperiosteal abscess of the orbit: Computed tomography and the clinical course. Ophthalmic Plastic and Reconstructive Surgery. Mar 1996;**12**(1):1-8

[27] Marchiano E, Raikundalia MD, Carniol ET, Echanique KA, Kalyoussef E, Baredes S, et al. Characteristics of patients treated for orbital cellulitis: An analysis of inpatient data. Laryngoscope. Mar 2016;**126**(3):554-559

[28] Pushker N, Tejwani LK, Bajaj MS, Khurana S, Velpandian T, Chandra M. Role of oral corticosteroids in orbital cellulitis. American Journal of Ophthalmology. Jul 2013;**156**(1): 178-183.e1

[29] Chen L, Silverman N, Wu A, Shinder R. Intravenous steroids with antibiotics on admission for children with orbital cellulitis. Ophthalmic Plastic and Reconstructive Surgery. May/Jun 2018;**34**(3):205-208

[30] Garcia GH, Harris GJ. Criteria for nonsurgical management of subperiosteal abscess of the orbit: analysis of outcomes 1988–1998. Ophthalmology. Aug 2000;**107**(8):1454-1456 (discussion 1457 8)

[31] Sharma PK, Saikia B, Sharma R. Orbitocranial complications of acute sinusitis in children. The Journal of Emergency Medicine. Sep 2014;**47**(3):282-285

[32] Traficante D, Riss A, Hochman S. Bifrontal brain abscesses secondary to orbital cellulitis and sinusitis extension. International Journal of Emergency Medicine. Dec 2016;**9**(1):23

Chapter 6

Sinonasal Cancers: Diagnosis and Management

Deepti Sharma, Neha Sharma and Vivek Sharma

Additional information is available at the end of the chapter

http://dx.doi.org/10.5772/intechopen.81161

Abstract

Sinonasal cancers are rare tumors constitute 3% of head and neck cancers. These include malignancies of the nasal cavity and paranasal sinuses (maxillary sinus, ethmoid sinuses, frontal sinus and sphenoid sinus). Patients are often asymptomatic until late in the course of their disease. Tumors of the maxillary sinus are more common than those of the ethmoid sinus or nasal cavity. The workup for patients with suspected paranasal sinus tumors includes complete head and neck CT/MRI with contrast. FDG-PET/CT may be considered in the workup of patients with clinically apparent stage III or IV disease. The most common histology for these tumors is squamous cell carcinoma, others reported includes adenocarcinoma, esthesioneuroblastoma, minor salivary gland tumors, or sinonasal neuroendocrine carcinoma [SNEC]). Surgical resection for all T stages (except T4b, any N) followed by postoperative therapy remains a cornerstone of treatment. However, definitive RT or systemic therapy/RT is recommended for T4b, any N. Locoregional control and incidence of distant metastasis are dependent on T stage, N stage, and tumor histology.

Keywords: sinonasal cancers, radiotherapy, surgery, maxilla, ethmoid

1. Introduction

Para-nasal sinuses are small air filled cavities occupying the facial and skull bones and along with nasal cavity, they form a small anatomical space but they are site of origin of histologically diverse group of tumors. These incorporate neoplasms derived from mucosal epithelium, seromucinous glands, soft tissues, bone, cartilage, neural/neuroectodermal tissue, haemato-lymphoid cells and the odontogenic apparatus.

2. Epidemiology

Nasal cavity and paranasal sinus cancers are a group of rare cancers, representing about 5% of all head and neck (H and N) cancer patients. They have an incidence of about 1 case every 100,000, with an average age between 50 and 60 years [1]. About 60% of sinonasal tumors originate in the maxillary sinus, 20–30% in the nasal cavity, 10–15% in the ethmoid sinus, and 1% in the sphenoid and frontal sinuses [2]. The incidence of cancer of the nasal cavity and paranasal sinuses (sinonasal cancer) is low in most of the populations (<1.5/100,000 in men and <1.0/100,000 in women), although higher incidence is seen in Japan and certain parts of China and India [3, 4]. Sinonasal squamous cell carcinoma and intestinal-type adenocarcinoma occur more commonly in men, with a male-to-female ratio of 2:1 in sinonasal squamous cell carcinoma, and up to 6:1 in intestinal-type adenocarcinoma [4, 5].

3. Anatomy

The paranasal sinuses are named according to the bones in which they are located: the ethmoid, maxilla, sphenoid, and frontal (**Figure 1**) [6].

3.1. Ethmoid complex

This paired complex of sinuses contains 3–18 cells that are grouped as anterior, middle, or posterior, according to the location of their ostia. The *posterior group* drains into the superior meatus above the middle nasal concha; sometimes one or more opens into the sphenoidal

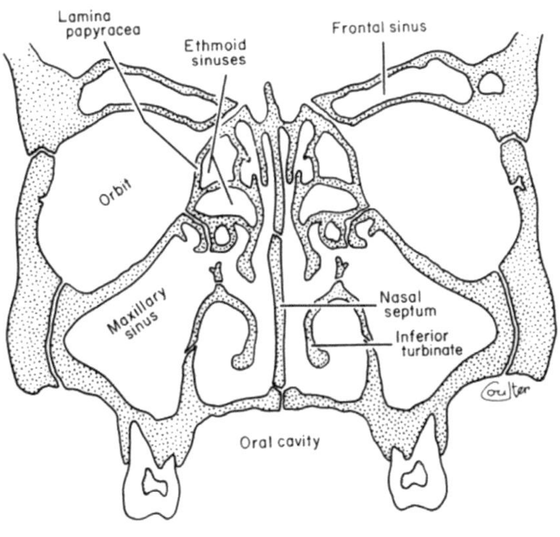

Figure 1. A schematic illustration of the relationship between the eye and the paranasal sinuses. The roof of the orbit, the medial wall, and the floor are shared by the frontal, ethmoid, and maxillary sinuses, respectively.

sinus. The *middle group* into the middle meatus of the nose on or above the bulla ethmoidalis and the *anterior group* drains into the middle meatus of the nose by way of the infundibulum.

Since ethmoid sinus is a paired structure, it is connected in midline by cribriform part of ethmoid bone, which also separates it from anterior cranial fossa. Direct extension of the tumor through cribriform plate causes involvement of frontal lobe. A pointed bony landmark called crista galli stretches out from the midline of the cribriform plate upward into the floor of the anterior cranial fossa. The perpendicular plate of the ethmoid bone descends from the cribriform plate forms superior two thirds of the nasal septum. Middle, superior, and supreme turbinates originate from medial wall of each ethmoid labyrinth. Lamina papyracea forms the thin lateral wall, separating the ethmoid cells from the orbit. It forms an easy conduit for tumor spread from ethmoid sinus to orbit. The fovea ethmoidalis is a segment of the ethmoid bone and represents its superior portion which is seen as a continuation of the superior orbital roof to the cribriform plate.

3.2. Maxillary sinus

The maxillary sinus is the largest sinus occupying the body of the maxillary bone. The sinus is pyramidal in shape and has three recesses. The alveolar recess lies inferiorly, the zygomatic recess pointing laterally and the infra-orbital recess pointing superiorly. The floor is formed by the alveolar process of the maxilla. The roof is formed by floor of the orbit. It is traversed by infraorbital nerves and vessels. The base of the maxillary sinus forms the inferior part of the lateral wall of the nasal cavity. Anterior wall of the pterygopalatine fossa, also known as the sphenopalatine fossa, forms posterior wall of the maxillary sinus. The anterior sinus wall is the facial surface of the maxilla that is perforated by the infraorbital foramen below the orbital rim. The maxillary sinus drains into the middle meatus by means of the semilunar hiatus. The floor of the maxillary sinus is slightly below the level of the nasal cavity, and it is related to the upper teeth [7].

3.3. Sphenoid sinus

Sphenoid sinus is a paired structure that lies in the body of sphenoid bone. They may vary in size and are usually asymmetrical, attributable to the parallel dislocation of the mediating septum. The relationship of the posterior extension of the sphenoid in relation to the sella turcica is variable. With the exception of the sinus roof, the other sinus walls are of variable thickness depending on the degree of pneumatization. The sphenoid sinus is related superiorly to cavernous sinus, sella turcica and its contents, inferiorly to nasal cavity and posteriorly to nasal cavity and posterior ethmoidal cells. Posteriorly it is related to middle cranial fossa and laterally to cavernous sinus and cranial cavity [7].

3.4. Frontal sinus

They are paired structures located between the inner and outer tables of the frontal bone. Each opening into the anterior part of the corresponding middle nasal meatus of the nose through the frontonasal duct. Medially associated with the contralateral frontal sinus, Superiorly, laterally and posteriorly with the frontal bone and frontal lobe and Inferiorly with the orbit [7].

4. Etio-pathogenesis

4.1. Etiology

The etiologic factors vary by tumor type and location. Occupational exposures to wood and leather dust have been strongly associated with sinonasal cancers [7]. The risk of developing sinonasal cancer also increases with exposure to formaldehyde, in the textile industry and to nickel/chromium compounds [8]. Adenocarcinomas have been associated with wood dust, leather dust, and formaldehyde [9]. The risk is strongest in cases of adenocarcinomas and in sinonasal malignancies. The impact is present after 40 or more years since first introduction and persists after discontinuation. Squamous cell carcinomas have been linked to arsenic and welding fumes [10].

High relative risks of sinonasal cancers (SNC) have been observed for specific chemical exposures and occupational settings, including farming, construction, miners, drillers, blasters, plumbers, machinists, bakers and pastry confectioners, metal industry (chromium and nickel compounds) [11–14]. In contrast to most head and neck cancers, tobacco smoking does not seem to have a key role in the development of sinonasal tumors; nevertheless, evidence suggests that smoking tobacco can increase the risk of SNSCC twofold to threefold [1].

4.2. Pathogenesis

Several studies have established a causal role of exposure to hard wood dust and leather in the development of sinonasal cancer. Wood dust is a complex mixture of organic and inorganic components, including genotoxic and carcinogenic factors [15]. Its capacity to induce DNA damage has been attributed in part to its particulate nature, which induces the generation of reactive oxygen species in the cells. Several studies have established a causal role of exposure to hard wood dust and leather in the development of sinonasal cancer, with particular association with intestinal-type adenocarcinoma.

Molecular alterations seen in intestinal-type adenocarcinoma (ITAC) mainly focused on TP53, K-ras and H-ras gene mutations and EGFR or HER2 over-expression. Ras genes were found to be mutated only in rare cases, with conflicting reports about a possible prognostic role [16]. EGFR and HER2 are over-expressed in about 30% of cases [17]. The rate of TP53 mutations in intestinal-type adenocarcinoma is about 60% and it is significantly higher than in squamous cell carcinomas; TP53 mutation rate in ITAC is directly correlated with duration, average and cumulative level of wood dust exposure [18].

In a study by Chernock et al. (81.8%) were diffusely positive for c-KIT, 27.3% cases were positive for EGFR, but none of the cases were positive for HER2/neu [19]. In contrast, in a

Malignant epithelial tumors

- Squamous cell carcinoma
  - Verrucous carcinoma
  - Papillary squamous cell carcinoma
  - Basaloid squamous cell carcinoma
  - Spindle cell carcinoma
  - Adenosquamous carcinoma
  - Acantholytic squamous cell carcinoma
- Lymphoepithelial carcinoma
- Sinonasal undifferentiated carcinoma
- Adenocarcinoma
  - Intestinal-type adenocarcinoma
  - Nonintestinal-type adenocarcinoma
- Salivary gland-type carcinomas
  - Adenoid cystic carcinoma
  - Acinic cell carcinoma
  - Mucoepidermoid carcinoma
  - Epithelial-myoepithelial carcinoma
  - Clear cell carcinoma N.O.S.
  - Myoepithelial carcinoma
  - Carcinoma ex pleomorphic adenoma
  - Polymorphous low-grade adenocarcinoma
- Neuroendocrine tumors
  - Typical carcinoid
  - Atypical carcinoid
  - Small cell carcinoma, neuroendocrine type

Benign epithelial tumors

- Sinonasal papillomas
  - Inverted papilloma
  - (Schneiderian papilloma, inverted type)
  - Oncocytic papilloma
  - (Schneiderian papilloma, oncocytic type)
  - Exophytic papilloma
  - (Schneiderian papilloma, exophytic type)
- Salivary gland-type adenomas
  - Pleomorphic adenoma
  - Myoepithelioma
  - Oncocytoma

Soft tissue tumors

- Malignant tumors
  - Fibrosarcoma
  - Malignant fibrous histiocytoma
  - Leiomyosarcoma
  - Rhabdomyosarcoma
  - Angiosarcoma
  - Malignant peripheral nerve sheath tumor
- Borderline and low malignant potential tumors
  - Desmoid-type fibromatosis
  - Inflammatory myofibroblastic tumor
  - Glomangiopericytoma
  - (Sinonasal-type haemangiopericytoma)
  - Extrapleural solitary fibrous tumor
- Benign tumors
  - Myxoma
  - Leiomyoma
  - Haemangioma
  - Schwannoma
  - Neurofibroma
  - Meningioma

Tumors of bone and cartilage

- Malignant tumors
  - Chondrosarcoma
  - Mesenchymal chondrosarcoma
  - Osteosarcoma
  - Chordoma
- Benign tumors
  - Giant cell lesion
  - Giant cell tumor
  - Chondroma
  - Osteoma
  - Chondroblastoma
  - Chondromyxoid fibroma
  - Osteochondroma (exostosis)
  - Osteoid osteoma
  - Osteoblastoma
  - Ameloblastoma
  - Nasal chondromesenchymal hamartoma

Haematolymphoid tumors

- Extranodal NK/T cell lymphoma
- Diffuse large B-cell lymphoma
- Extramedullary plasmacytoma
- Extramedullary myeloid sarcoma
- Histiocytic sarcoma
- Langerhans cell histiocytosis

Neuroectodermal

- Ewing sarcoma
- Primitive neuroectodermal tumor
- Olfactory neuroblastoma
- Melanotic neuroectodermal tumor of infancy
- Mucosal malignant melanoma

Germ cell tumors	Secondary tumors
• Immature teratoma • Teratoma with malignant transformation • Sinonasal yolk sac tumor (endodermal sinus tumor) • Sinonasal teratocarcinosarcoma • Mature teratoma • Dermoid cyst	

Table 1. Classification of nasal and paranasal sinus tumors (modified by the World Health Organization histological classification of nasal and paranasal sinus cancer) [23].

study by Takahashi et al., sinonasal squamous cell cancer (SCC) is associated with increase in number of EGFR and HER2 copies in about 40 and 20% of the cases, respectively, with their occurrence being mutually exclusive. Expression of these biomarkers is seen in 82% of the cases, usually indicating a worse outcome [20].

There is increasing evidence that the human papillomavirus (HPV) is associated with a subset of sinonasal carcinomas. HPV has been detected in about 30% of sinonasal carcinomas [21]. HPV 16 seems to be the most frequent HPV type. The identification of HPV in sinonasal carcinomas has important clinical implications, because the presence of HPV could be a prognostic factor associated with a favorable outcome [21].

4.3. Pathological classification

The most-common subtypes of epithelial tumor are sinonasal squamous cell carcinoma, which predominantly occur in the maxillary sinus and nasal cavity, and intestinal-type adenocarcinoma (ITAC), which almost exclusively arise in the ethmoid sinus (**Table 1**) [22].

5. Pattern of spread

The pattern of spread of maxillary sinus cancers varies with the site of origin. Suprastructure tumors extend into the nasal cavity, ethmoid cells, orbit, pterygopalatine fossa, infratemporal fossa, and base of skull. Infrastructure tumors often infiltrate the palate, alveolar process, gingivobuccal sulcus, soft tissue of the cheek, nasal cavity, masseter muscle, pterygopalatine space, and pterygoid fossa [24].

Lymphatic drainage from the nasal cavity and paranasal sinus occurs in two directions, anterior, and posterior [25]. The anterior mucosal and vestibular skin drainage is by way of lymphatic channels traveling to the facial, parotid, or submandibular groups of nodes, then to the superior deep cervical nodal chain, primarily level II. The posterior lymphatics course posteriorly to a plexus anterior to the torus tubarius, posterior to the retropharyngeal nodes, and inferiorly to the posterior and superior deep cervical nodes [26]. Studies have demonstrated that SCC is associated with a high incidence of nodal metastasis, neck failure and inferior disease-specific survival rate [27, 28].

6. Clinical presentation

The majority of maxillary sinus tumors present with nasal fullness, stuffiness, obstruction, epistaxis, rhinorrhea, pain, paresthesia to tooth mobility, tooth loss, proptosis, diplopia, and lacrimation [29].

Owing to the nonspecific and the often relatively mild nature of the symptoms at early stages of disease, sinonasal malignancies have a prolonged diagnostic latency [29].

7. Diagnostic evaluation

Inspection and palpation of the orbits, nasal and oral cavities, and nasopharynx can provide preliminary determination of tumor extent. Bimanual palpation is important in assessing contiguous extension of nasal vestibule lesions and in identifying buccinator and submandibular nodal involvement.

For a suspected sinonasal expansile mass, the clinical examination is incomplete without a nasal endoscopy by flexible and/or rigid endoscopes. Nasal endoscopy allows direct visualization of the lesion and may help in differentiating an inflammatory polyp from a neoplasm, benign or malignant. A unilateral expansile mass with an irregular surface, necrotic areas, and contact bleeding ought to be considered as suspicious and potentially suggestive of malignancy.

Endoscopic evaluation may also allow, especially in those cases not completely filling the nasal fossa, identification or suggestion of the possible site of origin of the lesion, its local extension and to assess the presence of satellite lesions. Oral cavity should also be examined to check for loosening of teeth to rule out involvement of alveolar process of maxilla in cases of maxillary sinus malignancy or any oro-nasal/oro-antral fistula; maxillary sinus tumours may also present as a submucosal swelling at level of the cheek, gingiva-buccal sulcus. A recent history of an otherwise unexplainable tooth extraction or mobility should also be considered.

Although the incidence of cervical lymph node involvement is relatively low in sinonasal malignancies, but all cervical lymph node stations must be palpated. The lesions involving the oral mucosa and/or with aggressive histologic behaviour show high risk of lymphatic spreading (i.e., sinonasal undifferentiated carcinoma, high-grade olfactory neuroblastoma). In these cases, clinical evaluation of the neck must be completed by ultrasound so as confirm any neck swelling and metastasis to neck nodes must be confirmed by fine needle aspiration cytology.

Clinical examination of cranial nerves (from I to VI) should be also performed. Malignancies of ethmoid sinus or maxillary sinus can present with alteration of eyeball positioning due to orbital invasion, which can present with proptosis with or without diplopia, due to orbit compression, intraorbital extension or extrinsic muscle involvement. The infraorbital nerve (branch of the maxillary division of the trigeminal nerve) can also be affected especially in lesions extending into the pterygopalatine fossa and/or masticatory space, resulting in sensory disturbances of the cheek. Involvement of cavernous sinus or orbital apex can lead to visual disturbances due to optic nerve infiltration.

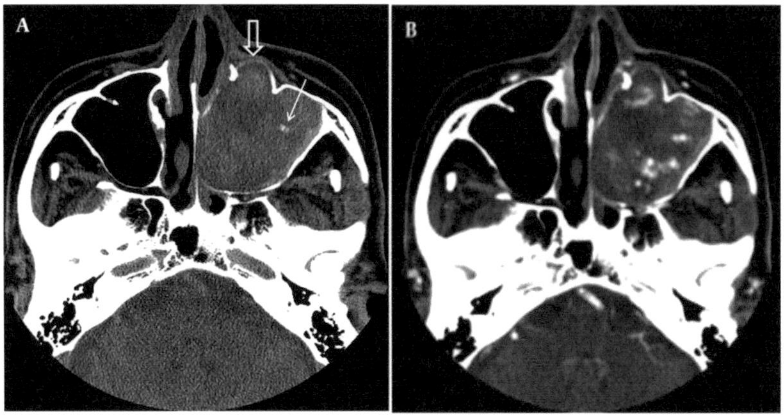

Figure 2. (A) Nonenhanced axial CT scan shows a large, soft tissue mass in the nasal cavity and maxillary sinus, on the left side. (B) Enhanced axial CT of the lesion shows an inhomogeneously enhancing soft tissue mass.

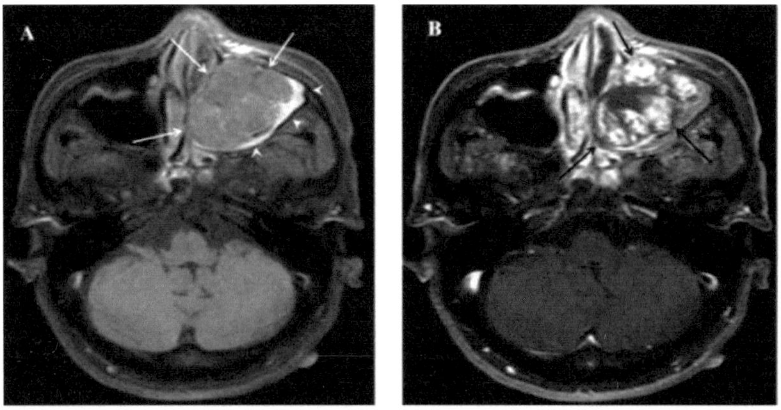

Figure 3. (A) Axial scan shows T1-weighted image with intermediate signal intensity lobulated mass lesion (white arrows) in the left maxillary sinus. Obstructed left maxillary sinus have high signal intensity sinonasal secretions (arrowheads). (B) Enhanced T1-weighted image shows heterogeneous intense enhancement (black arrows).

In the diagnosis of paranasal sinuses tumors MR imaging is a vital tool in the diagnosis of these lesions and is used in conjunction with computed tomography to precisely delineate the extent of neoplasms and involvement of the skull base, the orbits (**Figures 2** and **3**) [30]. The involvement of fine bone structures is best evaluated with contrast-enhanced computed tomography (**CECT**). CECT provides excellent details about the thin bony paranasal sinuses walls separating the ethmoid from the anterior skull base and the orbit [31].

7.1. Biopsy

Transnasal biopsy is preferred for tumors arising from or extending into the nasal cavity or nasopharynx. Some paranasal sinus tumors may be more easily sampled using transoral procedures or an open Caldwell-Luc approach.

8. Staging

The American Joint Committee on Cancer (AJCC) staging system for the nasal cavity and paranasal sinuses (8th edition, 2017) is depicted in **Tables 2–8** [32] (mucosal melanoma of the nasal cavity and paranasal sinuses are not included).

T category	T criteria for maxillary sinus
TX	Primary tumor cannot be assessed
Tis	Carcinoma in situ
T1	Tumor limited to maxillary sinus mucosa with no erosion or destruction of bone
T2	Tumor causing bone erosion or destruction including extension into the hard palate and/or middle nasal meatus, except extension to posterior wall of maxillary sinus and pterygoid plates
T3	Tumor invades any of the following: bone of the posterior wall of maxillary sinus, subcutaneous tissues. Floor or medial wall of orbit, pterygoid fossa, ethmoid sinuses
T4a	Moderately advanced local disease Tumor invades anterior orbital contents, skin of cheek, pterygoid plates, infratemporal fossa, cribriform plate, sphenoid or frontal sinuses
T4b	Very advanced local disease Tumor invades any of the following: orbital apex, dura, brain, middle cranial fossa, cranial nerves other than maxillary division of trigeminal nerve (V2), nasopharynx, or clivus

Table 2. T staging for maxillary sinus.

T category	T criteria for ethmoid sinus and nasal cavity
TX	Primary tumor cannot be assessed
Tis	Carcinoma in situ
T1	Tumor restricted to any one subsite, with or without bony invasion
T2	Tumor invading two subsites in a single region or extending to involve an adjacent region within the nasoethmoidal complex, with or without bony invasion
T3	Tumor extends to invade the medial wall or floor of the orbit, maxillary sinus, palate, or cribriform plate
T4a	Moderately advanced local disease Tumor invades any of the following: anterior orbital contents, skin of nose or cheek, minimal extension to anterior cranial fossa, pterygoid plates, sphenoid or frontal sinuses
T4b	Very advanced local disease Tumor invades any of the following: orbital apex, dura, brain, middle cranial fossa, cranial nerves other than (V2), nasopharynx, or clivus

Table 3. T staging for ethmoid sinus and nasal cavity.

N category	N criteria
NX	Regional lymph nodes cannot be assessed
N0	No regional lymph node metastasis
N1	Metastasis in a single ipsilateral lymph node, 3 cm or smaller in greatest dimension and ENE(−)

N category	N criteria
N2	Metastasis in a single ipsilateral node larger than 3 cm but not larger than 6 cm in greatest dimension and ENE(−); or metastases in multiple ipsilateral lymph nodes, none larger than 6 cm in greatest dimension and ENE(−); or in bilateral or contralateral lymph nodes, none larger than 6 cm in greatest dimension and ENE (−)
N2a	Metastasis in a single ipsilateral node larger than 3 cm but not larger than 6 cm in greatest dimension and ENE(−)
N2b	Metastasis in multiple ipsilateral nodes, none larger than 6 cm in greatest dimension and ENE(−)
N2c	Metastasis in bilateral or contralateral lymph nodes, none larger than 6 cm in greatest dimension and ENE (−)
N3	Metastasis in a lymph node larger than 6 cm in greatest dimension and ENE(−); or metastasis in any node(s) with clinically overt ENE(+)
N3a	Metastasis in a lymph node larger than 6 cm in greatest dimension and ENE(−)
N3b	Metastasis in any node(s) with clinically overt ENE (ENEC)

Table 4. Clinical regional lymph nodes.

N category	N criteria
NX	Regional lymph nodes cannot be assessed
N0	No regional lymph node metastasis
N1	Metastasis in a single ipsilateral lymph node, 3 cm or smaller in greatest dimension and ENE(−)
N2	Metastasis in a single ipsilateral lymph node, 3 cm or smaller in greatest dimension and ENE(+); or larger than 3 cm but not larger than 6 cm in greatest dimension and ENE(−); or metastases in multiple ipsilateral lymph nodes, none larger than 6 cm in greatest dimension and ENE (−); or in bilateral or contralateral lymph nodes, none larger than 6 cm in greatest dimension and ENE(−)
N2a	Metastasis in single ipsilateral or contralateral node 3 cm or less in greatest dimension and ENE(+); or a single ipsilateral node larger than 3 cm but not larger than 6 cm in greatest dimension and ENE(−)
N2b	Metastasis in multiple ipsilateral nodes, none larger than 6 cm in greatest dimension and ENE(−)
N2c	Metastasis in bilateral or contralateral lymph nodes, none larger than 6 cm in greatest dimension and ENE (−)
N3	Metastasis in a lymph node larger than 6 cm in greatest dimension and ENE(−); or in a single ipsilateral node larger than 3 cm in greatest dimension and ENE(+); or multiple ipsilateral, contralateral or bilateral nodes, any with ENE(+)
N3a	Metastasis in a lymph node larger than 6 cm in greatest dimension and ENE(−)
N3b	Metastasis in a single ipsilateral node larger than 3 cm in greatest dimension and ENE(+); or multiple ipsilateral, contralateral or bilateral nodes, any with ENE(+)

Table 5. Pathological regional lymph nodes.

M category	M criteria
M0	No distant metastasis (no pathologic MO; use clinical M to complete stage group)
M1	Distant metastasis

Table 6. Distant metastasis.

Stage 0	Tis	N0	Mo
Stage I	T1	N0	M0
Stage II	T2	N0	M0
Stage III	T3	N0	Mo
	T1–3	N1	M0
Stage IVA	T4a	N0–2	M0
	T1–3	N2	M0
Stage IVB	T4b	Any N	M0
	Any T	N3	M0
Stage IVC	Any T	Any N	M1

Table 7. Anatomic stage/prognostic groups.

GX	Grade cannot be assessed
G1	Well differentiated
G2	Moderately differentiated
G3	Poorly differentiated
G4	Undifferentiated

Table 8. Histologic grade (G).

9. Prognostic factors

Patient-specific factors (primarily prognostic for survival) include age and performance status. Disease specific factors (primarily prognostic for locoregional control) include location, histology, and locoregional extent (reflected in TNM stage), and perineural invasion. Independent of the treatment type used, the prognosis of patients with sinonasal carcinomas is poor, with an overall 5-year survival rate of 30–50% [33].The 5-year survival rates depend on disease stage and drops from 80% in patients with T1 disease to 30% in patients with T4 tumors [34]. Extensive local disease involving the nasopharynx, base of skull, or cavernous sinuses markedly increases surgical morbidity as well as increases local recurrence often within 2 years of follow up [35].

10. Treatment option overview

Treatment should be individualized based on location and extent of disease, patient performance status, stage of tumor, histopathologic subtype of tumor and availability of local expertise; because of the rarity of these tumors, consideration should be given to referring patients to centers with experience in their management.

Studies have shown that surgery gives the best results. Early infrastructure lesions may be cured by surgery alone, but, for most other cases, RT is given postoperatively even if margins are negative. Adjuvant Chemo-radiotherapy should be considered for a positive margin. The extension of cancer to the skull base, nasopharynx, or sphenoid sinus contraindicates excision [29, 30, 36].

10.1. Surgery

Surgery can produce excellent control rates for T1 and T2 tumors and is generally the mainstay of treatment.

However for T2 tumors, radiation therapy along with surgery is recommended. In patients undergoing radical surgery, it not only removes the bulk of the tumor but also re-establishes the drainage of involved sinus. It can be further followed by postoperative radiotherapy depending upon the stage of the tumor. Radical neck dissection or elective neck radiation therapy is prescribed only for the patients presenting with positive neck nodes. The incidence of lymph node metastases is generally low (approximately 20% of all cases).

Intracranial extension of tumor (i.e., anterior cranial fossa in cases of involvement of cribriform plate in ethmoid sinus tumors), cavernous sinus, or the pterygoid process; infiltration of the mucous membranes of the nasopharynx; or nonresectable lymph node metastases are relative contraindications to surgery [26, 27].

Maxillary sinus and ethmoid sinus tumors often present as locally advanced disease (large T3 or T4) and are commonly managed with surgery and postoperative radiation therapy. Ethmoid sinus carcinomas can be treated with radiation alone or with concurrent chemotherapy to avoid structural or functional deficits [37].

Surgical approaches include fenestration with removal of the bulk tumor, which is usually followed by radiation therapy or block resection of the upper jaw. Surgery generally involves medial maxillectomy and en bloc ethmoidectomy. A craniofacial approach is required if tumor extends superiorly to the ethmoid roof or olfactory region. A combined craniofacial approach, including resection of the floor of the anterior cranial fossa is used with success in selected patients [38].

Surgical exploration may be required to determine operability. Destruction of the base of skull (i.e., anterior cranial fossa), cavernous sinus, or the pterygoid process; infiltration of the mucous membranes of the nasopharynx; or nonresectable lymph node metastases are relative contraindications to surgery.

10.2. Chemotherapy

Few studies have investigated the role of neoadjuvant chemotherapy in the management of advanced cancer of the PNS [39, 40]. Intra-arterial cisplatin in combination with intravenous paclitaxel and ifosfamide in patients with locally advanced carcinoma of the PNS was studied at MD Anderson Cancer Center to determine the efficacy, organ-preservation rate, and safety. Despite better organ preservation rates, generous toxicity was also reported [41]. Further study of the role of neoadjuvant chemotherapy in patients with SCC of the PNS is warranted to determine whether the response (or lack of same) to neoadjuvant chemotherapy can help in the choice of definitive treatment [42].

Concurrent chemo-radiation therapy can also be used for patients with medical conditions that preclude surgery if those patients have good performance status. Depending on the patient's performance status and renal function, single-agent cisplatin or carboplatin can be used concurrently with external beam radiation for locally advanced, unresectable squamous cell carcinoma [43].

10.3. Radiation therapy

RT treatment planning includes the entire maxilla, the adjacent nasal cavity, the ethmoid sinus, the nasopharynx, and the pterygopalatine fossa. All or part of the orbit is included in patients with extension into or near the orbit. Target volume definition is aided by the use of treatment planning CT combined with image-fusion MRI.

When using conventional definitive fractionation, the primary tumor and involved lymph nodes (i.e., high-risk sites) generally require a total of 66 Gy (2.2 Gy/fraction) to 70 Gy (2.0 Gy/fraction) [44]. When using hyperfractionation, high-risk sites generally require up to 81.6 Gy (1.2 Gy/fraction) [45]. In contrast, elective irradiation to low-risk and intermediate-risk sites requires 44 Gy (2.0 Gy/fraction) to 63 Gy (1.6–1.8 Gy/fraction), depending on the estimated level of tumor burden, and on whether 3-D conformal RT or IMRT is used.

For 3-D conformal RT and sequentially planned IMRT, suggest 44–50 Gy (2.0 Gy/fraction). For concurrent chemoradiation the dose is typically 70–70.2 Gy (1.8–2.0 Gy/fraction) in 5 fractions. Higher doses of postoperative RT alone (60–66 Gy), or with systemic therapy, are recommended for the high-risk features of extracapsular disease and/or positive margins (**Table 9**) [46].

Postoperative RT	• T3-T4 primary disease • Microscopic margins < 5 mm (irrespective of intra-operative revision or additional postresection sampling of the surgical site) • >1 additional features at primary: 1. High-grade disease 2. Peri-neural invasion (PNI) 3. Lymph-vascular invasion (LVSI) • Lymph node involvement at pathology 1. ≥2 lymph nodes 2. Any lymph node > 3 cm (N2+) 3. Level IV-V LN positive 4. Extracapsular extension (ECE)
Preoperative RT	• Locally advanced cancer for downstaging of disease
Concurrent chemoradiotherapy	• Positive (inked) margin • Extracapsular extension

Table 9. Indications of radiation therapy.

10.3.1. Simulation and daily localization

The patient is simulated in supine position with head extended and the head and neck are immobilized. If possible, shoulders should also be immobilized to ensure accurate patient setup on a daily basis especially when an extended-field IMRT plan is used. To spare the tongue from high dose nasopharyngeal region, a bite block can be used.

CT scan with IV contrast using 3 mm thickness should be performed from the top of the head including the brain to the carina. 5 mm thickness can be reconstructed below the clavicle to the level of the carina.

Image registration and fusion applications with MRI and PET scans should be used to help in the delineation of target volumes, especially for regions of interest encompassing the gross tumor, skull base, brainstem, and optic chiasm.

10.4. Complication of treatment

Complications of surgery include failure of the split thickness skin graft to heal, trismus, CSF leak, meningities, parasinusities and hemorrhage.

The most frequent and significant complications of RT involve the eye [47, 48]. When only a portion of the ipsilateral eye is irradiated (the medial one third), it is possible to preserve vision in the majority of patients. When there is extensive disease in the orbit, however, the entire eye is irradiated to a high dose with almost certain loss of vision. A few patients will experience a transient CNS syndrome that includes vertigo, headaches, decreased cerebration, and lethargy [49]. Other rare complications are aseptic meningitis, chronic sinusitis, or serous otitis media.

11. Results of treatment

The management of PNS cancers remains a major challenge in oncology. A major problem in patients with carcinomas of the PNS is that most tumors are highly advanced at the time point of diagnosis.

For single-modality therapies, outcome is generally poor. Amendola et al. compared surgery versus definitive radiation on 39 patients and found no statistically significant differences in survival at 3 and 5 years, with a 5 year survival rate of 31 and 35% for resection and RT, respectively. Later, combined modality treatment was considered superior [50]. A number of reports have demonstrated some improvement in outcome with combined modality therapy. A report by St. Pierre and Baker based on treatment responses of 61 patients treated with surgical resection alone, definitive RT or combined treatment, showed a clear benefit for patients receiving combined surgery [51].

Clinical outcomes of postop patients with carcinomas of the paranasal sinuses and nasal cavity according to decade of radiation treatment were compared at Memorial Sloan-Kettering Cancer Center. In this study, 46% patients were treated by conventional radiotherapy; 35% patients by three-dimensional conformal radiotherapy; and 18% patients by intensity-modulated radiotherapy. The 5-year overall survival rates were 52%, local control rate was 62%, and disease-free survival was 54%, respectively. There were no significant differences in any of these parameters with respect to radiotherapy technique. The 5-year overall survival rate for patients treated in the 1960s, 1970s, 1980s, 1990s, and 2000s was 46, 56, 51, 53, and 49%, respectively. The observed incidence of severe late toxicity was 53, 45, 39, 28, and 16% among patients treated in the 1960s, 1970s, 1980s, 1990s, and 2000s, respectively [52].

In the past, the main concern in the radiotherapeutic treatment of PNS tumors was treatment-related toxicity. The introduction of IMRT now allows application of high doses to complex target volumes, while the surrounding OARs can be spared and toxicity may be reduced. Over the last years, IMRT has been implemented widely into the clinical routine. Duthoy et al. compared IMRT with conventional RT in 39 patients with PNS cancers. In the comparison between the IMRT and conventional RT groups, no significant differences were found for LC and OS [53].

Dose conformality to the target volume and conformal avoidance of the organs at risk achieved through IMRT may provide better local control and less optic toxicity compared to conventional radiotherapy technique. Image-guided radiation therapy (IGRT) has also been introduced to complement these approaches in ensuring the safe delivery of a highly conformal treatment, by facilitating convenient and frequent imaging of the patient anatomy throughout the treatment course [54].

Author details

Deepti Sharma*, Neha Sharma and Vivek Sharma

*Address all correspondence to: drdeeptisharma16@gmail.com

Department of Radiation Oncology, MAMC and LokNayak Hospital, New Delhi, India

References

[1] Youlden DR, Cramb SM, Peters S, Porceddu SV, Møller H, Fritschi L, et al. International comparisons of the incidence and mortality of sinonasal cancer. Cancer Epidemiology. 2013;**37**(6):770-779

[2] Robin PE, Powell D, Stansbie JM. Carcinoma of the nasal cavity and paranasal sinuses: Incidence and presentation of different histological types. Clinical Otolaryngology. 1979; **4**(6):431-456

[3] Boffetta P, Boccia S, La Vecchia C. A quick guide to cancer epidemiology. Epidemiology, Biostatistics and Public Health. Overview of the Major Causes of Human Cancer. 2014;**11**(1): 77-88

[4] Kuijpens JH, Louwman MW, Peters R, Janssens GO, Burdorf AL, Coebergh JW. Trends in sinonasal cancer in the Netherlands: More squamous cell cancer, less adenocarcinoma: A population-based study 1973–2009. European Journal of Cancer. 2012;**48**(15):2369-2374

[5] Sanghvi S, Khan MN, Patel NR, Yeldandi S, Baredes S, Eloy JA. Epidemiology of sinonasal squamous cell carcinoma: A comprehensive analysis of 4994 patients. The Laryngoscope. 2014;**124**(1):76-83

[6] Clemente MP. Surgical anatomy of the paranasal sinus. In: Sinus Surgery: Endoscopic and Microscopic Approaches. New York: Thieme; 2005. pp. 1-56

[7] IARC. IARC Monographs on the Evaluation of Carcinogenic Risks to Humans, Vol. 62. Lyon: Wood Dust and Formaldehyde; 1995. pp. 1-377. DOI: 978-92-832-1262-1

[8] Binazzi A, Ferrante P, Marinaccio A. Occupational exposure and sinonasal cancer: A systematic review and meta-analysis. BMC Cancer. 2015;**15**(1):49

[9] Demers PA, Kogevinas M, Boffetta P, Leclerc A, Luce D, Gérin M, et al. Wood dust and sinonasal cancer: Pooled reanalysis of twelve case-control studies. American Journal of Industrial Medicine. 1995;**28**(2):151-166

[10] d'Errico A, Pasian S, Baratti A, Zanelli R, Alfonzo S, Gilardi L, et al. A case-control study on occupational risk factors for sino-nasal cancer. Occupational and Environmental Medicine. 2009;**66**(7):448-455

[11] Leclerc A, Luce D, Demers PA, Boffetta P, Kogevinas M, Belli S, et al. Sinonasal cancer and occupation. Results from the reanalysis of twelve case-control studies. American Journal of Industrial Medicine. 1997;**31**(2):153-165

[12] Luce D, Leclerc A, Morcet JF, Casal-Lareo A, Gérin M, Brugère J, et al. Occupational risk factors for sinonasal cancer: A case-control study in France. American Journal of Industrial Medicine. 1992;**21**:163-175

[13] Leclerc A, Martinez Cortes M, Gérin M, Luce D, Brugère J. Sinonasal cancer and wood dust exposure: Results from a case-control study. American Journal of Epidemiology. 1994;**140**:340-349

[14] Comba P, Barbieri PG, Battista G, Belli S, Ponterio F, Zanetti D, et al. Cancer of the nose and paranasal sinuses in the metal industry: A case-control study. British Journal of Industrial Medicine. 1992;**49**:193-196

[15] Bhattacharyya N. Cancer of the nasal cavity: Survival and factors influencing prognosis. Archives of Otolaryngology—Head & Neck Surgery. 2002;**128**(9):1079

[16] Perrone F, Oggionni M, Birindelli S, Suardi S, Tabano S, Romano R, et al. TP53, p14ARF, p16INK4a and H-ras gene molecular analysis in intestinal-type adenocarcinoma of the nasal cavity and paranasal sinuses. International Journal of Cancer. 2003;**105**(2):196-203

[17] Franchi A, Fondi C, Paglierani M, Pepi M, Gallo O, Santucci M. Epidermal growth factor receptor expression and gene copy number in sinonasal intestinal type adenocarcinoma. Oral Oncology. 2009;**45**(9):835-838

[18] Holmila R, Bornholdt J, Heikkilä P, Suitiala T, Févotte J, Cyr D, et al. Mutations in TP53 tumor suppressor gene in wood dust-related sinonasal cancer. International Journal of Cancer. 2010;**127**(3):578-588

[19] Chernock RD, Perry A, Pfeifer JD, Holden JA, Lewis JS. Receptor tyrosine kinases in sinonasal undifferentiated carcinomas—Evaluation for EGFR, c-KIT, and HER2/neu expression. Head & Neck. 2009;**31**(7):919-927

[20] Takahashi Y, Bell D, Agarwal G, Roberts D, Xie TX, El-Naggar A, et al. Comprehensive assessment of prognostic markers for sinonasal squamous cell carcinoma. Head & Neck. 2014;**36**(8):1094-1102

[21] Syrjänen K, Syrjänen S. Detection of human papillomavirus in sinonasal carcinoma: Systematic review and meta-analysis. Human Pathology. 2013;**44**(6):983-991

[22] Slootweg PJ, Ferlito A, Cardesa A, Thompson LDR, Hunt JL, Strojan P, et al. Sinonasal tumors: A clinicopathologic update of selected tumors. European Archives of Oto-Rhino-Laryngology. 2012;**270**:5-20

[23] Barnes L, Eveson JW, Reichart P, Sidransky D, editors. World Health Organization Classification of Tumours. Pathology and Genetics. Head and Neck Tumours. Lyon: IARC Press; 2005

[24] Dooley L, Shah J. Management of the neck in maxillary sinus carcinomas. Current Opinion in Otolaryngology & Head and Neck Surgery. 2015;**23**(2):107-114

[25] Day TA, Beas RA, Schlosser RJ, Woodworth BA, Barredo J, Sharma AK, et al. Management of paranasal sinus malignancy. Current Treatment Options in Oncology. 2005;**6**:3-18

[26] Pan WR, Suarl H, Corlett RJ, Ashton MW. Lymphatic drainage of the nasal fossae and nasopharynx: Preliminary anatomical and radiological study with clinical implications. Head and Neck—Journal for the Sciences and Specialties of the Head and Neck. 2009;**31**: 52-57

[27] Scurry WC, Goldenberg D, Chee MY, Lengerich E, Liu Y, Fedok FG. Regional recurrence of squamous cell carcinoma of the nasal cavity—A systematic review and meta-analysis. Archives of Otolaryngology—Head & Neck Surgery. 2007;**133**:796-800

[28] Jiang GL, Ang KK, Peters LJ, Wendt CD, Oswald MJ, Goepfert H. Maxillary sinus carcinomas: Natural history and results of postoperative radiotherapy. Radiotherapy and Oncology. 1991;**21**:193-200

[29] Cantu G, Solero CL, Miceli R, Mattana F, Riccio S, Colombo S, et al. Anterior craniofacial resection for malignant paranasal tumors: A monoinstitutional experience of 366 cases. Head & Neck. 2011;**34**(1):78-87

[30] Raghavan P, Phillips CD. Magnetic resonance imaging of sinonasal malignancies. Topics in Magnetic Resonance Imaging. 2007;**18**:259-267

[31] Ariyoshi Y, Shimahara M. Magnetic resonance imaging of maxillary cancer: Possibility of detecting bone destruction. Oral Oncology. 2000;**36**:499-507

[32] AJCC Cancer Staging Manual. 2017. DOI: 10.1007/978-3-319-40618-3

[33] Ansa B, Goodman M, Ward K, Kono SA, Owonikoko TK, Higgins K, et al. Paranasal sinus squamous cell carcinoma incidence and survival based on surveillance, epidemiology, and end results data, 1973–2009. Cancer. 2013;**119**(14):2602-2610

[34] Turner JH, Reh DD. Incidence and survival in patients with sinonasal cancer: A historical analysis of population-based data. Head & Neck. 2011;**34**(6):877-885

[35] Haerle SK, Gullane PJ, Witterick IJ, Zweifel C, Gentili F. Sinonasal carcinomas: Epidemiology, pathology, and management. Neurosurgery Clinics. 2013;**24**(1):39-49

[36] Abu-Ghanem S, Fliss DM. Surgical approaches to resection of anterior skull band paranasal sinuses tumors. Balkan Medical Journal. 2013;**30**(2):136-141

[37] Waldron JN, O'Sullivan B, Warde P, Gullane P, Lui F, Payne D, et al. Ethmoid sinus cancer: Twenty-nine cases managed with primary radiation therapy. International Journal of Radiation Oncology, Biology, Physics. 1998;**41**(2):361-369

[38] Lund VJ, Howard DJ, Wei WI, et al. Craniofacial resection for tumors of the nasal cavity and paranasal sinuses. A 17-year experience. Head & Neck. 1998;**20**:97-105

[39] Lorusso P, Tapazoglou E, Kish JA, Ensley JF, Cummings G, Kelly J, et al. Chemotherapy for paranasal sinus carcinoma. A 10-year experience at Wayne state university. Cancer. 1988;**62**(1):1-5

[40] Lee MM, Vokes EE, Arie R, Ellen WM, Weichselbaum Ralph R, Haraf DJ. Multimodality therapy in advanced paranasal sinus carcinoma: Superior long-term results. International Journal of Radiation Oncology, Biology, Physics. 1998;**42**(1):327

[41] Papadimitrakopoulou VA, Ginsberg LE, Garden AS, Kies MS, Glisson BS, Diaz EM, et al. Intraarterial cisplatin with intravenous paclitaxel and ifosfamide as an organ-preservation approach in patients with paranasal sinus carcinoma. Cancer. 2003;**98**(10):2214-2223

[42] Hanna EY, Cardenas AD, Demonte F, Roberts D, Kupferman M, Weber R, et al. Induction chemotherapy for advanced squamous cell carcinoma of the paranasal sinuses. Archives of Otolaryngology–Head & Neck Surgery. 2011;**137**(1):78

[43] Iqbal MS, Chaw C, Kovarik J, Aslam S, Jackson A, Kelly J, et al. Primary concurrent chemoradiation in head and neck cancers with weekly cisplatin chemotherapy: Analysis of compliance, toxicity and survival. International Archives of Otorhinolaryngology. 2017; **21**(2):171-177

[44] Fu K, Pajak T, Trotti A, Jones C, Spencer S, Phillips T, et al. A radiation therapy oncology group (RTOG) phase III randomised study to compare hyperfractionation and two variants of accelerated fractionation to standard fractionation radiotherapy for head and neck squamous cell carcinomas; first report of RTOG 9003. Cancer/Radiothérapie. 2001;**5**(1):95-96

[45] Overgaard J, Hansen HS, Specht L, Overgaard M, Grau C, Andersen E, et al. Five compared with six fractions per week of conventional radiotherapy of squamous-cell carcinoma of head and neck: DAHANCA 6&7 randomised controlled trial. The Lancet. 2003; **362**(9388):933-940

[46] Cooper JS, Zhang Q, Pajak TF, Forastiere AA, Jacobs J, Saxman SB, et al. Long-term follow-up of the RTOG 9501/intergroup phase III trial: Postoperative concurrent radiation

Contents

Preface

Implantable cardiac pacemakers have been utilized for more than 50 years now. Continuous development transformed them from rudimentary, asynchronous pulse generators to sophisticated devices with advanced diagnostic and therapeutic capabilities. Implantable defibrillators and biventricular devices, treating malignant tachyarrhythmias and dyssynchrony, use a similar technology. As initial issues of bradycardia-related pacing got resolved, new issues have been recognized, such as the deleterious effects of chronic right ventricular pacing or high risk of complications due to utilization in a frail patient population.

Evidence-based practice guidelines were initially developed with a focus on indications and contraindications. Safe utilization of implantable antiarrhythmia devices begins with proper patient selection; implantation method and technique, device programming and follow up are also important aspects that determine the outcome. Lack of high quality data, which could guide these decisions, leads to large individual and geographical variations. Recently, expert consensus documents addressed several important topics, such as follow-up or end-of-life considerations, however, further research is still needed to provide a basis for a more uniform, safe therapy.

This book reviews several current issues and recent advances in pacemaker therapy. Improving safety of implantation is of utmost importance to decrease complications. Transvenous route became the standard approach for antiarrhythmic cardiac device implantation as it poses only a minimal burden to the patient. Cardiac resynchronization therapy can still be challenging from this approach due to highly variable individual anatomy – recently, interventional and minimally invasive surgical methods have been developed and studied in detail, with great success. Although the risk of severe periprocedural complications is low for pacemaker or defibrillator implants, there are still dreaded consequences, such as endocarditis or lead perforation, which may be lethal if not addressed in a timely and appropriate manner. Transvenous lead extraction revolutionized management of these complications. Other common issues encountered during follow up include unnecessary right ventricular pacing and atrial fibrillation, with its potential to interact with device function. Several new algorithms have been introduced lately to address these issues – familiarity with these may prevent misinterpreting appropriate device function as malfunction.

Patients are frequently seen by multiple healthcare providers in various settings, and questions may arise whether the implanted device contributes to, or is responsible for the clinical presentation. As device-specific programmers are not always immediately available, routine diagnostic modalities, such as a 12-lead ECG should be evaluated first as these may often identify or rule out a potential issue.

Multiple ongoing research projects address potential applications related to implantable cardiac arrhythmia devices: studies on nonlinear cardiac dynamics, mobile telemonitoring and phrenic nerve stimulation in patients with diaphragmatic paralysis will be reviewed, displaying the potential of the technology beyond antibradycardia pacing.

I am extremely grateful to the international group of authors who contributed this book - their expertise clearly shows the worldwide abundance of pacemaker technology and thriving research activity in this field. I would like to also appreciate the help of the wonderful InTech editorial staff – Ms. Tanja Skorupan and Mr. Hrvoje Pecotic, who expertly guided us through the publication process. A special thanks to my family – wife, Erika, and children, Fruzsina, Alice and Adam, who provided a supportive environment while working on this project.

Attila Roka MD, PhD
Hospital of St. Raphael, New Haven, CT,
USA

Section 1

Novel Implantation Techniques

Chapter 1

Techniques of Permanent Pacemaker Implantation

Majid Haghjoo

Additional information is available at the end of the chapter

http://dx.doi.org/10.5772/48639

1. Introduction

Currently available permanent pacemakers contain a pulse generator and one or more pacing leads. Early in the era of pacemaker implantation, this procedure was only performed by the cardiac surgeons because of the initial mandate for epicardial lead implantation. Further advancements in the pacing hardware and percutaneous venous catheterization simplified the implantation technique and made it feasible to implant the transvenous leads. Simultaneously, further innovations in the pulse generator and its circuitry extended the utility of the percutaneous technique even in the very young patients.

All device trainees will require basic skills in pacemaker implantation. However, first step is to identify whether a patient needs a permanent pacemaker. This chapter will summarize the necessary equipments, patient preparation, and implantation techniques. Like any practical skill it is only possible to give a flavor of the methodology in writing, and nothing can replace the practical tuition of an experienced implanter in the pacing theatre during a number of pacemaker implants.

2. Equipments

The pacemaker implantation can be performed in electrophysiology (EP) laboratory, catheterization laboratory, or operating room [1]. Pacemaker implantation by interventional electrophysiologist in EP lab or catheterization laboratory resulted in a significant reduction in medical cost and hospital stay [2].

Minimum required personnel for pacemaker implantation consist of implanting physician, scrub nurse, and circulating nurse or technician. Scrub nurse is required to help the implanter throughout the procedure. The circulating nurse or technician is required to prepare and administer medications, and to operate pacing system analyzer.

Fluoroscopy and electrocardiography (ECG) are necessary equipments in every device implant. Single-plane fluoroscopy via anteroposterior, 30° right anterior oblique, and 45° left anterior oblique views is usually adequate for transvenous implantation from either the right or the left pectoral approach. Currently, initial lead sensing and capture measurements are obtained by pacing system analyzers (Figure 1), which may be stand-alone or built into the pacer programmer.

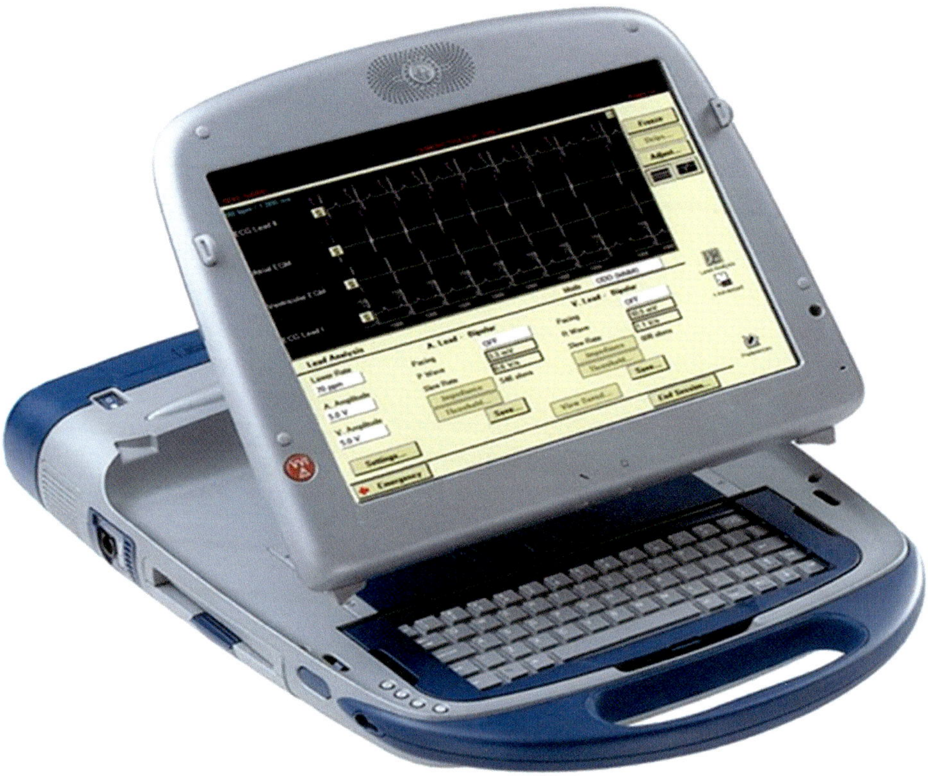

Figure 1. Built-in pacing system analyzer

Apart from the fluoroscopy equipment and vital observation monitors, there are a number of sterile surgical instruments and equipment that are needed (Figure 2). Suture materials include both nonabsorbable material for lead and device anchoring and absorbable material for pocket closure. Antimicrobial flush and saline for pocket irrigation should be available. If venography is to be performed, an appropriate intravenous contrast agent must be available.

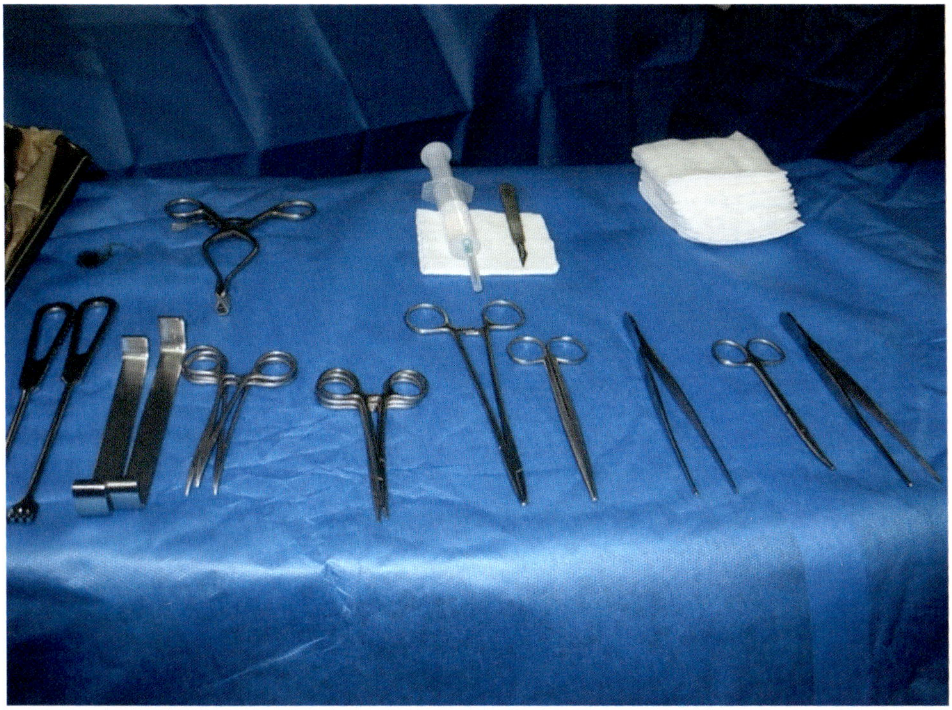

Figure 2. Minor surgical tray for permanent pacemaker implantation

3. Patient preparation

Before pacemaker implantation, an informed consent should be obtained. Any anticipated risks and benefits should be honestly discussed with patient or the patient's family. The indication for pacing should be thoroughly described to the patient. The need for lifelong follow-up should be emphasized and patient should be informed about the generator change and possible lead replacement in the future. Any physical or occupational restrictions related to the pacemaker implantation including rules regarding the driving should be discussed in detail with the patient.

Routine pre-implant lab tests are 12-lead ECG, chest x-ray, complete blood count, prothombin and partial thromboplastin times, serum electrolytes, blood urea nitrogen, and serum creatinine. Many of the patients requiring a pacemaker may be on oral anticoagulant [3]. Perioperative management of these patients is often challenging and needs special experience. In the past, standard practice was to discontinue warfarin 48 hours before the procedure, bridge with intravenous heparin, and then reinitiate warfarin the day of the procedure or even the night before. This practice has been associated with higher risk of hematoma formation compared with that encountered in unanticoagulated patients (up to 20%) [4]. Recently, there has been an increasing interest in performing the pacemaker implantation without reversal of the anticoagulant. This practice was associated with lower risk of pocket bleeding and shorter hospital stay [3, 5-7].

Antibiotic prophylaxis is a controversial issue, but most implanters prefer to give oral or intravenous (IV) antibiotics to decrease the incidence of local or systemic infections based on limited data available [8]. Although there is a distinct lack of either national or international guidance in this area, meta-analysis of the randomized trials suggests a benefit from pre-procedure intravenous antibiotics [9]. Our routine practice is to give 1 gram of cefazolin or vancomycin (in penicillin-allergic patients) one hour before the procedure.

Implantation of pacemaker usually involves a combination of local anesthesia and conscious sedation. Infiltration of skin and subcutaneous tissue at the implant site with 1-2% lidocaine provides sufficient local anesthesia for the majority of implant procedures. However, to obtain optimal anesthesia, conscious sedation in the form of carefully titrated IV midazolam and fentanyl is recommended. On rare occasions, general anesthesia may be required in an extremely uncooperative patient.

Implant area from the angle of jaw to the nipple line bilaterally should be completely cleansed and shaved. Placement of an IV line ipsilateral to the intended implant site is routine for administration of prophylactic antibiotics, administration of IV analgesia/sedation, and potentially to perform venography.

On entering the procedure room, the patient is usually placed on his or her back with the arms tucked and physiologic monitoring (ECG, pulse oximetry, and noninvasive blood pressure) should be quickly established to detect any arrhythmia or hemodynamic abnormality. Preparing the procedure field is also crucial to minimizing complications. Sterility is obviously of paramount importance; the chest is prepared with an antiseptic solution, and the area is covered with sterile drapes to keep the incision area as clean as possible.

4. Implant techniques

4.1. Central venous access techniques

A central vein (ie, the subclavian, internal jugular or axillary vein) is accessed via a percutaneous approach. Alternatively, target vein is accessed via direct visualization by a cut down technique (most commonly, cephalic vein). Figure 3 shows a standard prepackaged introducer set for implantation. In patients in whom this is technically difficult because skeletal landmarks are deviated, an initial brief fluoroscopic examination will greatly reduce the time and complications associated with obtaining the access (Figure 4).

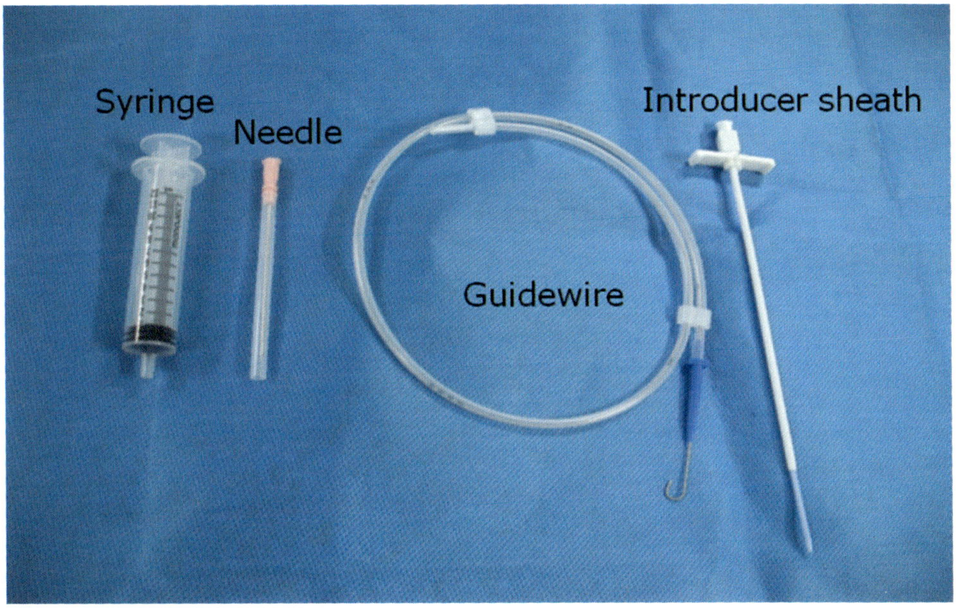

Figure 3. Introducer set used for percutaneous access to central veins

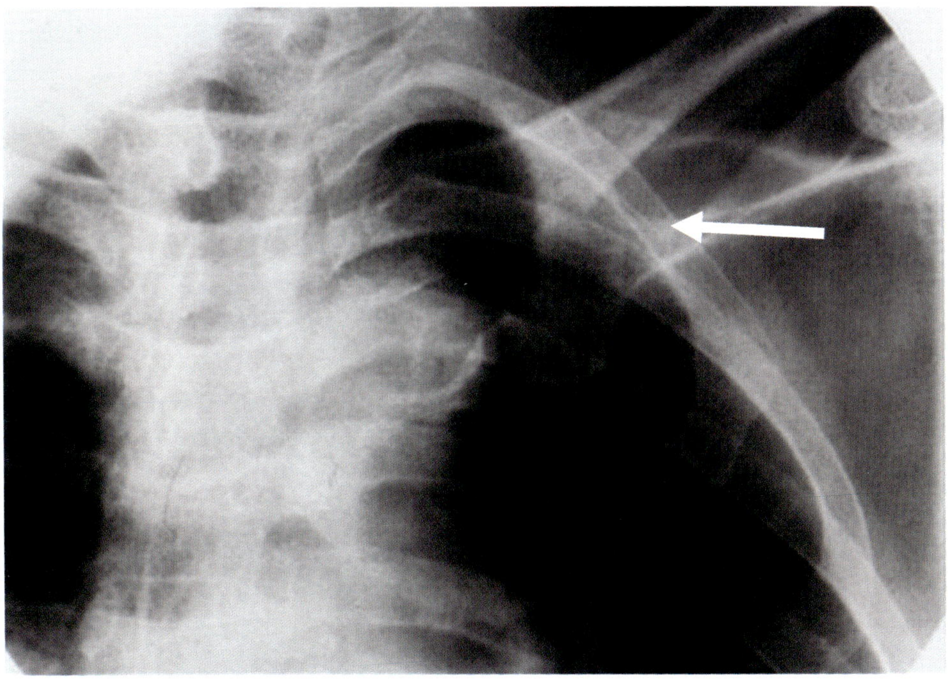

Figure 4. Target area for subclavian vein puncture is marked by white arrow.

Subclavian vein puncture is the first choice technique for most operators. The needle is advanced (gently aspirating on an attached syringe as with any other indirect puncture), aiming for the space below the clavicle and over the first rib until either the vein is cannulated or the rib is struck. The subclavian vein is typically accessed at the junction of the first rib and the clavicle. On occasion, venography may be required to visualize the vein adequately or to confirm its patency (Figure 5). This approach is associated with minimal incidence of pneumothorax.

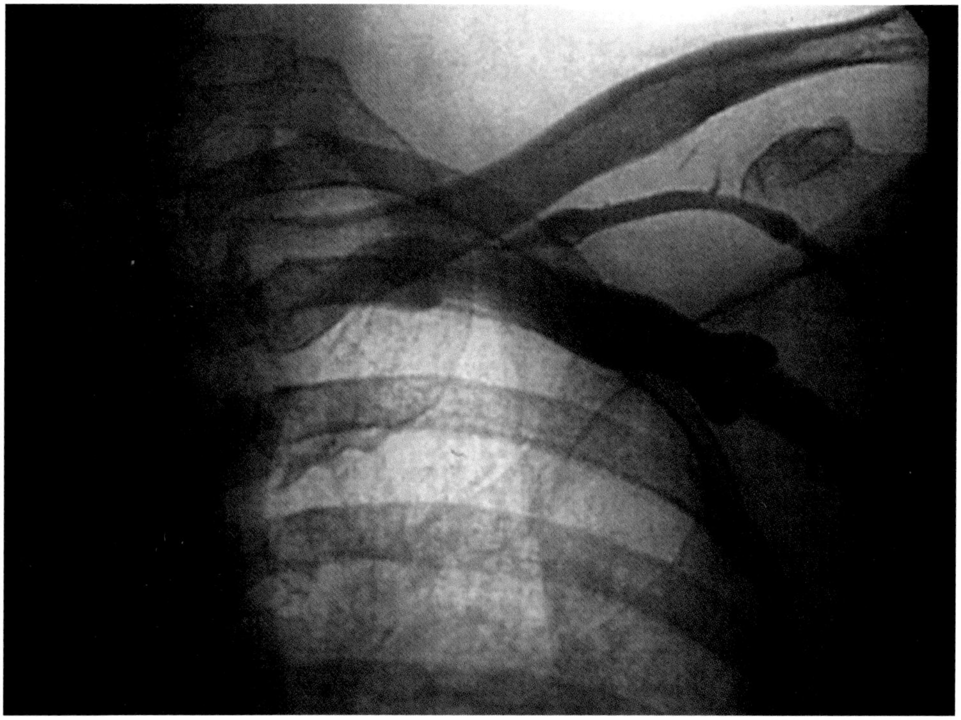

Figure 5. Contrast venography performed from left brachial vein. The figure clearly shows axillary vein, cephalic vein, subclavian vein

Other important alternative central vein techniques for lead implantation are cephalic vein cut down and axillary vein puncture. The cephalic vein resides in the sulcus between the deltoid and pectoral muscles. This area is easily identified by palpation and is occupied by loose connective tissue and fat, which can be dissected to identify the cephalic vein. Occasionally, the vein is deep or consists of a plexus of tiny veins. In these circumstances, other routes should be used for lead insertion. After vein isolation for 1 to 2 cm within the groove, it is ligated distally. A ligator is placed around the proximal part of the vein for hemostasis. The vein can be entered using venotomy or with 16- or 18-guage peripheral IV catheter. The axillary vein can be accessed by blind percutaneous puncture by entering the pectoral muscle just medial to the acromion process on anteroposterior fluoroscopy. The needle then is directed to the point at which the lateral border of the first rib appears to cross the inferior margin of the clavicle. Alternatively, the axillary vein can be accessed using contrast venography.

After venous access is obtained, a guide wire is advanced through the access needle, and the tip of the guide wire is positioned in the right atrium or the venacaval area under fluoroscopy. The needle is then withdrawn, leaving the guide wire in place. If indicated, a second access will be obtained in a similar fashion for positioning of a second guide wire.

Sometimes, a double-wire technique is used, whereby 2 guide wires are inserted through the first sheath and the sheath then withdrawn, so that 2 separate sheaths can be advanced over the 2 guide wires. This technique can cause some resistance or friction during sheath or lead advancement.

4.2. Pocket formation

Although the pocket may be formed in the axilla or in the abdomen (for epicardial or femoral systems), the most common site is the pectoral region. In the latter approach, a 1.5- to 2-inch incision is made in the infraclavicular area parallel to the middle third of the clavicle, and a subcutaneous pocket is created with sharp and blunt dissection where the pacemaker generator will be implanted. Some physicians prefer to make the pocket first and obtain access later through the pocket or via venous cutdown; once access is obtained, they position the guide wires as described above.

4.3. Positioning of atrial and ventricular leads

Over the guide wire, a special peel-away sheath and dilator are advanced. The guide wire and dilator are withdrawn, leaving the sheath in place. A stylet (a thin wire) is inserted inside the center channel of the pacemaker lead to make it more rigid, and the lead-stylet combination is then inserted into the sheath and advanced under fluoroscopy to the appropriate heart chamber. Usually, the ventricular lead is positioned before the atrial lead to prevent its dislodgment.

Making a small curve at the tip of the stylet renders the ventricular lead tip more maneuverable, so that it can more easily be placed across the tricuspid valve and positioned at the right ventricular apex.

Once correct lead positioning is confirmed, the lead is affixed to the endocardium either passively with tines (like a grappling hook) or actively via a helical screw located at the tip. The screw at the tip of the pacemaker is extended or retracted by turning the outer end of the lead with the help of a torque device. Adequate extension of the screw is confirmed with fluoroscopy. Each manufacturer has its own proprietary identification marks for confirming adequate extension of the screw.

Once the lead is secured in position, the introducing sheath is carefully peeled away, leaving the lead in place. After the pacing lead stylet is removed, pacing and sensing thresholds and lead impedances are measured with a pacing system analyzer, and pacing is performed at 10 V to make sure that it is not causing diaphragmatic stimulation. After confirmation of lead position and thresholds, the proximal end of the lead is secured to the underlying tissue (ie, pectoralis) with a nonabsorbable suture that is sewn to a sleeve located on the lead.

If a second lead is indicated, it is positioned in the right atrium via a second sheath, with the lead tip typically positioned in the right atrial appendage with the help of a preformed J-shaped stylet.

In a patient who is without an atrial appendage as a result of previous cardiac surgery, the lead can be positioned medially or in the lateral free wall of the right atrium. As with the ventricular lead, the atrial lead position is confirmed, impedance is assessed, the stylet is withdrawn, and the lead is secured to the underlying pectoralis with a nonabsorbable suture.

4.4. Lead connection and pulse generator insertion in the pocket

When the leads have been properly positioned and tested and sutured to the underlying tissue, the pacemaker pocket is irrigated with antimicrobial solution, and the pulse generator is connected securely to the leads. Many physicians secure the pulse generator to underlying tissue with a nonabsorbable suture to prevent migration or twiddler syndrome.

Typically, the pacemaker is positioned superficial to the pectoralis, but occasionally, a subpectoral or inframammary position is required. After hemostasis is confirmed, a final look under fluoroscopy before closure of the incision is recommended to confirm appropriate lead positioning.

4.5. Pocket closure

The incision is closed in layers with absorbable sutures and adhesive strips. Sterile dressing is applied to the incision surface. An arm restraint or immobilizer is applied to the unilateral arm for 12-24 hours to limit movement.

4.6. Post-procedural care

Pain levels are typically low after the procedure, and the patient can be given pain medication to manage breakthrough pain associated with the incision site. There is controversy over the routine use of IV or oral antibiotics after the procedure. A postoperative chest radiograph is usually obtained to confirm lead position and rule out pneumothorax. Before discharge on the following day, posteroanterior and lateral chest radiographs will be ordered again to confirm lead positions and exclude delayed pneumothorax. Pacemaker interrogation is also recommended to ensure proper pacing function before patient leaving the hospital.

Author details

Majid Haghjoo,
Cardiovascular Medicine, Cardiac Electrophysiology Research Center,
Department of Cardiac pacing and Electrophysiology, Rajaie Cardiovascular Medical Center,
Tehran University of Medical Sciences, Tehran, Iran

5. References

[1] Garcia-Bolao I, Alegria E [1999] Implantation of 500 consecutive cardiac pacemakers in the electrophysiology laboratory. Acta. Cardiol. 54: 339-343.

[2] Yamamura KH, Kloosterman EM, Alba J, Garcia F, Williams PL, Mitran RD, Interian A Jr [1999] Analysis of charges and complications of permanent pacemaker implantation in the cardiac catheterization laboratory versus the operating room. Pacing. Clin. Electrophysiol. 22: 1820-1824.

[3] Guidici MC, Barold SS, Paul DL, Bontu P [2004] Pacemaker and implantable cardioverter defibrillator implantation without reversal of warfarin. Pacing. Clin. Electrophysiol. 27:358-360.

[4] Chow V, Ranasinghe I, Lau J, Stowe H, Bannon P, Hendel N, Kritharides L [2010] Peri-procedural anticoagulation and the incidence of haematoma formation after permanent pacemaker implantation in the elderly. Heart. Lung. Circ. 19:706-712.

[5] Li HK, Chen FC, Rea RF, Asirvatham SJ, Powell BD, Friedman PA, Shen WK, Brady PA, Bradley DJ, Lee HC, Hodge DO, Slusser JP, Hayes DL, Cha YM [2011] No increased bleeding events with continuation of oral anticoagulation therapy for patients undergoing cardiac device procedure. Pacing. Clin. Electrophysiol. 34: 868-874.

[6] Cheng A, Nazarian S, Brinker JA, Tompkins C, Spragg DD, Leng CT, Halperin H, Tandri H, Sinha SK, Marine JE, Calkins H, Tomaselli GF, Berger RD, Henrikson CA [2011] Continuation of warfarin during pacemaker or implantable cardioverter-defibrillator implantation: a randomized clinical trial. Heart. Rhythm. 8: 536-540.

[7] Ahmed I, Gertner E, Nelson WB, House CM, Dahiya R, Anderson CP, Benditt DG, Zhu DW [2010] Continuing warfarin therapy is superior to interrupting warfarin with or without bridging anticoagulation therapy in patients undergoing pacemaker and defibrillator implantation. Heart. Rhythm. 7: 745-749.

[8] Mounsey JP, Griffith MJ, Tynan M, Gould FK, MacDermott AF, Gold RG, Bexton RS [1994] Antibiotic prophylaxis in permanent pacemaker implantation: a prospective randomized trial. Br. Heart. J. 72: 339-343.

[9] Da Costa A, Kirkorian G, Cucherat M, Delahaye F, Chevalier P, Cerisier A, Isaaz K, Touboul P [1998] Antibiotic prophylaxis for permanent pacemaker implantation: a meta-analysis. Circulation. 97:1796-1801.

Interventional and Minimally Invasive Surgical Techniques Facilitating Cardiac Resynchronization Therapy

Bela Merkely, Levente Molnar and Attila Roka

Additional information is available at the end of the chapter

http://dx.doi.org/10.5772/50291

1. Introduction

Cardiac resynchronization therapy (CRT) with atriobiventricular pacing has been utilized for more than a decade for severe congestive heart failure associated with intraventricular dyssynchrony. The primary objective of CRT is to coordinate myocardial contraction with stimulation via right atrial (RA), right ventricular (RV) and left ventricular (LV) leads, using a biventricular pacemaker (CRT-P) or defibrillator (CRT-D). Although it provides both morbidity and mortality benefits in addition to medical therapy and implantable cardioverter-defibrillator, several issues remain unresolved, most importantly the high number of non-responder patients (up to 30%) and the technically challenging implantation. These are linked, as optimal lead position is essential for successful resynchronization.

Atriobiventricular pacing is most commonly accomplished with transvenous placement of the system. Endocardial right atrial and right ventricular leads are conventional. The left ventricle is stimulated via a branch of the coronary sinus, performing epicardial stimulation. Unfavorable coronary sinus or vein anatomy, such as valves, tortuosity or focal stenosis may render left ventricular lead implantation very difficult. Even in the absence of these, there may be no appropriate vein in the area which would provide effective resynchronization. The average implantation time of CRT in high volume centers is under 2 hours, with a procedural success rate of 87%-96% (Alonso, 2009). Perioperative complications are seen in 10% and the rate of late complications is 5.5% (Khan, 2009).

Recent evidence suggests that LV lead position is crucial to ensure effective CRT. This chapter will review the indications for CRT, use of imaging modalities to facilitate targeted lead placement, perioperative issues and techniques shown to be useful in challenging cases.

2. Indications for CRT

Most clinical CRT trials were performed in patients with advanced heart failure: LVEF ≤35%, wide QRS, sinus rhythm, NYHA III-IV functional stage despite optimal medical treatment (COMPANION, CARE-HF, MIRACLE, MUSTIC SR etc.). Few studies included patients with less severe symptoms (MADIT CRT, REVERSE, RAFT) or who were in atrial fibrillation (MUSTIC-AF and partially RAFT). The guidelines for implantation were recently updated by the HFA and ESC (McMurray, 2012). (Figure 1)

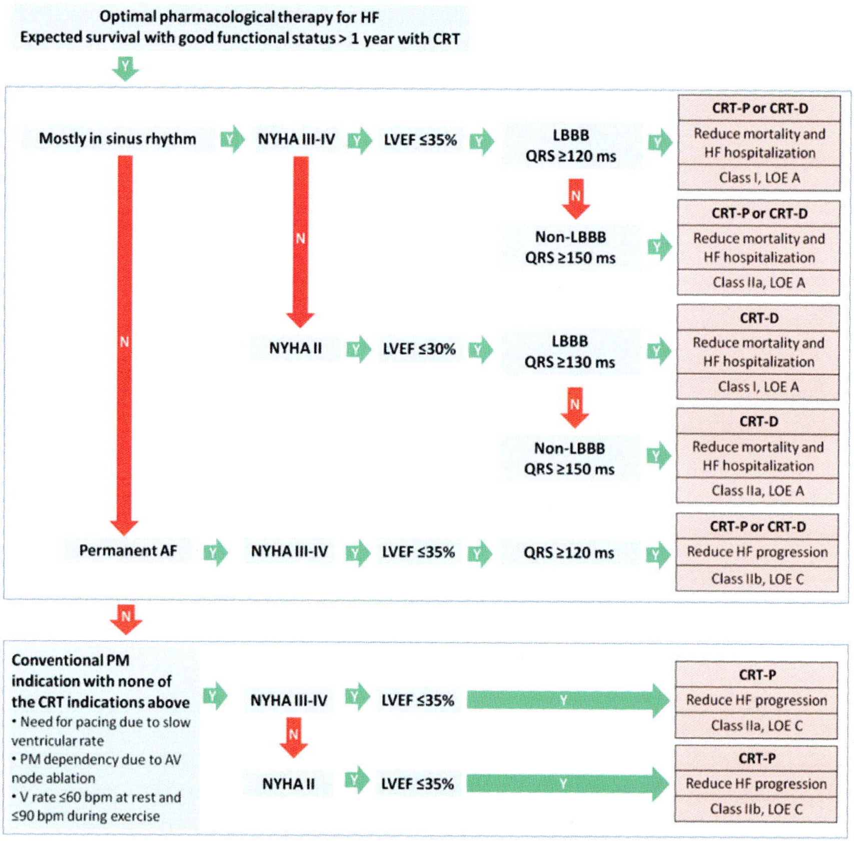

Figure 1. Indications for cardiac resynchronization therapy, Heart Failure Association and European Society of Cardiology, 2012 (McMurray, 2012). Stage IV heart failure patients should be "ambulatory" – pressor-dependent or acutely decompensated patients are generally not good candidates for CRT. *HF: heart failure. CRT: cardiac resynchronization therapy. NYHA: New York Heart Association functional class. LVEF: left ventricular ejection fraction. LBBB: left bundle branch block. CRT-P: cardiac resynchronization with biventricular pacemaker. CRT-D: cardiac resynchronization with biventricular implantable cardioverter defibrillator. PM: pacemaker. AV: atrioventricular. Class: strength of indication (class I – implantation recommended, class IIa – implantation should be considered, class IIb – implantation may be considered). LOE: level of evidence (A: multiple randomized trials or meta-analysis, C: expert opinion)*

3. Pre-implantation evaluation

Patient evaluation prior to implantation should include assessment of functional stage, left ventricular ejection fraction and 12-lead ECG to determine whether the patient is a candidate for CRT. Potentially reversible factors contributing to heart failure and cardiomyopathy should be looked for and corrected (ischemia, hypertension, suboptimal medical management etc.). Co-morbidities limiting life expectancy or decreasing possible benefits of CRT should be identified (cardiac cachexia, advanced renal disease, frailty etc.) (Theuns, 2011). Advanced age alone is not a contraindication to CRT. History of arrhythmias and eligibility for ICD should be also assessed to guide device and lead selection. The patient should not be in a decompensated condition at the time of implantation. Heart failure medications must be utilized at maximally tolerated doses for at least 3 months prior to considering the patient as a candidate for CRT implantation. In the immediate pre-implantation period, basic laboratory parameters should be checked and corrected as necessary to minimize surgical risks (complete blood cell count, electrolytes and kidney function, coagulation tests) (Epstein, 2008). A standardized evaluation of heart failure may help to assess response to CRT (serum BNP, 6 minute walking test).

Echocardiography is the most common test performed to assess severity of left ventricular dysfunction. Right ventricular dysfunction may affect response to CRT and should also be evaluated (Burri, 2010). Although multiple echocardiographic measurements exist to evaluate intraventricular or interventricular mechanical dyssynchrony, so far these were not proven to be helpful to guide patient selection for CRT. Absence of echocardiographic dyssynchrony should not defer utilization of CRT if the patient would otherwise be a candidate, however, the risk of deterioration is higher in these cases (Mullens, 2009).

Cardiac MRI with delayed enhancement imaging may be considered when the presence and location of myocardial scar is relevant and echocardiography is non-diagnostic (Bleeker, 2006).

4. Assessment of coronary vein anatomy

Transvenous endovascular left ventricular lead placement is limited by the anatomic constraints of the coronary veins. Patients with history of thoracic irradiation or cardiac surgeries may be at high risk for unsuccessful left ventricular lead implantation. Imaging studies prior to implantation may help to determine if the patient is suitable for transvenous implantation.

Coronary angiography is routinely performed during the workup of heart failure. Delayed images after contrast injection into the coronary arteries may outline the anatomy of the coronary sinus and its main branches. A major advantage of this method is that it does not provide any additional burden to the patient. The position of the orifice, the angle of the proximal CS, tortuousity and diameter of the vein are valuable clues for the selection of target vessel and the implantation approach. Most useful projections are anteroposterior and left anterior oblique, as these are common working views during CRT implantation.

Although the image quality is rarely good enough to assess terminal branches of the CS, the data obtained during coronary angiography may be used to identify fluoroscopic markers for CS cannulation as the ostium is almost always visualized. Another limitation is that this approach provides only two dimensional data (Kovacs, 2004) (Figure 2).

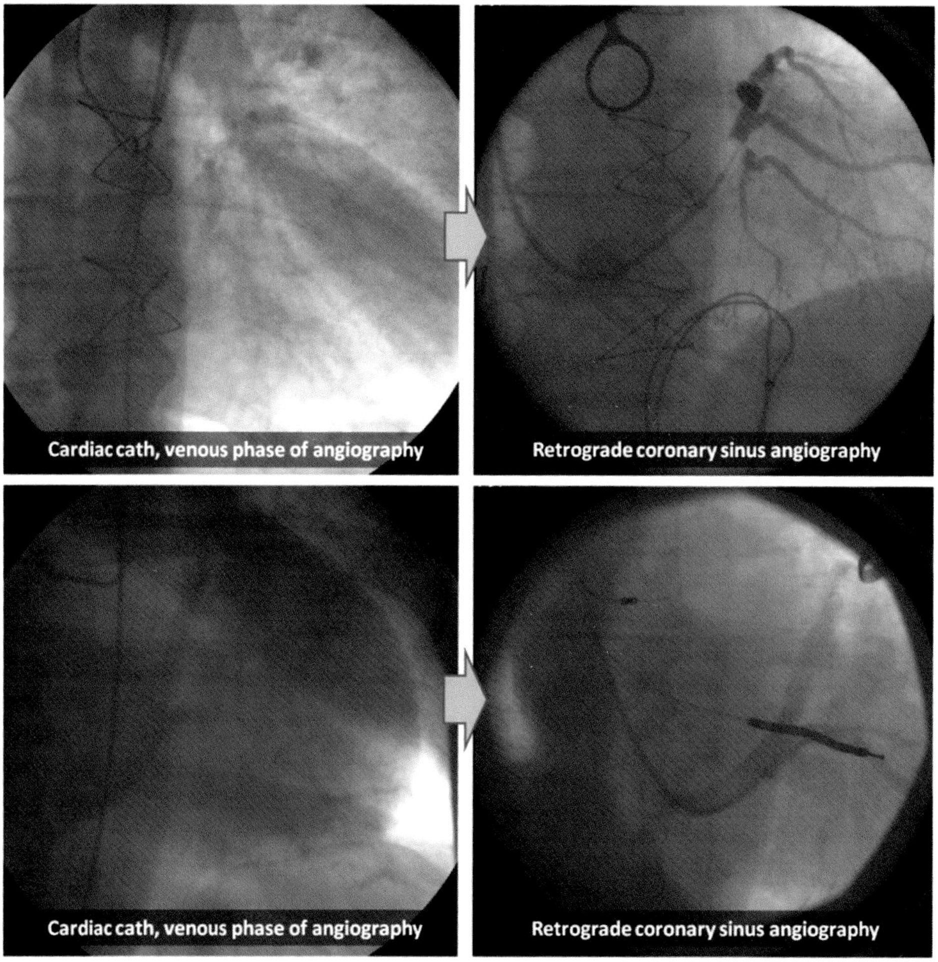

Figure 2. Evaluation of coronary vein anatomy during cardiac catheterization. The venous phase after contrast injection into the left coronary artery shows the coronary sinus and its major branches. Although the smaller branches are not visualized, the images are helpful to localize the CS ostium, the angle of the CS and origin of its major branches. The images correlate with those obtained during retrograde CS angiography.

Cardiac CT angiography provides detailed assessment of coronary arterial and venous anatomy, but requires x-ray radiation and contrast. Pre-implantation evaluation of the coronary venous anatomy can facilitate CRT, leading to decreased procedure time (Girsky,

2010 and Doganay, 2011). Area of latest mechanical activation may be correlated with echocardiographic images and veins in this region should be targeted for LV lead implantation – this approach correlates with improved acute response to CRT, however, no long term data available yet (Van de Veire, 2008). The phrenic nerve may also be visualized to identify high risk regions for inadvertent diaphragmatic stimulation (Matsumoto, 2007). Fusion of CT and fluoroscopic images may be of even greater benefit (Auricchio, 2009). Contrast allergy and advanced renal disease are contraindications for cardiac CT.

Cardiac MRI can also be used to assess coronary veins. These images may be overlayed with other MRI data, such as scar distribution or area of latest activation (Duckett, 2011a; White, 2010 and Kronborg, 2012). Imaging of scar burden improves prediction of response to CRT: in ischemic cardiomyopathy, less than 15% of total myocardium infarcted and absence of significant posterolateral scar is associated with better response (Bilchick, 2008 and Chalil, 2007). Real time MRI-guided intubation of the coronary sinus is being investigated (Neizel, 2010). Cardiac MRI requires gadolinium-based contrast and is contraindicated in patients with advanced renal dysfunction. Previously implanted non-MRI compatible hardware may also limit its utilization. The scanning times are longer and image acquisition requires some patient cooperation, which may be poorly tolerated in severe heart failure.

Although these advanced imaging modalities have improved both implantation success rate and responder rate in small studies, currently it is not known whether routine application in all patients undergoing CRT would be cost-efficient. In patients undergoing CRT, review of all existing relevant imaging data is recommended for implant strategy planning. Advanced modalities should be reserved for cases where difficult anatomy is anticipated or if the patient had an unsuccessful implantation attempt. If cardiac CT and MRI will be shown to predict and facilitate CRT in a cost-efficient manner, these modalities may potentially be implemented on a more routine basis in the future.

5. Perioperative period

The patient should be on a stable heart failure medication regimen for at least 3 months before CRT implantation. Vasopressor-dependent or significantly fluid overloaded/congested patients are not good candidates for the procedure. Following implantation, careful monitoring is required as occasionally significant diuresis is observed with initiation of CRT, leading to electrolyte imbalances. The dose of heart failure medications should be titrated as tolerated after recovery from the implantation procedure. Bradycardia may not be a limiting factor after CRT implantation when considering utilization of higher dose of beta-blockers. Hypotensive side effects of ACE inhibitors and other vasodilators may be less pronounced, however, individual responses vary significantly. The dose of diuretics should be decreased if significant improvement in volume status is observed with CRT, to avoid prerenal azotemia and hypotension.

Almost all patients undergoing CRT implantation are on antiplatelet or anticoagulation therapy, which increases bleeding risks. Compared to untreated patients, the likelihood of bleeding complications is doubled in patients on aspirin and quadrupled with dual antiplatelet therapy (1.6%, 3.9% and 7.2%, respectively) (Jamula, 2008). Antiplatelet medications for primary prevention can be safely discontinued for a period of 5–7 days prior to the implantation. Dual antiplatelet therapy following PCI should not be discontinued in patients high risk for subacute stent thrombosis (such as early after coronary stent implantation, with timing dependent on stent type) (Tompkins, 2011). Bridging anticoagulation with heparin is associated with higher bleeding risk (up to 20%), where short-term discontinuation of anticoagulation is not an option – in these cases, continuation of coumadin is recommended (Tompkins, 2010). Continuation of coumadin has a risk of postoperative pocket bleeding of 1.9–6.6% (Wiegand, 2004).

After decades of debate, now there is evidence that perioperative antibiotic prophylaxis decreases risk of infectious complications. Although these complications are rare (generally <1%), their consequences are devastating, leading to significant morbidity, mortality and costs (Klug, 2007 and Da Costa, 1998). Iv. cephazolin administered immediately before the procedure reduced the risk of infection from 3.28% to 0.63% in a large randomized trial (de Oliveira, 2009). Although some implant centers continue antibiotic utilization after the implantation, there is no proven benefit for this approach. Data regarding antibiotic prophylaxis for non-transvenous CRT implantation is scarce – generally, cardiothoracic surgical guidelines should apply as the optimal duration and selection of antibiotics may be affected by the given surgical approach (Mertz, 2011; Edwards, 2006 and Engelman, 2006).

Most interventional techniques may be safely utilized in the pacemaker laboratory. It is preferable that the physician attempting a complex implantation or a device upgrade is well trained and current in the appropriate interventional and surgical techniques, or a physician with this training is immediately available. In case lead extraction is planned, a hybrid operating room or prompt access to surgical backup is mandatory. The incidence of unsuccessful implantations is declining, which is partly due to the advances in lead technology and implanting tools, however, interventional cardiology techniques have also been increasingly utilized with excellent efficacy and safety records. Minimally invasive surgical options are rapidly evolving and should be considered in case transvenous implantation is not feasible.

Most common perioperative complications are failure to implant the LV lead, pocket hematoma, hemothorax or pneumothorax, CS dissection, cardiac perforation or tamponade, extracardiac stimulation, complete heart block, LV lead dislodgement, exacerbation of HF, acute renal failure, and death. Overall perioperative complication rates range from 4% in more recent trials to 28% in earlier CRT trials (Leon, 2005 and Linde, 2008).

6. Targeting LV lead placement

There is considerable variability in the ventricular activation pattern and distribution of mechanical dyssynchrony even in the LBBB population, and consequently inter-individual variability in the most optimal pacing site (Auricchio, 2004 and Derval, 2010). In addition, a significant number of patients don't even have typical LBBB. Lead placement via endocardial and surgical epicardial approach may have more potential for individualized targeted pacing. Targeting methods include those assessing electrical, mechanical and anatomic parameters, but there is no consensus yet regarding the best method to improve long term outcomes (Ansalone, 2002; Merchant, 2010; Gold, 2011 and Ypenburg, 2008).

Apically positioned LV lead location is associated with a worse clinical outcome in the REVERSE and MADIT-CRT trials (Thebault, 2012 and Singh, 2011). The COMPANION and MADIT-CRT studies showed a comparable response between lateral, anterior or posterior LV lead locations, while patients in REVERSE benefited from a lateral lead location (Saxon, 2009). Imaging may help to select specific sites for left ventricular pacing based on anticipated optimization of electromechanical effects (Toumoux, 2010). Echocardiography (tissue Doppler or tissue synchronization imaging) may identify LV sites with marked mechanical delay (Cannesson, 2006 and Murphy, 2006). Pacing these sites may result in greater ventricular remodeling and improved clinical outcomes. Currently there is not enough data supporting the role of acute hemodynamic measurements during implantation to target lead implantation (Duckett, 2011b).

Multisite ventricular stimulation (more than one LV lead) may provide even greater benefits with more homogenous ventricular activation. More clinical data will be needed to evaluate whether it is superior to biventricular stimulation.

7. Transvenous CRT implantation and reinterventions

The standard approach to CRT is to implant three endovascular leads for cardiac stimulation: endocardial RV and RA leads, and an epicardial LV lead into a coronary vein through the CS. Transvenous implantation should be the preferred way for CRT as most evidence is with this approach. The standard transvenous approach has significant drawbacks as it is dependent on the highly variable venous anatomy. Main reasons of failed LV lead implantations are inability to cannulate the CS due to RA dilatation or prominent Thebesian valve, diminutive CS, severe kinking of the vein or venous valve in the CS. Even with successful lead placement, unstable position, high pacing threshold or phrenic nerve stimulation may hinder effective delivery of LV pacing. Implantation success rate is above 90% in experienced centers, most failures are due to unsuccessful placement of the LV lead. In case of an unsuccessful procedure, repeat transvenous procedure with a more experienced operator or with interventional backup is recommended, if the venous anatomy seems to be suitable for implantation. In unsuitable cases, alternative approaches (surgical epicardial, transseptal endocardial) should be considered.

The EHRA and HRS has recently published guidelines for recommended approach for transvenous CRT implantation (Daubert, 2012). Implantation should be performed from the left subclavian vein system, unless preexisting pathology (venous occlusion, infection) makes this approach unfeasible. The right ventricular lead should be placed first as it is less likely to dislodge during manipulation of other leads and provides information about the position of the tricuspid valve and right atrial size.

New guidelines emphasize the role of cardiac resynchronization therapy in subgroups of patients who already have conventional pacemakers, to avoid pacing-induced dyssynchrony and remodeling. Upgrading an existing device may pose difficulties due to the necessity to operate in a previously scarred area and the presence of previously implanted leads in the venous system. The perioperative risks in these patients are significantly higher: the 6-month major complication rate was 18.7% in the REPLACE registry in patients undergoing upgrade to a CRT device with addition of a new endocardial LV lead to the existing leads (Poole, 2010). The risk of subclavian vein thrombosis is related to the number of leads implanted, among recipients of CRT devices severe obstruction or occlusion can be observed in 30% (Bulur, 2010). Subclavian venography with injection through the upper extremity veins is a simple and effective technique to evaluate venous anatomy prior to an upgrade or lead revision. Venoplasty may be performed if ipsilateral implantation is favored (Worley, 2011).

Extraction of non-used leads during an upgrade or revision has to be considered as the risk of long-term complications from abandoned leads is not negligible and correlates with the number of leads implanted and the number of prior procedures performed (Diemberger, 2011). Implantation via the jugular or contralateral subclavian vein, with subcutaneous tunneling is required if the anatomy does not permit ipsilateral addition of a new lead. Although primary transvenous device implantations are routinely performed using conscious sedation without much patient discomfort, deep sedation or general anesthesia may be required for lead tunneling (Fox, 2007). In case lead extraction has to be performed prior to the upgrade, general anesthesia, invasive monitoring and availability of immediate surgical backup is recommended (Kratz, 2010).

For CS cannulation, a wide array of sheaths are available. The ostium may be probed with a standard angiographic soft-tip wire, an angiographic catheter (such as Amplatz) may be inserted into the sheath to adjust its distal curve. Alternatively, a steerable CS EP catheter may also be used for mapping, individual practices vary significantly. Mapping with stiff catheters should be performed very cautiously as after overcoming any resistance from the Thebesian valve, the catheter may advance to the CS at an oblique angle, dissecting it, rendering continuation of the implantation procedure extremely difficult. This is most commonly encountered during insertion or advancement of the occlusion balloon catheter, as it has a relatively stiff distal portion. Transesophageal echocardiography may facilitate CS cannulation when traditional methods have proven ineffective (Bashir, 2003). In difficult cases intracardiac echocardiography may be more tolerable in patients under conscious sedation (Shalaby, 2005).

Cannulation of the CS is followed by coronary sinus angiography using an occluder balloon. Fluoroscopic acquisition should allow time to image late filling terminal branches, due to collateral flow. Some centers perform a single venography image, however, two orthogonal views (RAO and LAO) are preferred for better visualization of 3 dimensional anatomy. A minority of centers perform rotational venography, which may provide more detailed information (Blendea, 2007). The location and takeoff of the ostium may vary considerably, can be distorted by right atrial enlargement or prior surgery. Distally in the CS, the valve of

Vieussens (typically 3-5 cm from the ostium) may hinder cannulation of the distal vessel (Ho, 2004).

LV pacing leads may be implanted over a guidewire or directly. The guidewire may help to achieve more distal position by providing a rail when advancing the lead in a tortuous vein. Care should be taken to place the preformed fixation mechanism (curves, spiral or tags) with adequate distal penetration, to have a large area of contact with the vein wall (Hansky, 2002). Most current leads are at least bipolar with size and flexibility similar to previous unipolar leads. The advantage of multiple electrodes is the possibility of electrical "repositioning" when high pacing threshold or phrenic nerve stimulation is encountered (Gurevitz, 2005 and Forleo, 2011). (Figure 3)

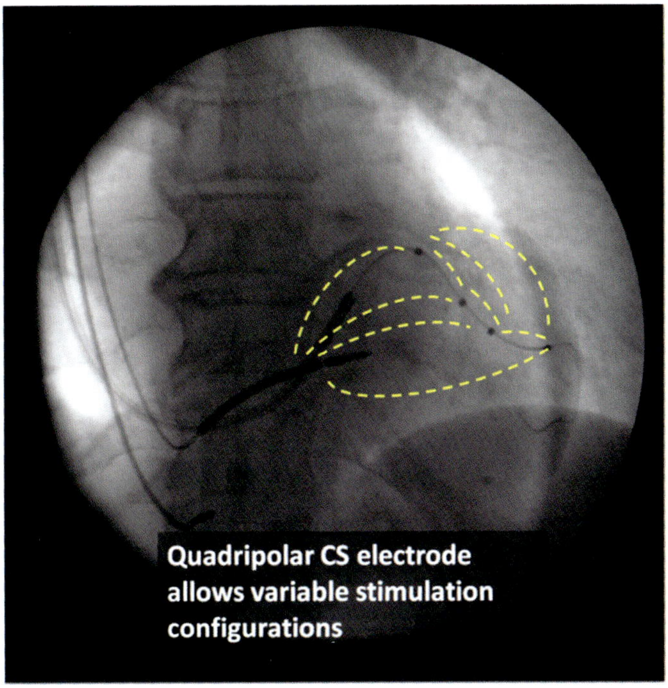

Figure 3. A quadripolar CS lead allows multiple pacing configurations, providing options to avoid phrenic nerve stimulation or sites with high threshold. It also enables a more stable distal lead position, while still allowing pacing on the proximal electrodes if desired.

If the vein is tortuous, a stiffer wire or buddy wire may be used with caution, as the wall thickness and tear resistance of coronary veins is much less compared to coronary arteries. In case severe tortuosity or kinking of the vein does not allow adequate force transition to advance the lead, use of telescopic guides may be considered (Russo, 2009). Inflated venogram (occluder) and coronary balloons can also be used as anchors to facilitate CS cannulation and left ventricular lead placement and help to recover lost CS and target vein access (Worley, 2009).

In case the target vein is stenotic, balloon angioplasty may be attempted. Although the pathophysiological basis for coronary artery stenoses and coronary sinus/vein abnormalities are different, in most cases these obstacles can be overcome with the use of conventional interventional cardiology techniques. The required instrumentation is the same as for coronary artery angioplasties. In the majority of cases with a focal stenosis or valve, balloon angioplasty is a safe method to facilitate passage of the lead. In selected cases coronary atherectomy or stent implantation may be required (Soga, 2007). Angioplasty may also be used as a rescue when dissection of the coronary sinus or the target vein is observed during implantation, which would otherwise prohibit further attempts for lead placement (Bosa, 2008 and Gutleben, 2008). In case of unfavorable coronary vein anatomy in the target area, dilatation and use of collateral veins may be considered (Abben, 2010). Complications from venoplasty are rare, however, venous rupture has been reported (Worley, 2008). With access to these techniques, implantation success rate may be as high as 99%: a retrospective single center analysis showed that 3.5% of patients required venoplasty for LV implantation (of these, 77% coronary vein, 13% subclavian vein, 10% valvular structures within the CS or a Marshall vein). The required inflation pressures for ring-like structures were high (16 ±3 atm), complications were rare. Mostly short balloons with 3 mm diameter were used (Luedorff, 2008). The presence of a persistent left superior vena cava may prohibit successful CRT implantation due to severely dilated CS and distorted anatomy, however, successful use of angioplasty in this case was reported (Cagin, 2010).

High pacing threshold or phrenic nerve stimulation may require repositioning of the lead from a stable to a less optimal position, where its fixation mechanism may not be as effective. In these cases, a coronary stent implanted near the distal end of the lead may stabilize the new position. A large single center study of 312 patients treated with stent implantation showed that the method was safe and effective in long term to prevent lead dislocation. 95% of patients had stenting due to intraoperative lead instability or phrenic nerve stimulation, while 5% required it due to previous lead disclocation. The bare metal stents were implanted 5-35 mm proximal to the most proximal electrode (unipolar and bipolar LV leads). There was no evidence of mechanical damage to the lead or CS perforation. During the follow-up of average 28.4 months, a significant increase in the left ventricular pacing threshold was found in four cases and reoperation was necessary in two patients (0.6%). Phrenic nerve stimulation was observed in 18 instances, and closed repositioning with an ablation catheter was performed in seven cases. In three cases the leads were extracted without complication after 3-49 months (infection, heart transplant) (Geller, 2011). (Figure 4)

Coronary sinus dissection is a rare complication of LV lead placement. It may be recognized as inability to pass instruments though a previously accessible area, and pooling of contrast after angiography. Although complete perforation is even less common and the pressure in the CS is low, cardiac tamponade may occasionally develop. If the dissection is small, it may be possible to finish the implantation, although balloon angioplasty or stenting of the dissected segment may be necessary. In these cases, patients need to be monitored after the implantation, however, the exact duration that is required before a safe discharge is unknown (Figure 5).

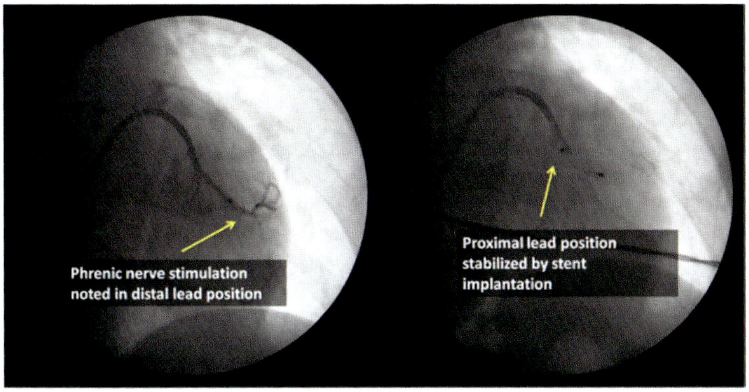

Figure 4. Phrenic nerve stimulation was encountered in the distal lateral vein. In a more proximal position, the pacing threshold was acceptable with no diaphragmatic stimulation, however, the lead position was unstable. A bare metal coronary stent was implanted just proximal to the proximal electrode, after which the lead position stabilized.

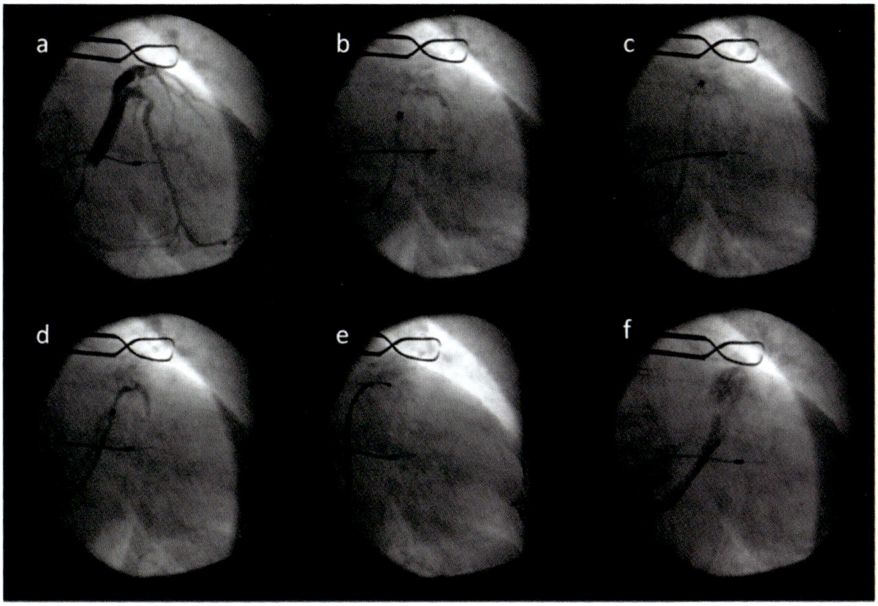

Figure 5. Complicated CS anatomy may prohibit transvenous lead implantation even with extensive use of interventional techniques. The targeted lateral vein has a narrowed proximal segment with a kink, which did not allow lead advancement (a). After passing a coronary guidewire, a bare metal stent was deposited into this region (b). Although the guidewire easily passed through this area, lead advancement was still not feasible, the stent is clearly visible (c). Selective venography shows dissection proximal to the stent (d). Even after multiple attempts with balloon angioplasty in this area, lead advancement was still not possible (e). After multiple attempts with a selective guide and buddy wire, repeat venography shows dissection of CS with distal occlusion and staining, at this point the procedure was aborted (f). No significant pericardial effusion or further sequelae were noted.

Epicardial left ventricular stimulation poses a unique challenge as the electrode position has to be stable to provide effective cardiac resynchronization with low energy output, while avoiding phrenic nerve stimulation. The coronary veins lack trabeculation and the thin wall prohibits the use of conventional screw-in active fixation leads. The majority of coronary sinus leads are passive fixation, which try to maintain stability with pre-shaped tips. Recently, built-in active lead fixation mechanisms became available. Up to 7% of transvenously placed LV leads may require revision (Borleffs, 2008) over long-term follow up (2 years). One third of the interventions are required more than 6 months after the implantation. A dislodged coronary sinus lead can be the source of multiple complications, such as inadvertent stimulation of extracardiac structures, arrhythmia or perforation, and loss of effective cardiac resynchronization. Repositioning most of the time requires access to the lead via a device pocket revision. As open revision carries a higher risk of system infection, minimally invasive procedures should be considered when appropriate. In some cases, the dislocation may be resolved by catheter-based techniques. In each case, an attempt has to be made to provide a more stable final lead position. A transfemoral approach was effective for the retraction of the LV lead from distal dislocation in a single center case series, where distal dislocation of the electrode lead to intolerable phrenic nerve stimulation (Szilagyi, 2008). The CS was cannulated with an Amplatz catheter, then a coronary stent was introduced over a guidewire besides the lead into the side branch in 7 patients or in 2 patients, into the CS. A steerable ablation catheter was looped around the LV lead in the atrium with bent tip and was drawn backwards together. The stent was then inflated to stabilize the lead tip in a new position. During follow-up of median 7.7 months, stable pacing thresholds and impedances were measured; transient and avoidable phrenic nerve stimulation was present in only one patient. There were no procedural complications or infections.

Stabilizing the lead position with retained stylets is not recommended due to high risk of late lead failure (Nagele, 2007). With active fixation of the CS leads, lead extraction may be an issue if the device has to be explanted. In the above mentioned case series, the few leads that had to be explanted and were previously stabilized with stent implantation, came out with manual traction most of the time, however, more data will be needed to assess if active anchoring of LV leads into the coronary veins poses any long-term risk.

8. Transseptal endocardial left ventricular pacing

Transseptal approach through the interatrial septum has been used for multiple interventional and electrophysiological procedures for decades. It is a relatively safe procedure in experienced hands, however, the facility should be prepared to address potential complications (mainly pericardiocentesis and emergent periocardiotomy). Using the transseptal approach, a conventional endocardial PM lead may be implanted into the LV cavity for endocardial stimulation. The thromboembolic risks are not negligible and these patient require long term anticoagulation. Mitral valve damage and endocarditis are rare, but serious compliations.

The transseptal implantation begins with a standard transseptal puncture via the femoral vein (van Gelder, 2007). After the successful puncture, full anticoagulation with iv. heparin is initiated. A 0.035-inch guidewire is inserted into one of the pulmonary veins and then the dilator and the sheath is removed. The puncture site is dilated with a 6-8 mm balloon. A steerable EP catheter is advanced from the subclavian area towards the interatrial septum, then into the left ventricle after deflating the balloon. A sheath is then advanced into the LA over the EP catheter. The endocardial surface of the LV may be mapped with the EP catheter to localize a site most suitable for lead implantation, then a standard endocardial bipolar pacemaker lead is implanted. Using a modified technique, electroanatomical mapping may be used to precisely identify the area of latest activation in the LV (Kutyifa, 2012).

The main disadvantage of this technique is the unknown long term thromboembolic risk, which may be similar to a mechanical valve, with INR goals in the higher range (3-4). Over an average of 85 month follow up of 6 patients in a case series, one patient had LV lead dislodgment at 3 months requiring reintervention. One patient had a transient ischemic attack, when anticoagulation was accidentally interrupted (Pasquie, 2007). The need to start full dose anticoagulation immediately after the implantation increases the risk of periprocedural bleeding complications.

This technique is a feasible and safe second option with a benefit of endocardial pacing site and implantation procedure with no more burden to the patient than conventional transvenous CRT implantation. Main disadvantage is the need for long term anticoagulation. Patients who are ineligible for surgical epicardial implantation and have no contraindications for lifelong oral anticoagulation can be selected for this approach. Biventricular pacing with endocardial stimulation may provide more homogenous intraventricular resynchronization than with epicardial stimulation, and is associated with better LV filling and systolic performance (Garrigue, 2001).

9. Surgical epicardial LV lead placement

In early cases of CRT, the LV lead was surgically placed via thoracotomy. This approach was associated with considerable morbidity, requiring general anesthesia and longer recovery time. Long term electrical stability of surgically placed electrodes is inferior when compared to transvenous leads (Lau, 2009). Major advantage of the surgical implantation is that it is not constrained by the venous anatomy and the latest contracting segment may be visually identified. Phrenic nerve stimulation may also be more easily avoided and there is no need for fluoroscopy. As transvenous implantation has a high success rate with excellent long-term stability, surgical implantation should not be considered are first line therapy. The risk of failed transvenous implant is higher in patients with prior cardiac surgeries (however, this also increases the risk of consecutive sternotomy/thoracotomy). In patients eligible for CRT, undergoing cardiothoracic surgical procedure, implantation of epicardial LV lead may be considered, which may be tunneled to the planned PM/ICD generator site. Surgical implantation may also be preferred in patients with complex congential heart disease, where the venous anatomy may interfere with the transvenous approach.

Usually, there is no need for full left thoracotomy for epicardial LV lead implantation as minimal thoracotomy provides adequate window for the procedure. The surgery is performed using single-lung ventilation on a beating heart. Transeosophageal echocardiography (TEE) control is needed throughout the procedure. A 3 to 5 cm incision is made over the 4th or 5th intercostal space anterior to the midaxillary line. The lung is pushed back and the pericardium is opened anterior to the phrenic nerve. The left ventricle is mapped for optimal pacing site and an epicardial lead placement device is used to attach the electrode (unipolar or bipolar) (Mair, 2005). The leads are tunneled to the PM/ICD generator site, usually in the left infraclavicular region. Short-term chest drainage is required postoperatively. A recent investigation described this technique as a safe and acceptable option, with benefits comparable to transvenous CRT: in 33 patients, functional and echocardiographic parameters showed similar improvement, however, with a delayed onset of peak VO2 improvement (Patwala, 2009).

Instead of minimal thoracotomy, video assisted thoracoscopy may be used for lead placement. It uses two incisions for the ports in the 4th or 5th intercostal space along the anterior and midaxillary line. General anaesthesia and single lung ventilation enables the deflation of the left lung. The camera and the manipulating instruments are inserted through the ports, the pericardium is opened laterally to the phrenic nerve under visual control, then the epicardial lead is screwed into the lateral wall of the LV. The lead is passed through the medial incision and then tunneled subcutaneously to the generator site. The procedure is well tolerated, it has minimal postoperative recovery and very good cosmetic results. In a series of 15 patients, who previously failed transvenous implantation, mean skin-to-skin operating time was 55±16 min, no conversion to thoracotomy was necessary. All patients were extubated in the operating room and remained in the intensive care unit for less than 24h. Chest tubes were removed after a mean of 1.6±0.5 days and the patients were discharged after a mean of 4±1.3 days. Intraoperative and postoperative pacing thresholds at 1 and 7 months were satisfactory in all cases and there was no lead dislocation. All but two patients had an improvement of their NYHA function class. There was neither surgical morbidity nor mortality (Gabor, 2005).

Endoscopic robotic surgery is rapidly evolving and has been investigated for CRT. This technique also needs general anesthesia, single lung intubation and TEE. The left and right arms for the DaVinci system are placed in the 5th and 9th intercostal space. The pericardium is opened posterior to the phrenic nerve and the region of the obtuse marginal is identified to find the latest activating area with a temporary pacing electrode, the procedure is similar to the endoscopic approach. The patient is extubated immediately after the procedure and there is no need for a chest tube. Patients are usually discharged on the first postoperative day. Follow-up results of 42 patients showed a procedure time on the plateau of the learning curve of 45±13 minutes, with a responder rate of 81% and 70% at 3 and 6 month follow up. Three patients experienced loss of LV capture at 1, 9, and 14 months (a second lead, which was simultaneously implanted with the first one and also tunneled to the generator site had to be activated in these patients) (Joshi, 2005). With growing experience and availability of surgical robotic system, this method may gain more widespread utilization.

10. Transapical endocardial lead implantation

This technique combines the minimally invasive surgical approach with the advantages of endocardial pacing. This may be the only option for patients with extensive epicardial adhesions prohibiting access to the pericardial space (Kassai, 2008). After induction of general anaesthesia and selective bronchial intubation, the LV apex is localized with transthoracic echocardiography, then a small left thoracotomy is performed. The apex of the left ventricle is punctured and an active fixation lead is inserted into the cavity, using Seldinger technique. The bleeding is controlled with purse-string sutures. The lead is guided into its final position with a guide, using fluoroscopy. As transapical endocardial lead implantation does not involve the mitral valve, the risk of mitral valve endocarditis is reduced. The lead is subcutaneously tunneled to the infraclavicular pocket to be connected to the generator. Long term anticoagulation is required, similar to patients with transseptal endocardial leads. Advantages of this technique are the accessibility of the endocardial segments without limitations of the CS anatomy and absence of phrenic nerve stimulation (Kassai, 2009).

11. Conclusion

Transvenous implantation of CRT systems is the preferred way as it poses the least risk for the patient, has excellent long term results and is supported by large amount of evidence from clinical trials. Familiarity with interventional angioplasty methods may facilitate the implant procedure. Although newer left ventricular leads have better maneuverability and improved fixation mechanisms, interventional techniques are useful adjuncts if difficult anatomy is encountered. In case of unsuitable anatomy of failed implantation, minimally invasive surgical procedures should be considered for LV lead placement.

Author details

Bela Merkely and Levente Molnar
Heart Center, Semmelweis University, Hungary

Attila Roka
Hospital of St. Raphael, New Haven, CT, USA

12. References

Abben, R.P., et al., V.Traversing and dilating venous collaterals: a useful adjunct in left ventricular electrode placement. J Invasive Cardiol, 2010. 22(6): p. E93-6.

Alonso, C., In the field of cardiac resynchronization therapy is left ventricular pacing via the coronary sinus a mature technique. Europace. 2009. 11(5): p. 544-5.

Ansalone, G., et al., Doppler myocardial imaging to evaluate the effectiveness of pacing sites in patients receiving biventricular pacing. J Am Coll Cardiol, 2002. 39(3): p. 489-99

Auricchio, A., et al., Characterization of left ventricular activation in patients with heart failure and left bundle-branch block. Circulation, 2004. 109(9): p. 1133-9.
Auricchio, A., et al., Accuracy and usefulness of fusion imaging between three-dimensional coronary sinus and coronary veins computed tomographic images with projection images obtained using fluoroscopy. Europace, 2009. 11(11): p. 1483-90.
Bashir, J.G., et al., Combined use of transesophageal ECHO and fluoroscopy for the placement of left ventricular pacing leads via the coronary sinus. Pacing Clin Electrophysiol, 2003. 26(10): p. 1951-4.
Bilchick, K.C., et al., Cardiac magnetic resonance assessment of dyssynchrony and myocardial scar predicts function class improvement following cardiac resynchronization therapy. JACC Cardiovasc Imaging, 2008. 1(5): p. 561-8.
Bleeker, G.B., et al., Effect of postero-lateral scar tissue on clinical and echocardiographic improvement following cardiac resynchronization therapy. Circulation, 2006. 113 p. 969-976.
Blendea, D., et al., Variability of coronary venous anatomy in patients undergoing cardiac resynchronization therapy: a high-speed rotational venography study. Heart Rhythm, 2007. 4(9): p. 1155-62.
Bosa, F., et al., Prolonged inflation of coronary angioplasty balloon as treatment for subocclusive dissection of the coronary sinus during implantation of a coronary sinus pacing lead. J Interv Card Electrophysiol, 2008. 23(2): p. 139-41.
Borleffs, C.J., et al., Requirement for coronary sinus lead interventions and effectiveness of endovascular replacement during long-term follow-up after implantation of a resynchronization device. Europace, 2008. 11(5): p. 607-11.
Bulur, S., et al., Incidence and predictors of subclavian vein obstruction following biventricular device implantation. J Interv Card Electrophysiol, 2010. 29(3): p. 199-202.
Burri, H., et al., Right ventricular systolic function and cardiac resynchronization therapy. Europace, 2010. 12(3): p. 389-94.
Cagin C., et al.,, Coronary venoplasty-assisted implantation of cardiac resynchronization device in a patient with persistent left superior vena cava. Heart Rhythm. 2010. 7(1): p.141-2.
Cannesson, M., et al., Velocity vector imaging to quantify ventricular dyssynchrony and predict response to cardiac resynchronization therapy. Am J Cardiol, 2006. 98(7): p. 949-53.
Chalil, S., et al., Effect of posterolateral left ventricular scar on mortality and morbidity following cardiac resynchronization therapy. Pacing Clin Electrophysiol, 2007. 30(10): p. 1201-9.
Da Costa, A., et al., Antibiotic prophylaxis for permanent pacemaker implantation: a meta-analysis. Circulation, 1998. 97(18): p. 1796-801.
Daubert, J.C., et al., 2012 EHRA/HRS Expert Consensus Statement on Cardiac Resynchronization Therapy Implant and Follow-up Considerations. Europace 2012, in press
de Oliveira, J.C., et al., Efficacy of antibiotic prophylaxis before the implantation of pacemakers and cardioverter-defibrillators: results of a large, prospective, randomized, double-blinded, placebo-controlled trial. Circ Arrhythm Electrophysiol, 2009. 2(1): p. 29-34.

Derval, N., et al., Optimizing hemodynamics in heart failure patients by systematic screening of left ventricular pacing sites: the lateral left ventricular wall and the coronary sinus are rarely the best sites. J Am Coll Cardiol, 2010. 55(6): p. 566-75.

Diemberger, I., et al., From lead management to implanted patient management: indications to lead extraction in pacemaker and cardioverter-defibrillator systems. Expert Rev Med Devices, 2011. 8(2): p. 235-55.

Doganay, S., et al., Usefulness of multidetector computed tomography coronary venous angiography examination before cardiac resynchronization therapy. Jpn J Radiol, 2011. 29(5): p. 342-7.

Duckett, S.G., et al., Cardiac MRI to investigate myocardial scar and coronary venous anatomy using a slow infusion of dimeglumine gadobenate in patients undergoing assessment for cardiac resynchronization therapy. J Magn Reson Imaging, 2011. 33(1): p. 87-95.

Duckett, S.G., et al., Invasive acute hemodynamic response to guide left ventricular lead implantation predicts chronic remodeling in patients undergoing cardiac resynchronization therapy. J Am Coll Cardiol, 2011. 58(11): p. 1128-36.

Edwards, F.H., et al., Society of Thoracic Surgeons. The Society of Thoracic Surgeons Practice Guideline Series: Antibiotic Prophylaxis in Cardiac Surgery, Part I: Duration. Ann Thorac Surg, 2006. 81(1): p. 397-404.

Engelman, R., et al.. Workforce on Evidence-Based Medicine, Society of Thoracic Surgeons. The Society of Thoracic Surgeons practice guideline series: Antibiotic prophylaxis in cardiac surgery, part II: Antibiotic choice. Ann Thorac Surg, 2007. 83(4): 1569-76.

Epstein, A.E., et al., ACC/AHA/HRS 2008 Guidelines for Device-Based Therapy of Cardiac Rhythm Abnormalities: a report of the American College of Cardiology/American Heart Association Task Force on Practice Guidelines (Writing Committee to Revise the ACC/AHA/NASPE 2002 Guideline Update for Implantation of Cardiac Pacemakers and Antiarrhythmia Devices) developed in collaboration with the American Association for Thoracic Surgery and Society of Thoracic Surgeons. J Am Coll Cardiol, 2008. 51(21): p. e1-62.

Forleo, G.B., et al., Left ventricular pacing with a new quadripolar transvenous lead for CRT: early results of a prospective comparison with conventional implant outcomes. Heart Rhythm, 2011. 8(1): p. 31-7.

Fox, D.J., et al., Safety and acceptability of implantation of internal cardioverter-defibrillators under local anesthetic and conscious sedation. Pacing Clin Electrophysiol, 2007. 30(8): p. 992-7.

Gabor, S., et al., A simplified technique for implantation of left ventricular epicardial leads for biventricular re-synchronization using video-assisted thoracoscopy (VATS). European Journal of Cardio-thoracic Surgery, 2005. 28(6), p. 797-800.

Garrigue, S., et al. Comparison of chronic biventricular pacing between epicardial and endocardial left ventricular stimulation using Doppler tissue imaging in patients with heart failure American Journal of Cardiology, 2001. 88(8), p. 858-862.

Geller L., et al., Long-term experience with coronary sinus side branch stenting to stabilize left ventricular electrode position. Heart Rhythm. 2011. 8(6): p. 845-50.

Girsky, M.J., et al., Prospective randomized trial of venous cardiac computed tomographic angiography for facilitation of cardiac resynchronization therapy. Pacing Clin Electrophysiol, 2010. 33(10): p. 1182-7. 49.

Gold, M.R., et al., The relationship between ventricular electrical delay and left ventricular remodelling with cardiac resynchronization therapy. Eur Heart J, 2011. 32(20): p. 2516-24.

Gurevitz, O., et al., Programmable multiple pacing configurations help to overcome high left ventricular pacing thresholds and avoid phrenic nerve stimulation. Pacing and clinical electrophysiology : PACE, 2005. 28(12): p. 1255-9.

Gutleben, K.J., et al., Rescue-stenting of an occluded lateral coronary sinus branch for recanalization after dissection during cardiac resynchronization device implantation. Europace, 2008. 10(12): p. 1442-4.

Hansky, B., et al., Left heart pacing--experience with several types of coronary vein leads. J Interv Card Electrophysiol, 2002. 6(1): p. 71-5.

Ho, S.Y., et al., A review of the coronary venous system: a road less travelled. Heart Rhythm, 2004. 1(1): p. 107-12.

Jamula, E., et al., Perioperative anticoagulation in patients having implantation of a cardiac pacemaker or defibrillator: a systematic review and practical management guide. J Thromb Haemost, 2008. 6(10): p. 1615-21.

Joshi, S., et al., Follow-up of robotically assisted left ventricular epicardial leads for cardiac resynchronization therapy. Journal of the American College of Cardiology. 2005. 46(12): p. 2358-2359.

Kassai, I., et al. New method for cardiac resynchronization therapy: transapical endocardial lead implantation for left ventrical free wall pacing. Europace, 2008. 10(7): p. 882-3.

Kassai, I., et al., A Novel Approach for Endocardial Resynchronization Therapy: Initial Experience with Transapical Implantation of the Left Ventricular Lead. Heart Surg Forum, 2009. 12(3): p. 137-40.

Khan, F.Z., et al., Left ventricular lead placement in cardiac resyncrnisation therapy: where and how? Europace, 2009. 11(5), p. 554-61.

Klug, D., et al., Risk factors related to infections of implanted pacemakers and cardioverter-defibrillators: results of a large prospective study. Circulation, 2007. 116(12): p. 1349-55. 93

Kovacs, B., et al., Anatomy of the coronary veins can be assessed with left coronary angiography (abstract). European Journal of Heart Failure, 2004. 5(Suppl 1): 820.

Kratz, J.M., et al., Pacemaker and internal cardioverter defibrillator lead extraction: a safe and effective surgical approach. Ann Thorac Surg, 2010. 90(5): p. 1411-7.

Kronborg, M.B., et al., Non-contrast magnetic resonance imaging for guiding left ventricular lead position in cardiac resynchronization therapy. J Interv Card Electrophysiol, 2012. 33(1): p. 27-35.

Kutyifa, V., et al., Usefulness of electroanatomical mapping during transseptal endocardial left ventricular lead implantation. Europace, 2012. 14(4): p. 599-604.

Lau, W.E. Achieving permanent left ventricular pacing – options and choice. Pacing Clinical Electrophysiology, 2009. 32(11), p. 1466-77.

Leon, A.R., et al., Safety of transvenous cardiac resynchronization system implantation in patients with chronic heart failure: combined results of over 2,000 patients from a multicenter study program. J Am Coll Cardiol, 2005. 46(12): p. 2348-56.

Linde, C., et al., Randomized trial of cardiac resynchronization in mildly symptomatic heart failure patients and in asymptomatic patients with left ventricular dysfunction and previous heart failure symptoms. J Am Coll Cardiol, 2008. 52(23): p. 1834-43.

Luedorff, G., et al. Different venous angioplasty manoeuvres for successful implantation of CRT devices. Clin Res Cardiol, 2009. 98(3): p. 159-64.

Mair, H., et al. Surgical epicardial left ventricular lead versus coronary sinus lead placement in biventricular pacing. European Journal of Cardiothoracic Surgery, 2005. 27(2), p. 235-42.

McMurray, J.J.V., et al. ESC Guidelines for the diagnosis and treatment of acute and chronic heart failure 2012. Eur Heart J, 2012. doi:10.1093/eurheartj/ehs104 (in press)

Merchant, F.M., et al., Interlead distance and left ventricular lead electrical delay predict reverse remodeling during cardiac resynchronization therapy. Pacing Clin Electrophysiol, 2010. 33(5): p. 575-82.

Mertz, D., et al. Does duration of perioperative antibiotic prophylaxis matter in cardiac surgery? A systematic review and meta-analysis. Ann Surg, 2011. 254(1): p. 48-54.

Matsumoto, Y., et al., Detection of phrenic nerves and their relation to cardiac anatomy using 64-slice multidetector computed tomography. Am J Cardiol, 2007. 100(1): p. 133-7.

Mullens, W., et al., Insights from a cardiac resynchronization optimization clinic as part of a heart failure disease management program. J Am Coll Cardiol, 2009. 53(9): p. 765-73. 42. Knappe, D., et al., Dyssynchrony, contractile function, and response to cardiac resynchronization therapy. Circ Heart Fail, 2011. 4(4): p. 433-40.

Murphy, R.T., et al., Tissue synchronization imaging and optimal left ventricular pacing site in cardiac resynchronization therapy. Am J Cardiol, 2006. 97(11): p. 1615-21.

Nagele, H., et al., Coronary sinus lead fragmentation 2 years after implantation with a retained guidewire. Pacing Clin Electrophysiol, 2007. 30(3): p. 438-9.

Neizel, M., et al., Magnetic resonance imaging of the cardiac venous system and magnetic resonance-guided intubation of the coronary sinus in swine: a feasibility study. Invest Radiol, 2010. 45(8): p. 502-6.

Pasquie, J.L., et al. Long-Term Follow-Up of Biventricular Pacing Using a Totally Endocardial Approach in Patients with End-Stage Cardiac Failure. Pacing Clinical Electrophysiology, 2007. 30(1), p. S31-33.

Patwala, A., et al. (2009) A prospective longitudinal evaluation of the benefits of epicardial lead placement for cardiac resynchronization therapy. *Europace, 2009.* 11(10): p. 1323-9.

Poole, J.E., et al., Complication rates associated with pacemaker or implantable cardioverter-defibrillator generator replacements and upgrade procedures: results from the REPLACE registry. Circulation, 2010. 122(16): p. 1553-61.

Russo, V., et al. Superselective cannulation of coronary sinus branch with telescopic system during left ventricular lead placement. Acta Biomed, 2009. 80(2):p. 153-5.

Saxon, L.A., et al., Influence of left ventricular lead location on outcomes in the COMPANION study. J Cardiovasc Electrophysiol, 2009. 20(7): p. 764-8.

Shalaby, A.A., Utilization of intracardiac echocardiography to access the coronary sinus for left ventricular lead placement. Pacing Clin Electrophysiol, 2005. 28(6): p. 493-7.

Singh, J.P., et al., Left ventricular lead position and clinical outcome in the multicenter automatic defibrillator implantation trial-cardiac resynchronization therapy (MADIT-CRT) trial. Circulation, 2011. 123(11): p. 1159-66.

Soga, Y., et al., Efficacy of coronary venoplasty for left ventricular lead implantation. Circ J, 2007. 71(9): p. 1442-5.

Szilagyi, S., et al. Minimal invasive coronary sinus lead reposition technique for the treatment of phrenic nerve stimulation. Europace, 2008. 10(10): p. 1157-60.

Thebault, C., et al., Sites of left and right ventricular lead implantation and response to cardiac resynchronization therapy observations from the REVERSE trial. Eur Heart J, 2012, in press.

Theuns, D.A., et al. The prognosis of implantable defibrillator patients treated with cardiac resynchronization therapy: comorbidity burden as predictor of mortality. Europace, 2011. 13(1): p. 62-9.

Tompkins, C., et al., Dual antiplatelet therapy and heparin "bridging" significantly increase the risk of bleeding complications after pacemaker or implantable cardioverter-defibrillator device implantation. J Am Coll Cardiol, 2010. 55(21): p. 2376-82.

Tompkins, C., et al. Optimal strategies for the management of antiplatelet and anticoagulation medications prior to cardiac device implantation. Cardiol J, 2011. 18(1): p. 103-9.

Tournoux, F., et al., Integrating functional and anatomical information to guide cardiac resynchronization therapy. Eur J Heart Fail, 2010. 12(1): p. 52-7.

Van de Veire, N.R., et al., Noninvasive imaging of cardiac venous anatomy with 64-slice multi-slice computed tomography and noninvasive assessment of left ventricular dyssynchrony by 3-dimensional tissue synchronization imaging in patients with heart failure scheduled for cardiac resynchronization therapy. Am J Cardiol, 2008. 101(7): p. 1023-9.

Van Gelder, B.M., et al. Transseptal endocardial left ventricular pacing: An alternative technique for coronary sinus lead placement in cardiac resynchronization therapy. Heart Rhythm, 2007. 4(4), p. 454–60.

White, J.A., et al., Fused whole-heart coronary and myocardial scar imaging using 3-T CMR. Implications for planning of cardiac resynchronization therapy and coronary revascularization. JACC Cardiovasc Imaging, 2010. 3(9): p. 921-30.

Wiegand, U.K., et al., Pocket hematoma after pacemaker or implantable cardioverter defibrillator surgery: influence of patient morbidity, operation strategy, and perioperative antiplatelet/anticoagulation therapy. Chest, 2004. 126(4): p. 1177-86.

Worley, S.J., Implant venoplasty: dilation of subclavian and coronary veins to facilitate device implantation: indications, frequency, methods, and complications. J Cardiovasc Electrophysiol, 2008. 19(9): p. 1004-7.

Worley, S.J. How to use balloons as anchors to facilitate cannulation of the coronary sinus left ventricular lead placement and to regain lost coronary sinus or target vein access. Heart Rhythm, 2009. 6(8): p. 1242-6.

Worley, S.J., et al., Subclavian venoplasty by the implanting physicians in 373 patients over 11 years. Heart Rhythm, 2011. 8(4): p. 526-33.

Ypenburg, C., et al., Optimal left ventricular lead position predicts reverse remodeling and survival after cardiac resynchronization therapy. J Am Coll Cardiol, 2008. 52(17): p. 1402-9.

Section 2

Follow Up and Optimization of Device Function

Chapter 3

Electrocardiographic Troubleshooting of Implanted Cardiac Electronic Devices

Attila Roka

Additional information is available at the end of the chapter

http://dx.doi.org/10.5772/50983

1. Introduction

1.1. Evaluation of CIED function

Pacemakers, ICDs and cardiac resynchronization devices are implanted and followed mostly by cardiac electrophysiologists. Detailed diagnostic data (pacing statistics, lead function, arrhythmia episode intracardiac electrograms etc.) are available using manufacturer-specific programmer devices or remote follow-up (Figure 1). However, patients may present with suspected cardiac or arrhythmia-related symptoms when these measures are not immediately available. Using conventional diagnostic methods basic device function can be evaluated and correlation with the clinical presentation may be assessed (McPherson, 2004). In certain cases, such as with transient events, these may be the only diagnostic clues available as current CIEDs do not have full Holter capability – only episodes of significance, as determined by the device, are stored.

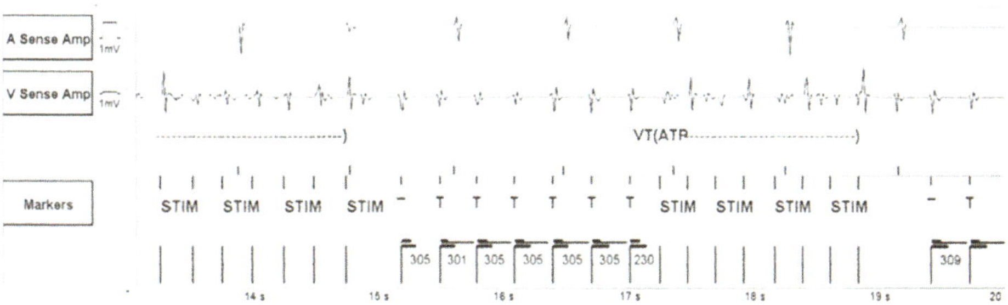

Figure 1. Device interrogation provides detailed information about intracardiac signals, their interpretation and device response. The tracing depicts an episode of ventricular tachycardia, where the implanted cardioverter-defibrillator attempted burst antitachycardia stimulation.

Basic evaluation of CIED function requires a 12-lead ECG and review of past medical records to identify device type and settings. If prior records are not available, a simple chest X-ray may provide important clues (pacemaker, ICD, or CRT; lead locations) (Jacob, 2011). In case intermittent or transient malfunction is detected and device interrogation does not provide clear answer, Holter monitoring or an event recorder may be required. If a programmer is available, diagnostic tests should be performed according to the guidelines (Wilkoff, 2008). Patient symptoms, if any, should be assessed, whether they can be signs of a possible device malfunction.

2. Electrocardiographic evaluation of device function

A 12-lead ECG may raise the suspicion of device malfunction. Careful evaluation of patient-related factors is required as these interact with device function (Table 1). Occasionally, very advanced forms of electrophysiological abnormalities may be identified as the devices generally do not prevent natural progression of underlying pathophysiology. In case an arrhythmia or device malfunction is suspected on a telemetry recording, a full 12-lead ECG is recommended to avoid misinterpretation (Figures 2-6). Artifacts may severely impact interpretation and tracings with good technical quality should be obtained (Figures 7-10). Atrial rhythm and characteristics of atrioventricular/ventriculoatrial conduction should also be assessed (Figures 11-17).

ECG feature	Importance – diagnostic clues and possible interaction with devices
Atrial rhythm	
Bradycardia	Should be paced unless there is oversensing or no atrial lead present
Premature beats	Blocked PACs should elicit different response than sinoatrial block if atrial sensing is present
Atrial flutter	May be tracked with high ventricular rate
Atrial fibrillation	May be undersensed, leading to ineffective atrial pacing
Atrioventricular conduction	
Variable AV conduction interval	May lead to fusion and pseudofusion beats
Complete heart block	May be intermittent or unidirectional
Retrograde conduction	May lead to pacemaker-tachycardia or pacemaker syndrome
Ventricles	
Native QRS morphology	Assess biventricular capture during cardiac resynchronization If atrial pacing only, may be used to identify ischemia, etc.
Premature beats	May trigger safety or sense response pacing or activate rate smoothing algorithms

Table 1. Important ECG features that should be assessed when evaluating CIED function.

Certain conditions, such as acute heart failure may require adjustment of device settings, even without device malfunction – pacemaker algorithms do not provide optimal hemodynamics for all situations. Unfortunately, evidence-based approach is limited due to scarcity of data (Lahiri, 2011).

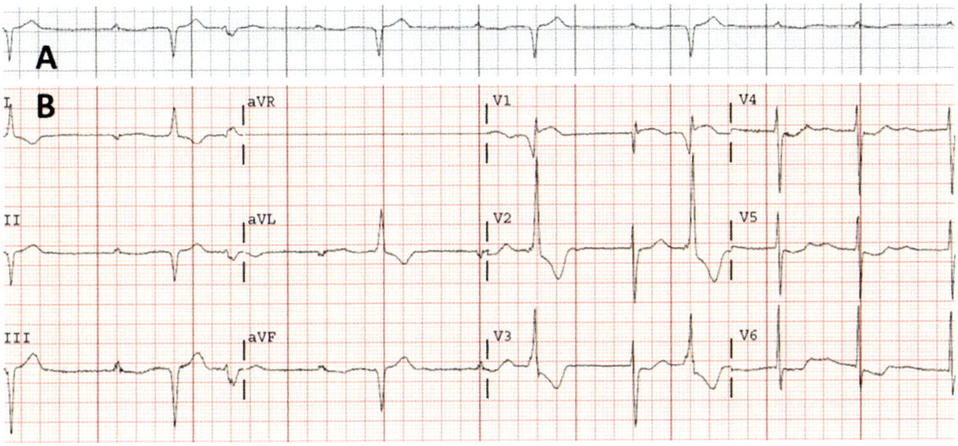

Figure 2. Rhythm strip suggestive of high degree AV block (A). 12 lead ECG obtained at the same time actually shows that the low amplitude signals are QRS complexes and the higher amplitude ones are PVCs (B).

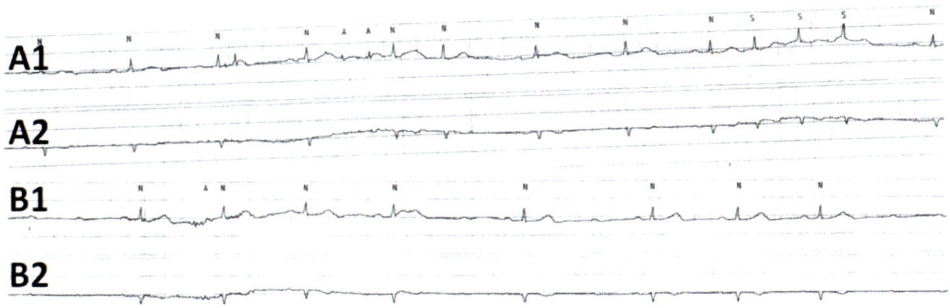

Figure 3. Artifacts masking AV block. High frequency artifacts mimic fast, irregular ventricular rate, resembling atrial fibrillation (A1). However, these artifacts are not present on the simultaneous tracing in a different lead (A2). Once the artifacts disappear, P waves are easily recognizable with high degree AV block (B1, B2).

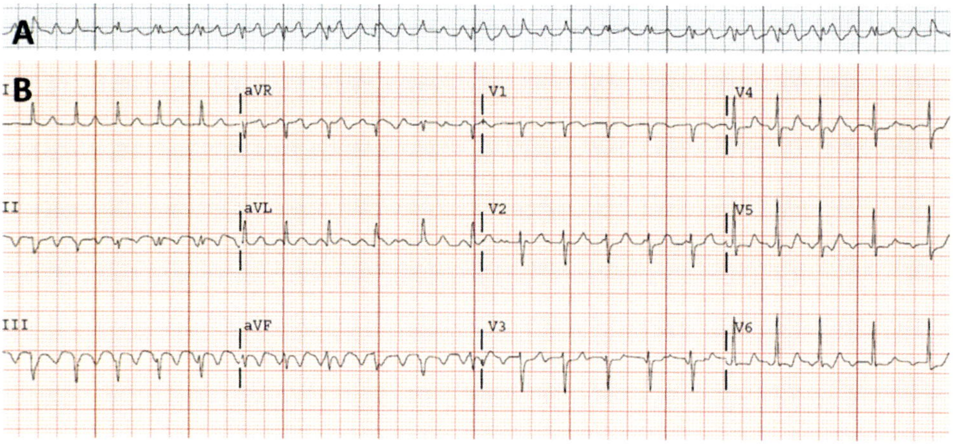

Figure 4. Atrial flutter may mimic ventricular tachycardia in a rhythm strip (A), however, 12-lead ECG clearly identifies the flutter with dominantly 2:1 conduction (B).

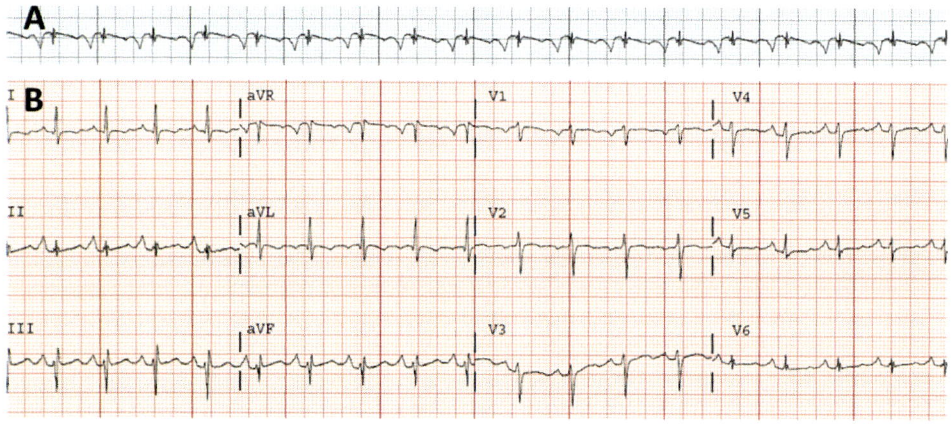

Figure 5. Rhythm strip suggestive of atrial pacing with prolonged AV interval (A). 12 lead ECG shows no evidence of pacing, however, P pulmonale is present and the QRS is low amplitude in II (B).

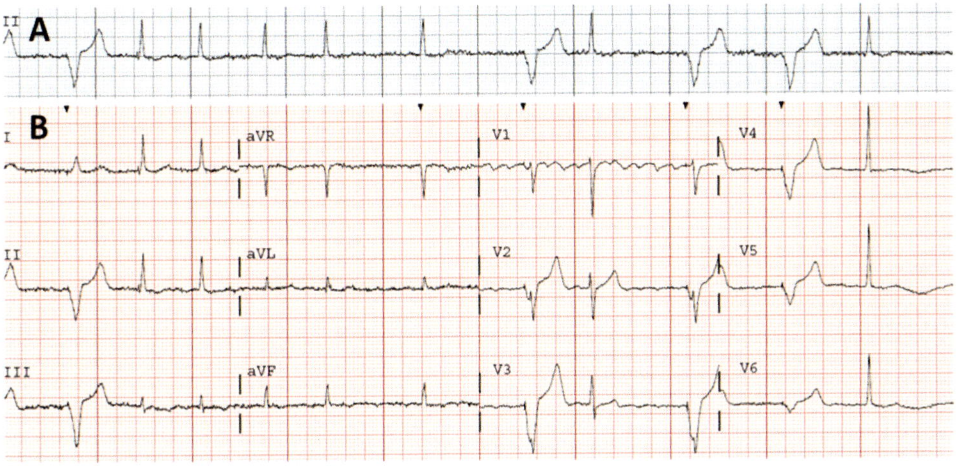

Figure 6. The rhythm strip suggests atrial fibrillation with PVCs or escape beats (A). Simultaneous 12 lead ECG shows evidence of VVI pacing at 60/minute (B). Even when pacing spikes are not visible, wide QRS beats with constant coupling interval, and no R-R cycle longer than this interval should suggest ventricular demand pacing.

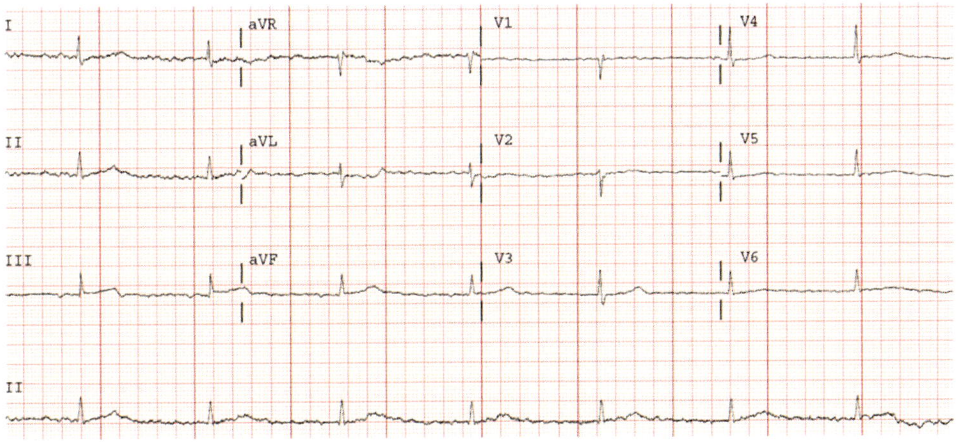

Figure 7. Low amplitude, high frequency artifact masking sinus or ectopic atrial bradycardia. The rhythm may be confused with atrial fibrillation and junctional rhythm, however, P waves can be identified in III and aVF.

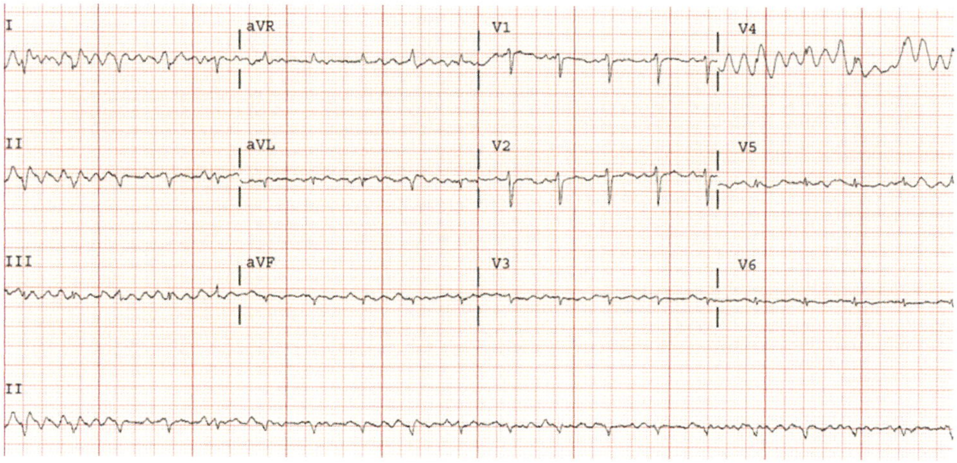

Figure 8. High amplitude artifacts with low ECG voltage may be misinterpreted as atrial flutter of fibrillation. However, sinus tachycardia is easy to recognize in V1 and V2.

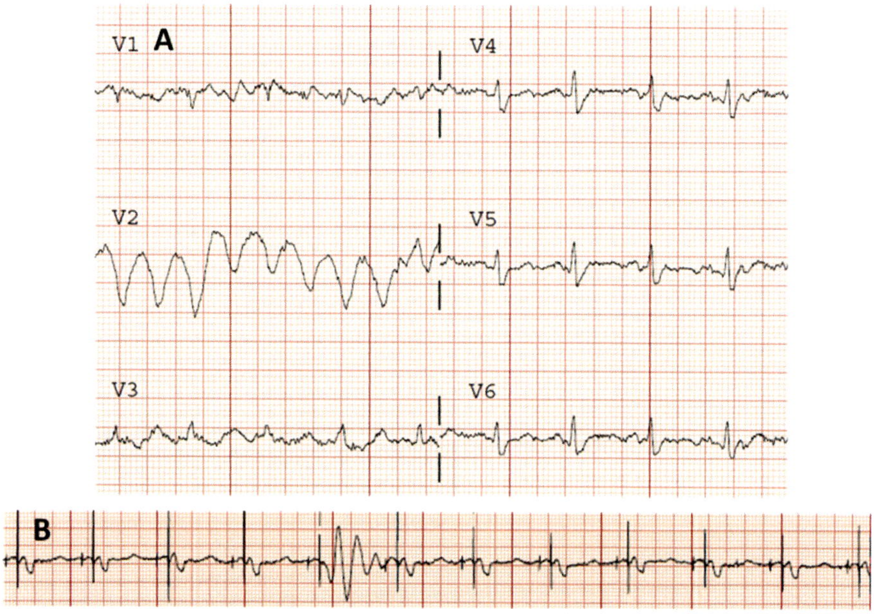

Figure 9. Artifacts suggestive of NSVT. However, the simultaneous V1 and V3, and the following V4-6 leads show that the underlying rhythm is sinus (A). Biventricular pacing is not affected by the artifact – this would be unlikely with any true ventricular arrhythmia (B).

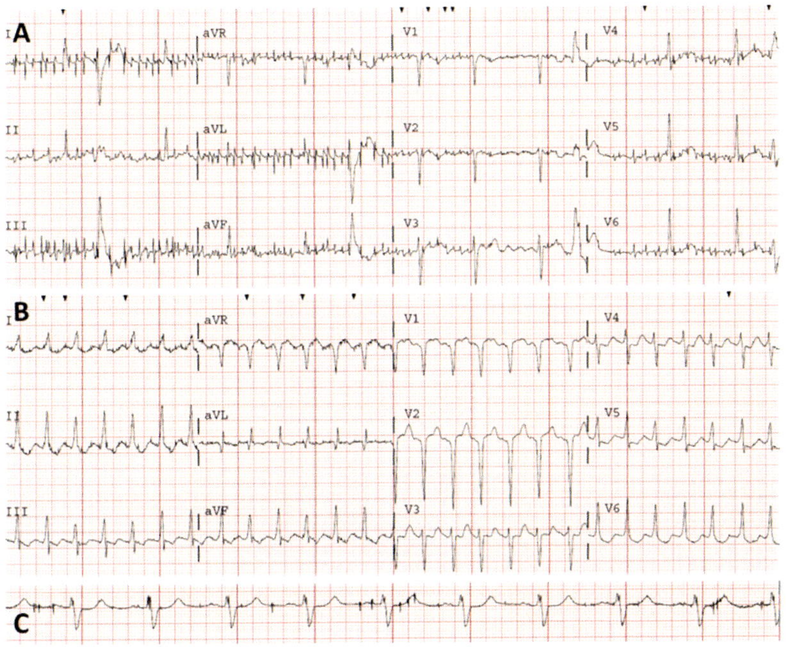

Figure 10. High frequency artifacts causing false detection of pacing in automated ECG device. Although the pacemaker-spike gain and marker functions of the ECG systems may be very helpful to identify small pacing spikes, these systems may be overcalling artifacts. This patient does not have a pacemaker, the ECG improperly identifies some artifacts as pacing (black triangles on top (A). In some cases, the artifacts may be less obvious (B), or may closely resemble pacing spikes (C).

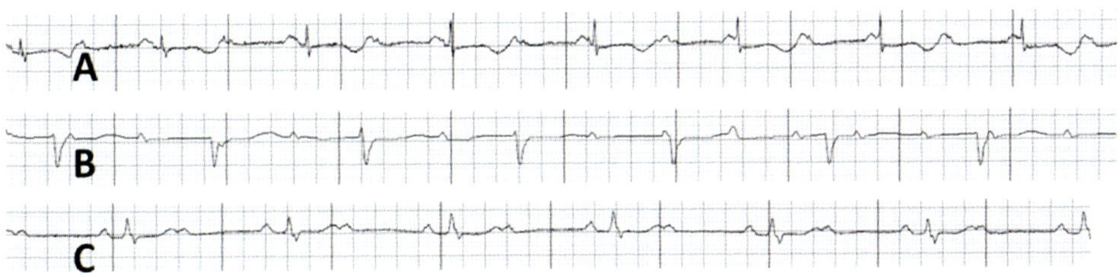

Figure 11. Rhythm strip suggestive of 2:1 AV block (A). However, the QRS complexes are „creeping in" on the preceding P waves – there is complete AV dissociation, more typical for complete heart block with junctional escape rhythm. A similarly difficult tracing (B), suggestive of first degree AV block. As the atrial rate accelerates, complete AV dissociation becomes apparent. (C) True 2:1 AV block – the PR interval following the conducted P waves is constant. Note that the P-P interval slightly irregular (short-long), which may represent ventriculophasic sinus arrhythmia or atrial bigeminy.

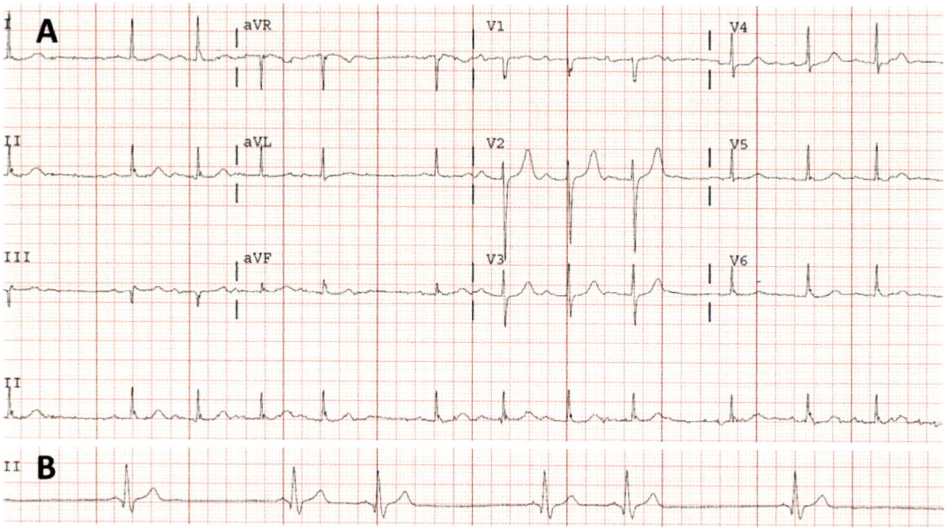

Figure 12. Blocked premature atrial beats (PACs) should be identified as they elicit a different response during atrial pacing (inhibition) than sinus arrest (pacing). In (A), V1 gives the clue for the arrhythmia mechanism – blocked PACs. In (B), there are no visible early P waves – this is 3:2 sinoatrial block.

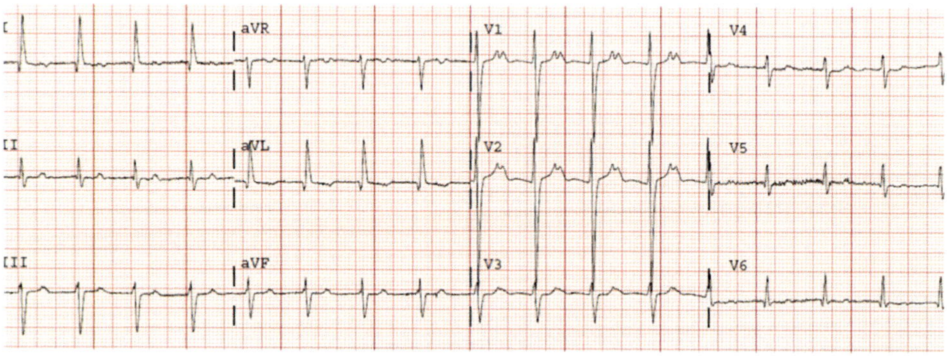

Figure 13. Sinus tachycardia with 1st degree AV block resembling junctional tachycardia. P waves with constant PR interval can be seen in V1-2.

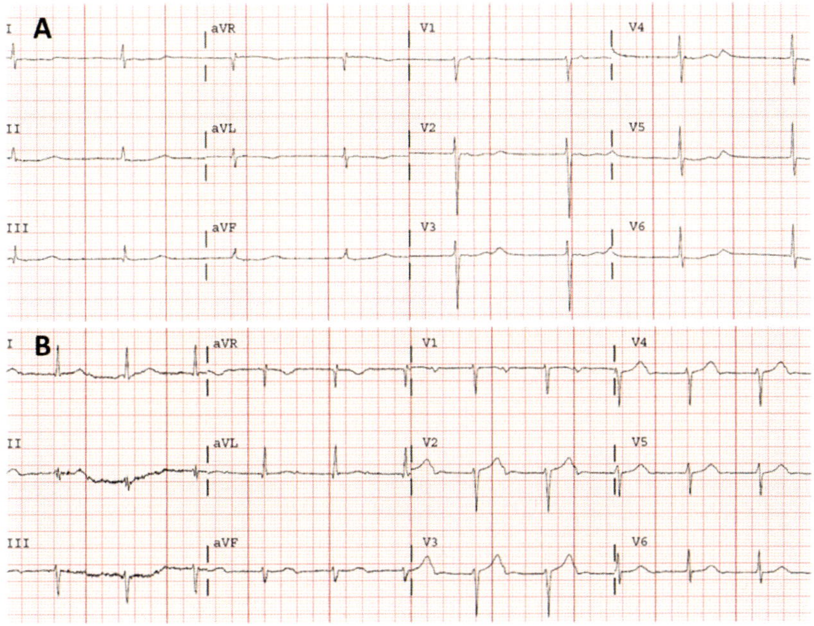

Figure 14. Junctional rhythm with 1:1 VA conduction. Retrograde P waves are visible in V1, which may be misinterpreted as T waves. Note, however, the prolonged QT in all other leads (A). Very long (640 ms) first degree AV block may be confused with junctional rhythm, however, P waves are seen in V1 (B).

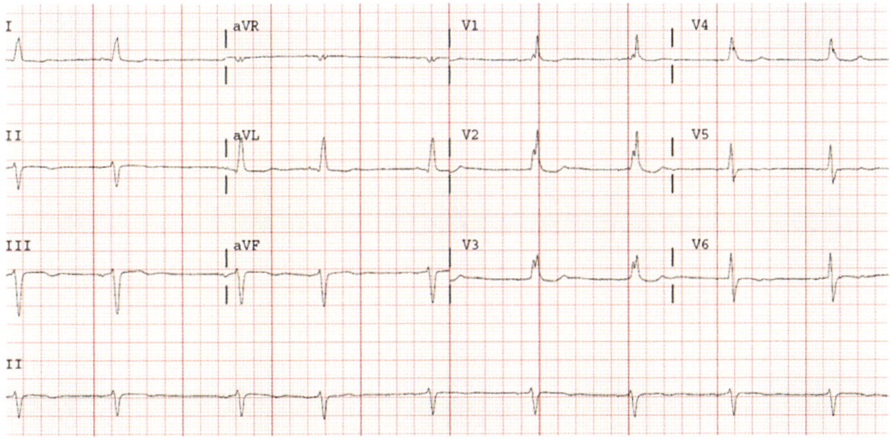

Figure 15. Irregular atrial rhythm resembling atrial fibrillation. The actual rhythm is most likely sinus with PACs, The P waves are of low amplitude, however, they can be identified in III and aVL with 1:1 relationship to QRS and with constant AV delay.

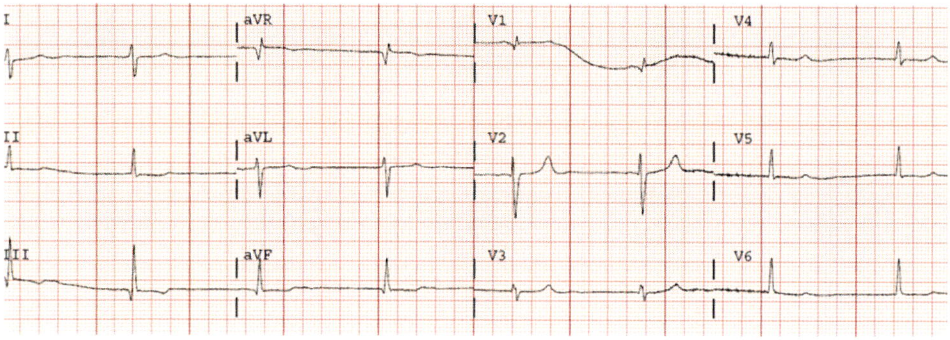

Figure 16. Regular bradycardia with narrow QRS would suggest junctional rhythm, however, P waves are seen before each QRS in V1 – the driving focus is atrial. Advanced atrial conduction disease is not uncommon in pacemaker recipients, leading to low amplitude, fragmented P waves.

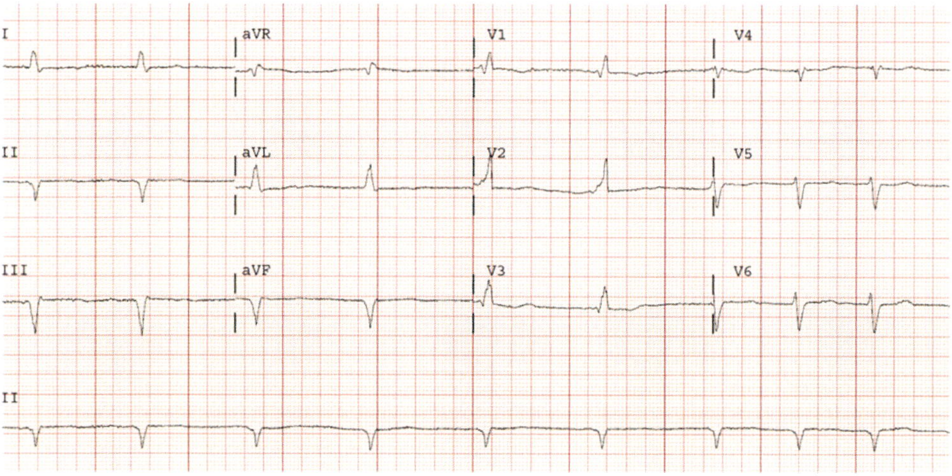

Figure 17. Atrial fibrillation with junctional escape. The regular rhythm may be misinterpreted as pure junctional rhythm, however, the ventricular rate changes when atrioventricular conduction improves and conducted activity overtakes junctional escape. Proper identification of atrial rhythm is important when evaluating pacemaker function – atrial fibrillation should suppress atrial pacing, while atrial pacing should take place with pure junctional rhythm, if an atrial lead is present.

3. Unexpected findings with normal device function

Certain artifacts or interaction of pacemaker algorithms with underlying rhythm may lead to electrocardiographic findings, which may be difficult to distinguish from abnormal function (Balachander, 2011). P/QRS morphology, timing and response to pacing spikes should be addressed, when analyzing the ECG. With ubiquity of bipolar systems, spikes may be difficult to identify (Figure 18). In addition, myocardial depolarization has a vector, which may be isoelectric in certain leads, or may be delayed by intraatrial or intraventricular conduction delay, suggesting ineffective stimulation (Figure 19). Spike morphology may be affected be automatic signal gain function of the ECG system or issues with digital sampling (Figure 20). „Anticipated" spikes may be missing due to very small variations in heart rate, inhibiting demand pacing (Figure 21).

Variable signal morphology may be caused by fusion beats (when the resulting signal morphology is the sum of activation from the pacemaker and spontaneous/conducted activation) or pseudofusion beats (pacing occurs when the myocardium is already refractory from spontaneous/conducted activation, Figures 22-24). Identification of the pacing site is crucial to prove appropriate device function (Figures 25-28).

Occasionally, pacing mode may be difficult to identify based solely on the ECG (Figure 29). It may change due to algorithms trying to minimize right ventricular stimulation (Figures 30-32), rate smoothing function (Figure 33), or arrhythmia – mainly, atrial fibrillation (Israel, 2002).

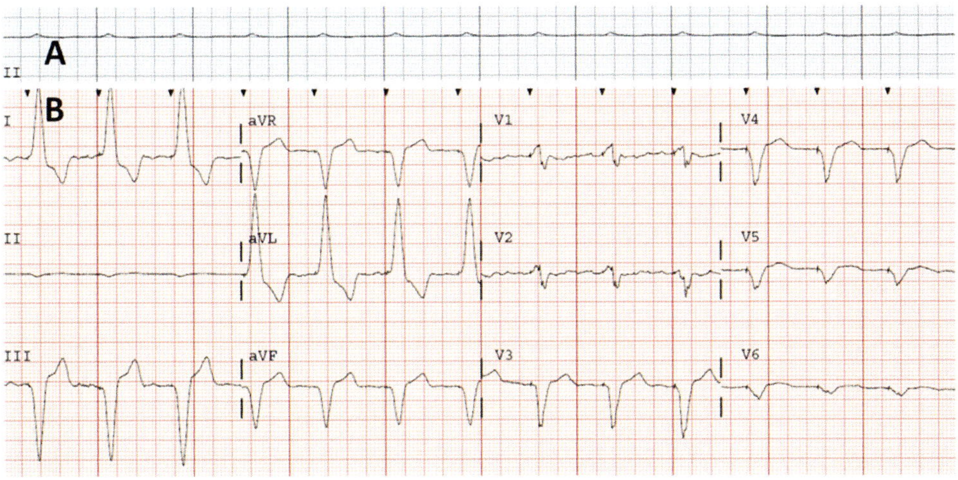

Figure 18. Rhythm strip suggestive of complete heart block and absence of pacing (A). Simultaneous 12 lead ECG shows appropriate ventricular stimulation – the vector of the myocardial activation is close to isoelectric in II.

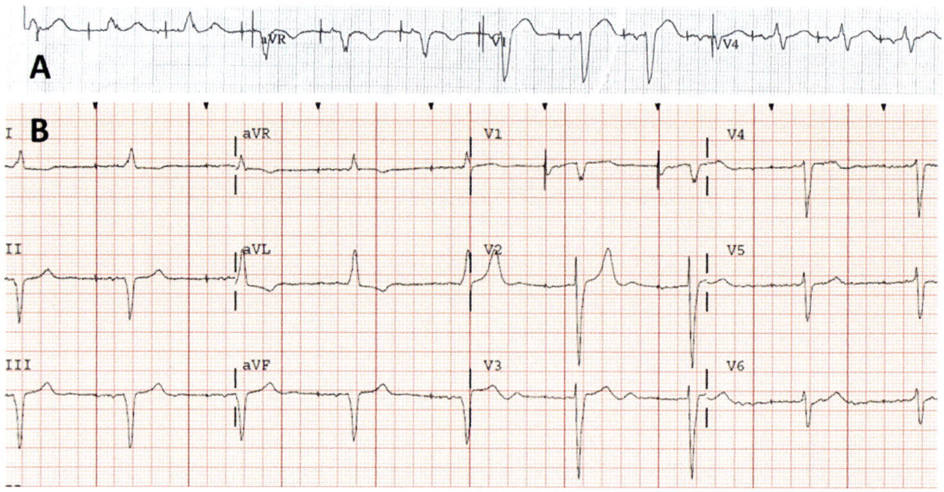

Figure 19. P waves are not seen in I despite effective atrial pacing – the atrial depolarization vector may be isoelectric in certain leads, depending on the atrial pacing site and pathologic conditions. Note that there is a delay in each lead from the atrial spike to the P wave, suggestive of conduction delay (A). Intra-atrial conduction delay may present even in regions far from the pacing electrode – note instant capture in V1, however, significantly prolonged, fragmented P wave in the frontal leads (200 ms) (B).

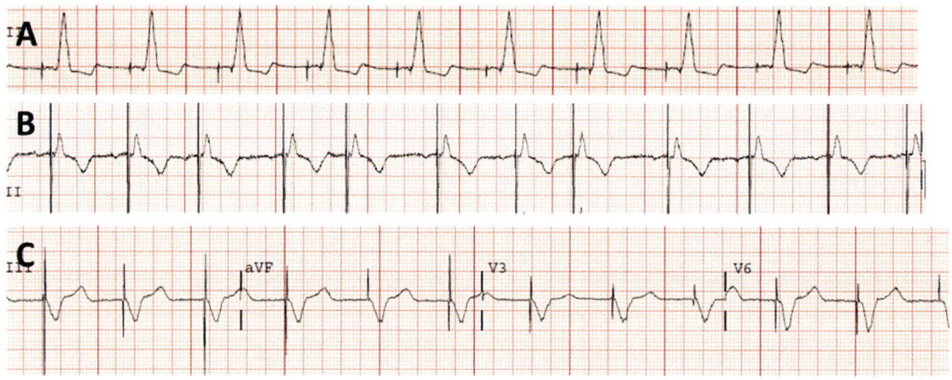

Figure 20. Variable spike morphology (A). This is a normal finding as the spike morphology is affected by the digital sampling of the ECG system and whether it uses pacemaker signal identification/amplification. There is no clinically useful correlation between the spike height and pacing energy. Generally, unipolar pacing (B) leads to much higher amplitude signals than bipolar (A). Spike height may vary not just between different ECG leads, but even with each beat (C).

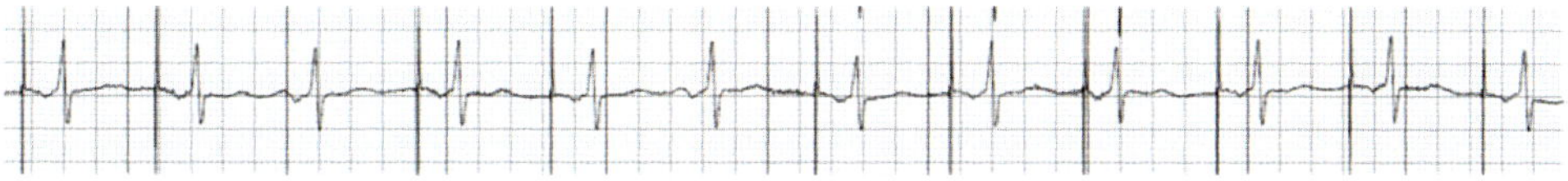

Figure 21. Sinus rhythm competing with AAI pacemaker – there is appropriate inhibition of atrial pacing when the P-P interval is shorter than the basic pacing cycle length.

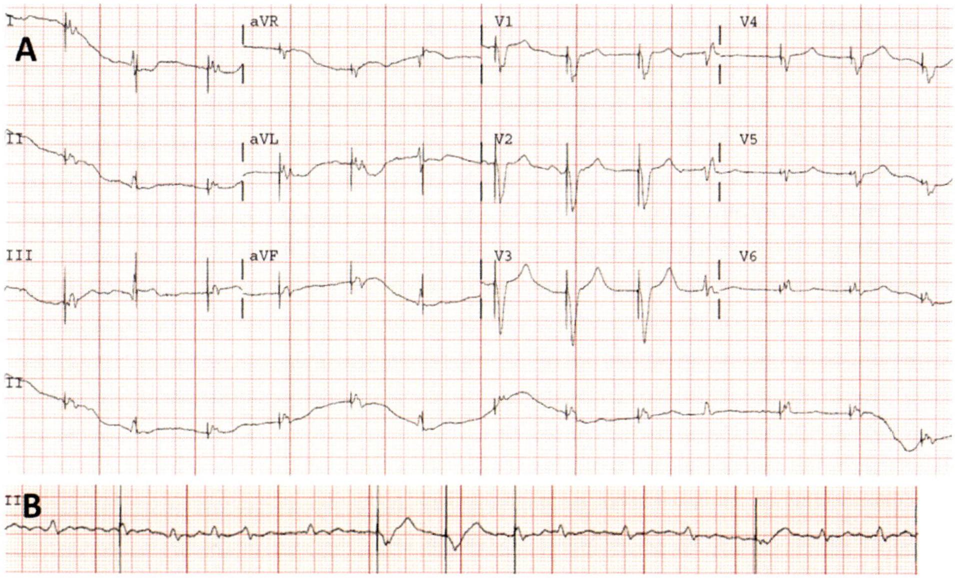

Figure 22. Pseudofusion beats during ventricular stimulation – this is a normal phenomenon as detection of ventricular activation is delayed due to lead tip position (usually right ventricular apex – the ventricles may be partially depolarized, when signal is sensed in this region). Beats 2 and 6 show pseudofusion, ventricular pacing is delivered after the ventricles are depolarized and refractory to further stimuli. Beat 10 is sensed appropriately and pacing is inhibited, as the coupling interval is somewhat shorter - this makes ventricular undersensing very unlikely as the cause for pseudofusion (A). Fusion and pseudofusion beats are very common during atrial fibrillation due to the wide range of coupling intervals (B).

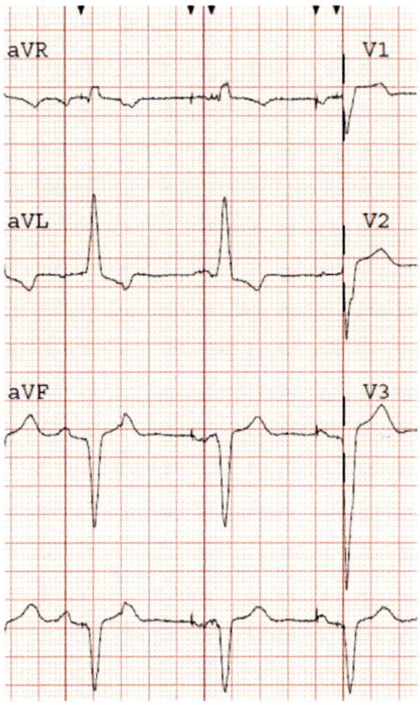

Figure 23. Fusion can be also encountered in the atria, although may be more difficult to identify due to lower signal amplitudes. Undersensing of PACs should be excluded and may require longer tracings or device interrogation.

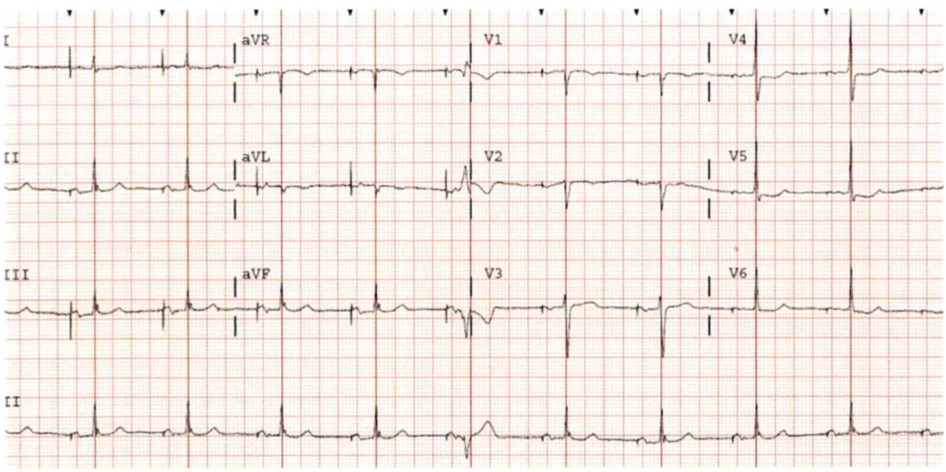

Figure 24. Wide QRS beat encountered during regular atrial pacing with short PR interval. This is most likely a premature ventricular contraction (PVC), fusing with the atrial paced, spontaneously conducted beat.

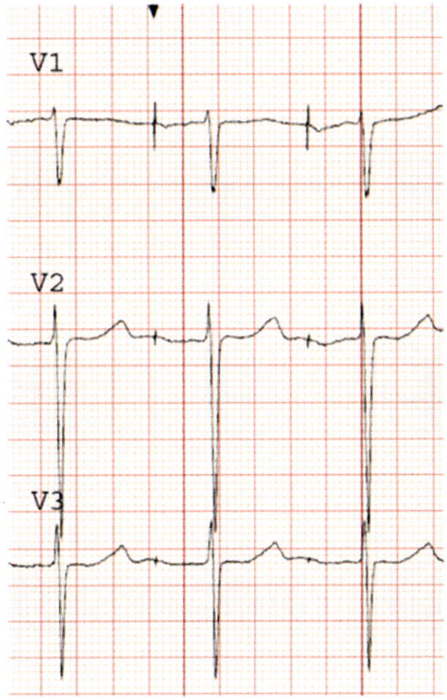

Figure 25. Pacing spikes fall into the U waves in V2 and V3 and are not followed by apparent capture. However, in V1 atrial capture is clear.

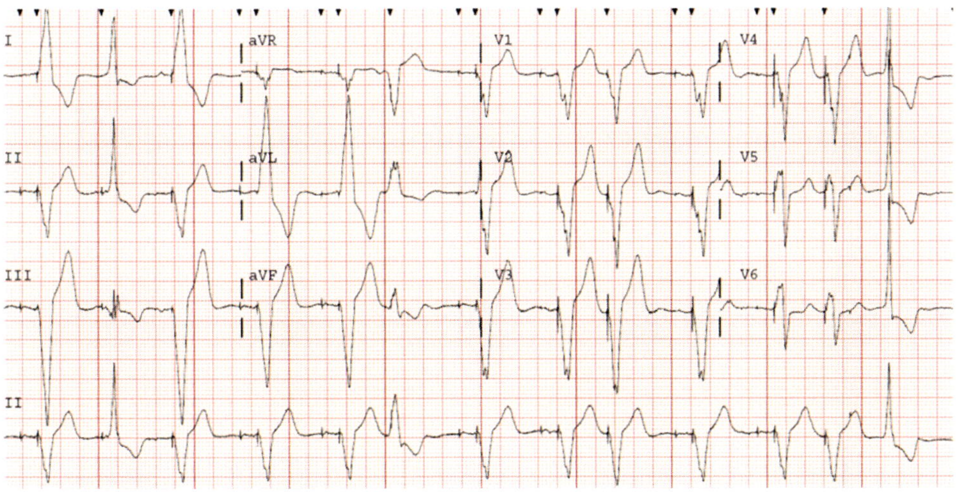

Figure 26. Pseudo pseudofusion – a spike appears immediately before (3rd spike) or within a QRS (9th spike). However, these are atrial spikes and the tracing represents appropriate DDD pacemaker response to frequent premature ventricular and atrial beats. Origin of pacing spikes should be identified based on their timing and sequence to avoid misinterpretation as undersensing or ineffective capture.

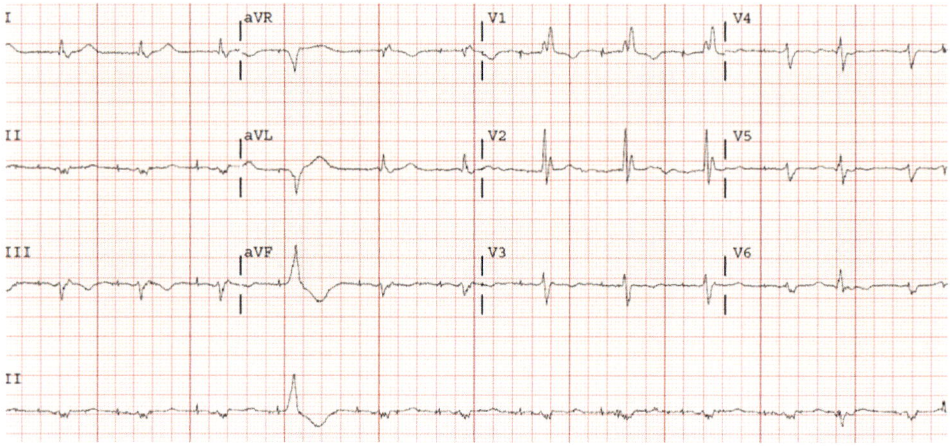

Figure 27. Identification of pacing site is important to avoid misinterpretation. The 4th spike seems to be non-capturing and is followed by a wide QRS beat with an 80 ms delay. However, this is an atrial stimulus as it is apparent by reviewing the consecutive beats. The wide QRS beat is a PVC, which does not have any correlation with atrial pacing. The P waves are of low amplitude and difficult to identify, however, regular atrial pacing followed by regular ventricular activation with the same atrioventricular delay suggests consistent atrial capture.

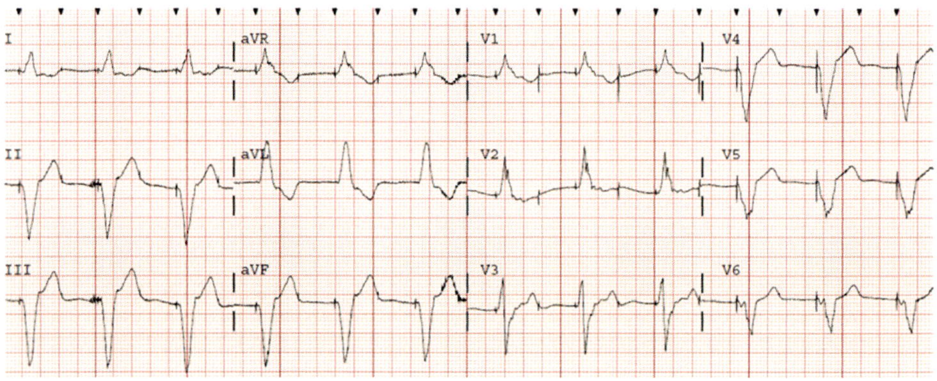

Figure 28. High frequency pacing may occasionally be a sign of serious pacemaker malfunction (runaway pacemaker) or appropriate response to an arrhythmia (tracked sinus/atrial tachycardia). In dual chamber systems, proper identification of pacing spikes is necessary for troubleshooting. In this tracing, 150/minute pacing seems to be capturing 2:1. Note, however, that the pacing is regularly irregular (short-long) and the spike morphology is alternating in V1 – every other one is an atrial spike. The patient is in atrial fibrillation, which is undersensed and the DDD pacemaker is delivering dual chamber stimulation at 70/minute with an AV delay of 400 ms.

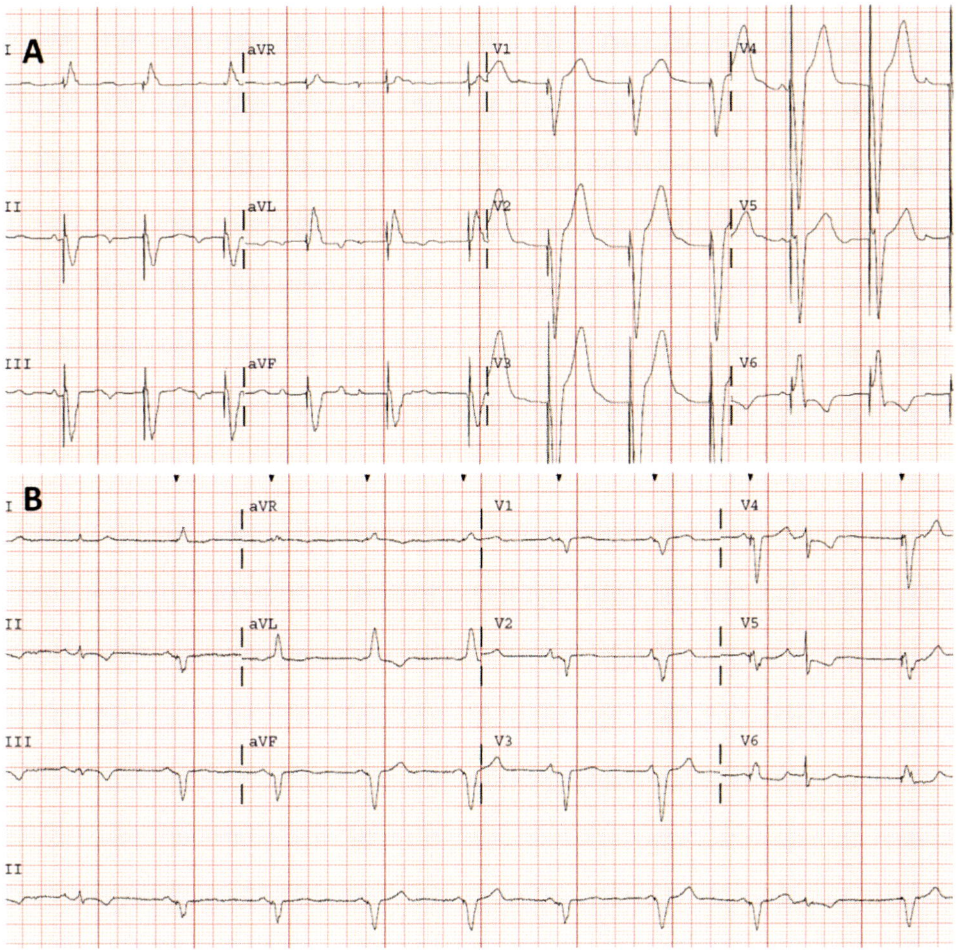

Figure 29. Pacing mode may be difficult to identify from surface ECG. (A) In III and aVF it may appear that the atrial activity is tracked to the ventricles. However, the ventricular rate is completely regular despite variable P-P intervals. AV dissociation is seen in V4 and V5. This device is a VVI pacemaker in a patient with complete heart block. (B) Isorhythmic dissociation between sinus rhythm and VVI pacing – close inspection of the PR intervals reveals that the atrial activity is not tracked

If pacing spikes are seen during tachycardia, most common causes are atrial tachyarrhythmia tracked by the pacemaker, or true PM mediated tachycardia (caused by retrograde conduction or atrial oversensing of ventricular events, leading to endless loop tachycardia). Rate response function may also cause transient increase in pacing rate. The differential is usually difficult based on surface ECG alone, unless initiation and termination can be clearly identified. Device interrogation is strongly recommended (Ip, 2011). Transient changes in rhythm may elucidate the mechanism of a suspected malfunction (Figure 34).

Both atrial and ventricular tachyarrhythmias may raise the concern of device malfunction. If no spikes are seen, the rhythm is likely not related to pacing and patient-related issues should be suspected (Figures 35-38). Underlying rhythm should be identified: atrial fibrillation/flutter may be difficult to recognize with asynchronous pacing, but still pose a thromboembolic risk (Figures 39-40).

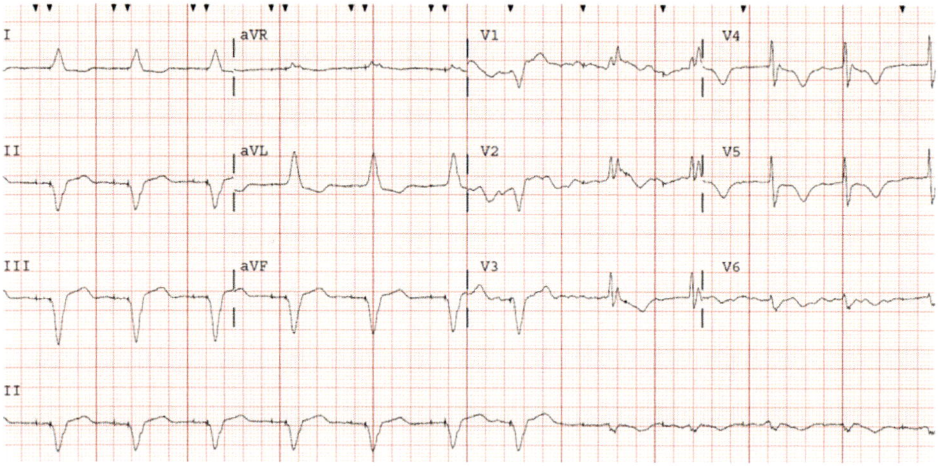

Figure 30. Response to a premature atrial beat with managed ventricular pacing algorithm (Medtronic, Inc). The DDD pacemaker is delivering atrioventricular stimulation, then an atrial-sensed ventricular pace following a premature atrial beat. Following this beat, an atrial stimulus is delivered with mode switch to ADI. As atrioventricular conduction is detected, the device continues with atrial stimulation and allows spontaneous conduction with prolonged AV delay.

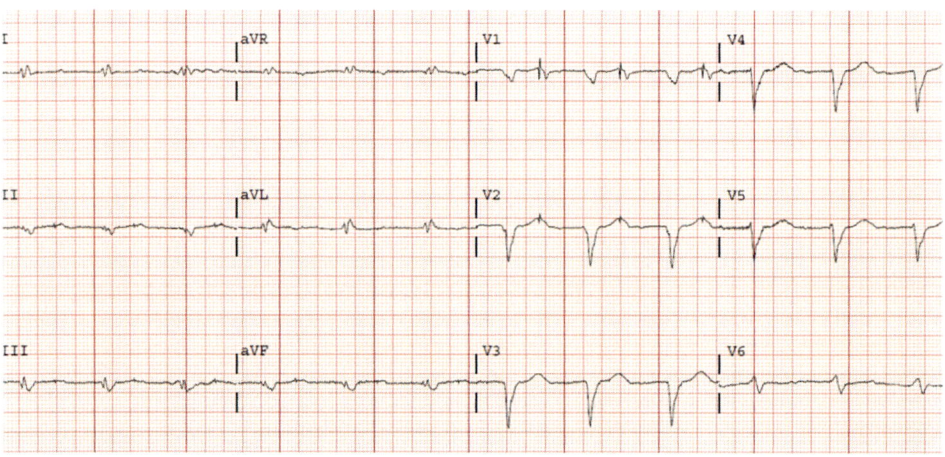

Figure 31. Managed ventricular pacing may maintain very long AV interval, if the 1:1 atrial:ventricular ratio is maintained. In this case, atrial pacing spikes occur after the QRS, in the T waves. V1 shows atrial capture with an AV delay of 460 ms.

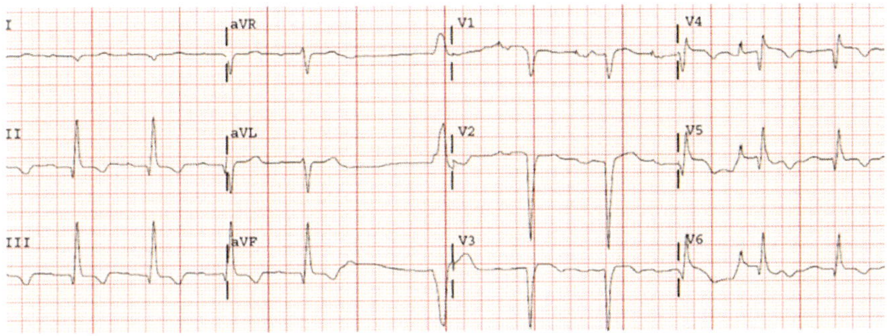

Figure 32. Heart rate may drop down to ≈50% of the basic rate for one cycle with managed ventricular pacing – in this case a late blocked PAC is followed by an atrial stimulus, followed by a ventricular stimulus with very short AV delay (wide QRS beat, the spikes are not visualized in these leads). V1 gives the clue that the rhythm is paced at 70/minute. The artifact in V4-6 is not related to pacing.

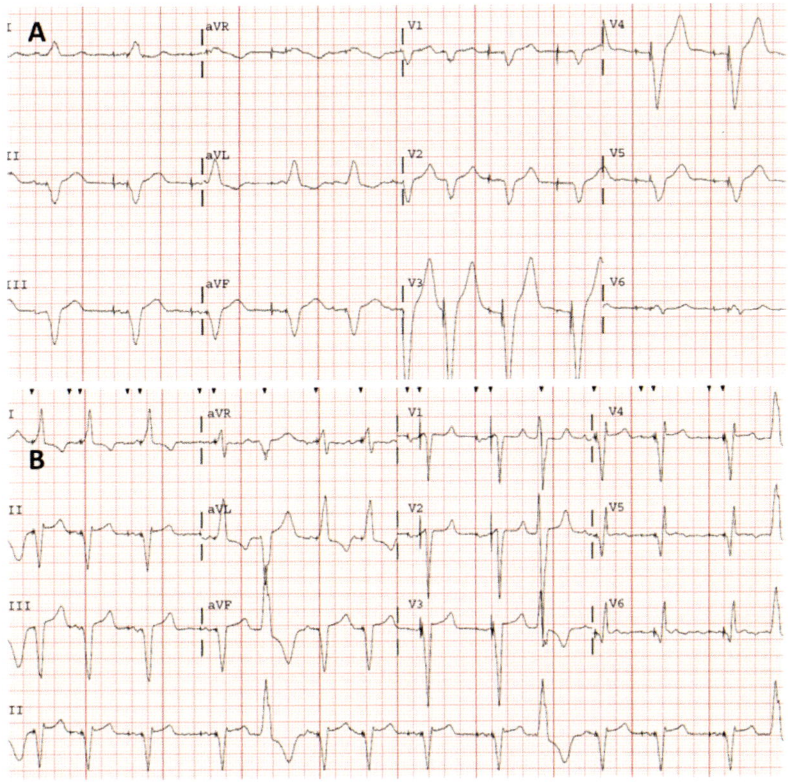

Figure 33. Rate smoothing with a DDD pacemaker (A). Following the premature beats, the atrial pacing rate is gradually decreased to the basic pacing rate. Irregular pacing caused by rate smoothing in a biventricular system (B). All premature beats are sensed (ventricular and atrial), and either a sense response pace or an tracked biventricular pace is delivered. The basic pacing rate is gradually decreased after these over a few cycles, the lowest pacing rate on this tracing is 65/minute.

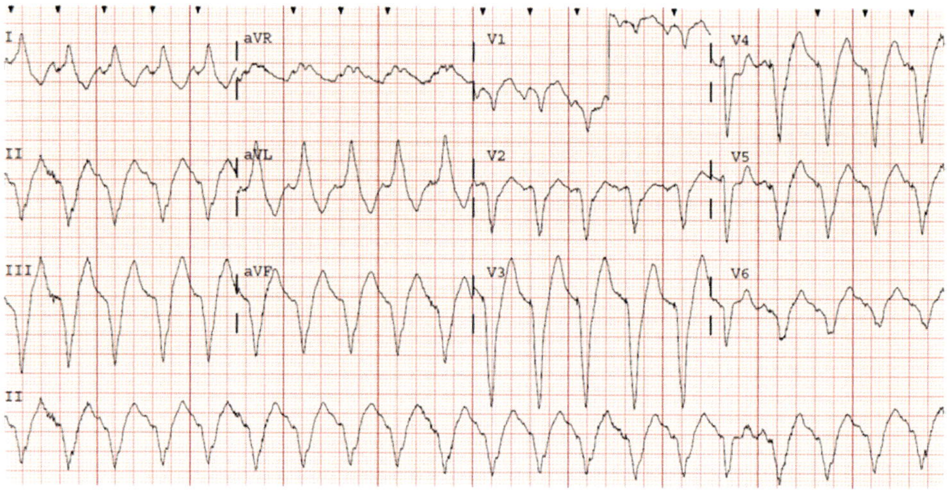

Figure 34. Sudden changes in regular tachycardia may elucidate the mechanism. The premature beat unmasks a P wave, followed by a ventricular paced beat – this is a supraventricular tachycardia tracked by the dual chamber pacemaker.

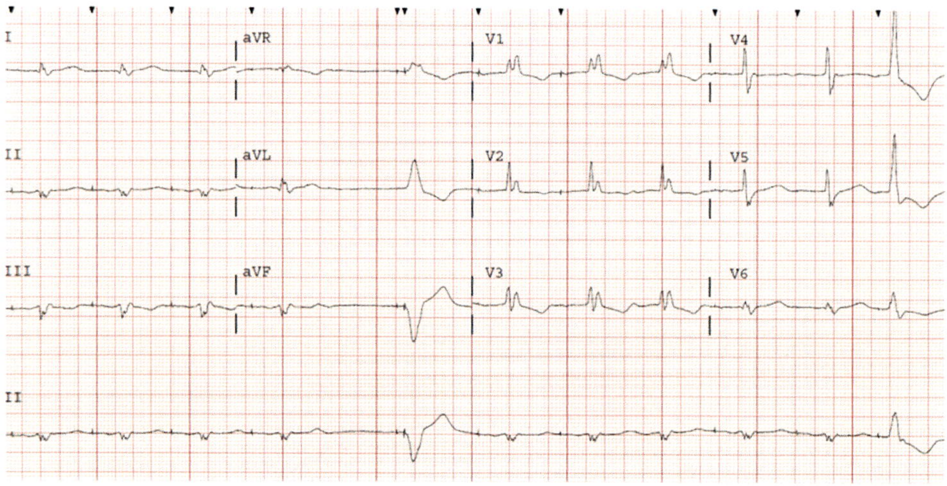

Figure 35. Hidden premature atrial beat mimics pacemaker malfunction. The 5th atrial spike is delayed, suggestive of oversensing, however, the 4th T wave in the rhythm strip is different from the previous three, suggestive of a buried premature atrial beat, with AV block. The 5th atrial spike actually comes right on time as the pacing cycle was reset by the premature atrial beat. Additionally, a ventricular pace is delivered by the managed ventricular pacing algorithm.

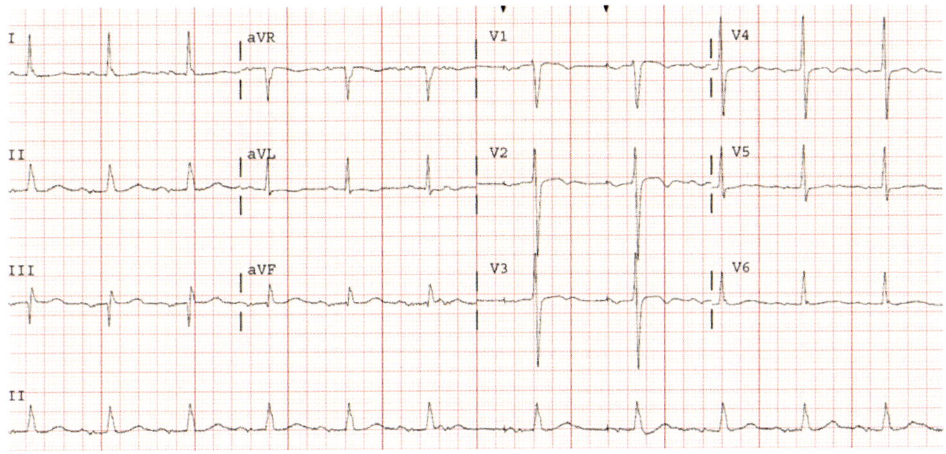

Figure 36. Blocked PAC without tracking with a DDD pacemaker. This is normal function, as the blocked PAC (after the 6th QRS) comes very early and was sensed in the post-ventricular atrial refractory period. Instead, an atrial stimulus is delivered later to maintain the basic rate. As there is spontaneous AV conduction, ventricular pacing is inhibited. After 2 atrial paced beats, sinus rhythm takes over again.

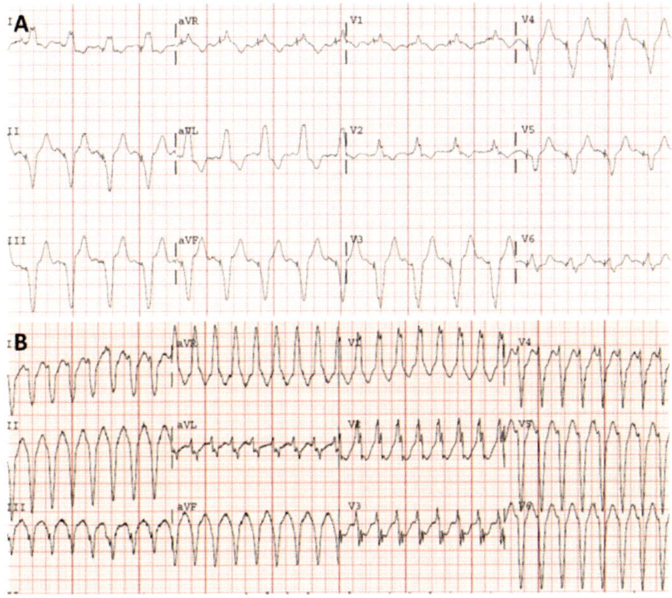

Figure 37. Wide QRS tachycardia in pacemaker recipients. Sinus tachycardia with appropriate sensing and ventricular pacing (A). With bipolar pacing the spikes may not be visible in all leads and the rhythm may be misinterpreted as ventricular tachycardia – especially in telemetry tracings. When ventricular rate is higher than the upper tracking rate (if known) or the QRS morphology is not compatible with usual pacing sites, VT (B) or SVT with aberrancy should be suspected.

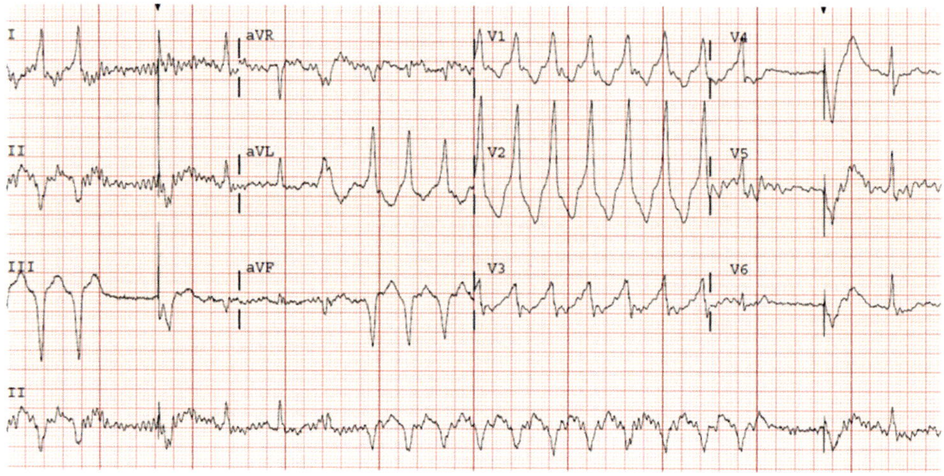

Figure 38. Non-sustained wide QRS tachycardia in a patient with a VVI pacemaker. Note appropriate demand pacing and the absence of spikes during the tachycardia – this is not pacing-related, but a true non-sustained ventricular tachycardia.

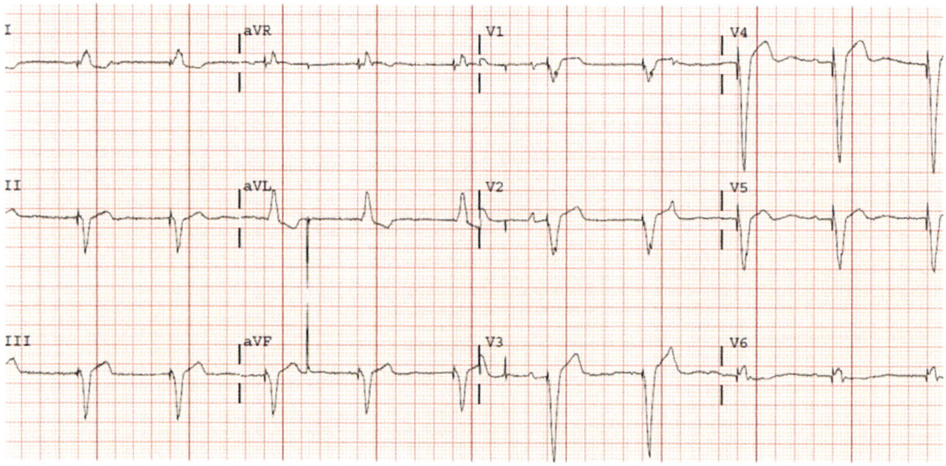

Figure 39. VVI pacing without retrograde conduction. An underlying, slow regular atrial rhythm is seen in V2 and V5. The spikes after the 3rd and 5th beats are artifacts.

ECG analysis should always include assessment of QRS and ST-T, even in patients with paced rhythms. Atrial pacing preserves normal ventricular activation, so it may be interpreted without interference from the device. Underlying conduction blocks may mimic paced beats (Figures 41-42). If artifacts limit interpretation, comparing multiple simultaneous ECG leads may be helpful (Figure 43).

In patients presenting with symptoms suspicious for pacemaker syndrome (hypotension, shortness of breath, dizziness, most commonly in an intermittent pattern), atrioventricular activation sequence and presence of ventriculoatrial conduction should be assessed. If these are compatible with PM syndrome, device settings should be adjusted (or the device should be upgraded), to restore AV synchrony and avoid atrial contraction during ventricular systole (Figures 44-45).

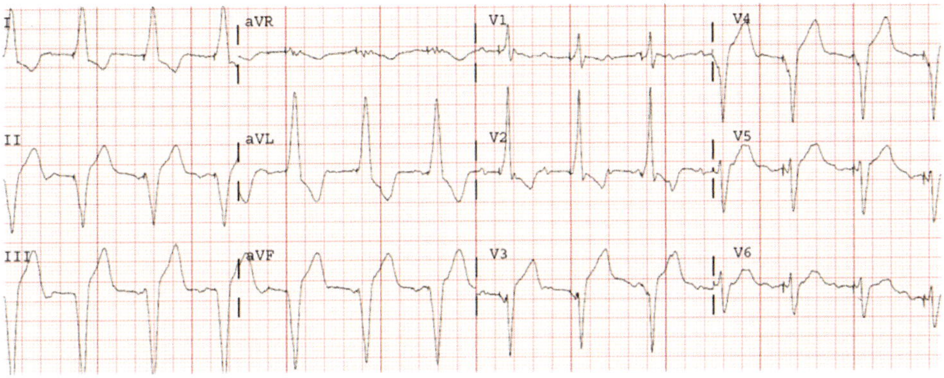

Figure 40. Underlying rhythm is atrial tachycardia or slow atrial flutter with a cycle length around 320 ms. This is neither spontaneously conducted, nor tracked by the pacemaker to the ventricles, 80/minute ventricular stimulation is seen.

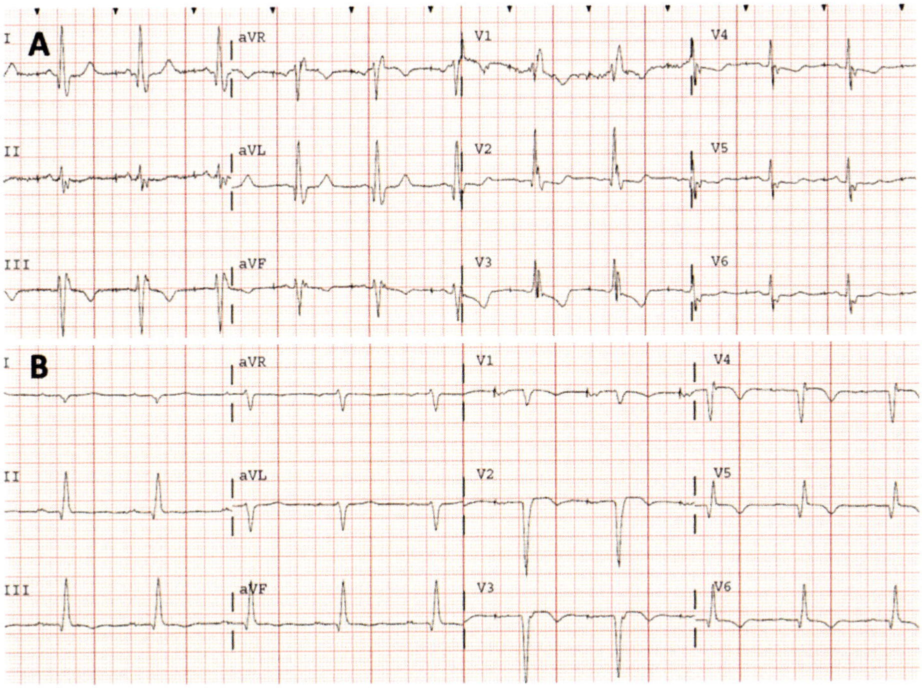

Figure 41. Atrial pacing preserves normal ventricular activation sequence, conventional ECG criteria may be used to identify ischemia, blocks, hypertrophy. RBBB (A), remote anterior MI (B).

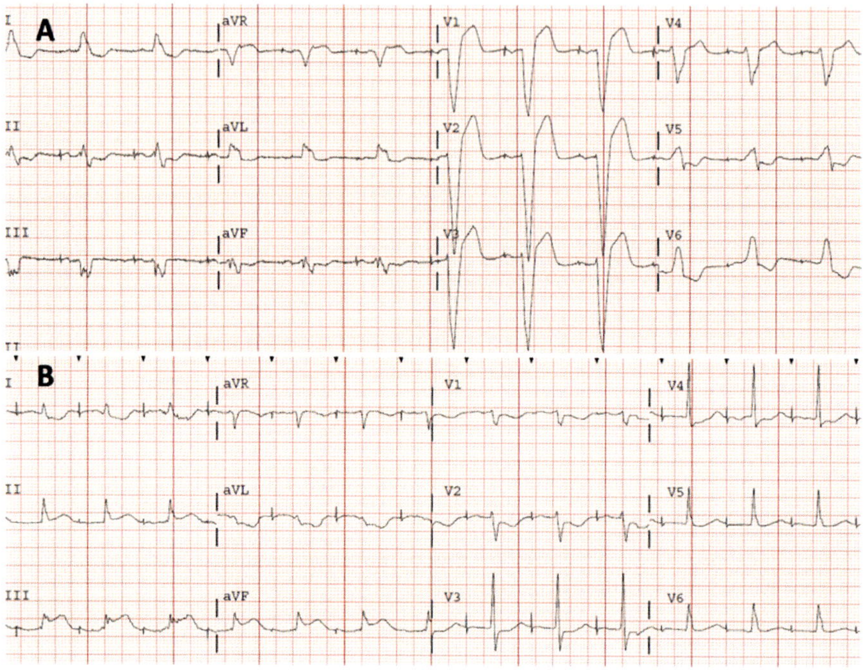

Figure 42. Preexisting LBBB may be confused with dual chamber pacing. Close inspection of the QRS complexes reveals atrial pacing and typical LBBB (A). Acute inferior MI with atrial pacing – typical ST elevation with reciprocal changes (B).

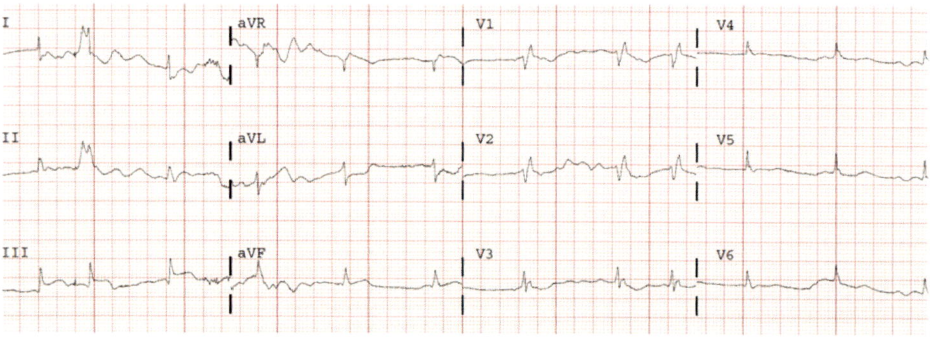

Figure 43. Artifact suggestive of ventricular undersensing with a recently placed temporary right ventricular lead. There appears to be a pacemaker spike shortly after the first QRS with a captured beat, suspicious for undersensing. However, the morphology of this "paced" beat is not typical and note that in III there is a 120 ms delay between the "spike" and the QRS and no change in depolarization/repolarization compared to non-paced beats – this would be impossible with a ventricular paced beat. This phenomenon was caused by an artifact causing a high amplitude, positive deflection in I and II, imitating a LBBB pattern, and there was actually no pacing – the artifact was gained as a spike by the ECG. There are multiple artifacts in I, II and aVR, suggestive of noise coming from the right upper extremity ECG electrode.

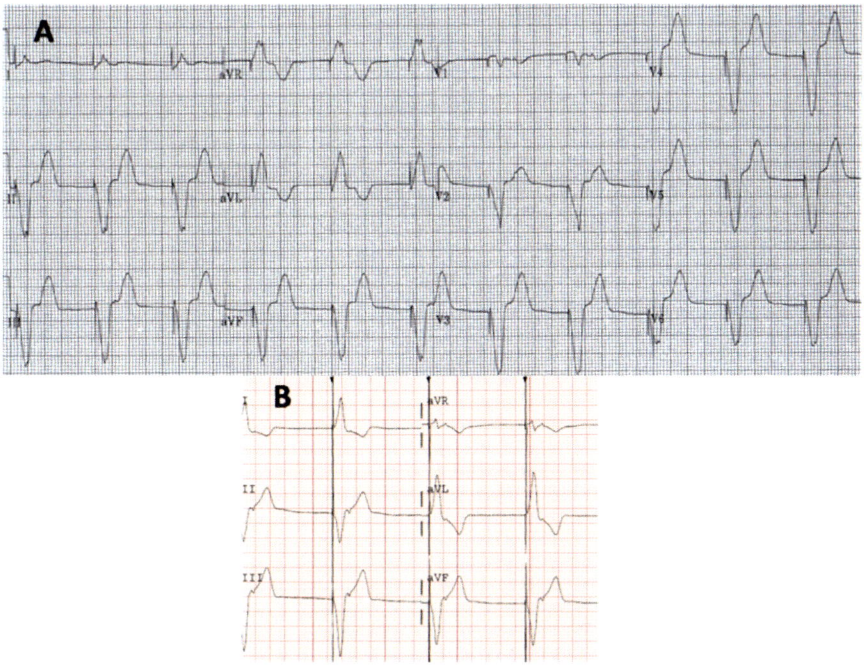

Figure 44. Mode switch due to battery depletion (A). The patient with a DDD PM presented with sudden onset complaints typical for pacemaker syndrome. ECG shows 65/minute ventricular stimulation with 1:1 VA conduction (best seen in V1) – this pacemaker converted to VVI 65/min backup mode when battery condition reached end-of-service. (B) is a more typical presentation of VVI stimulation with 1:1 retrograde conduction – without significant atrial conductive system disease, retrograde P waves are easily recognized

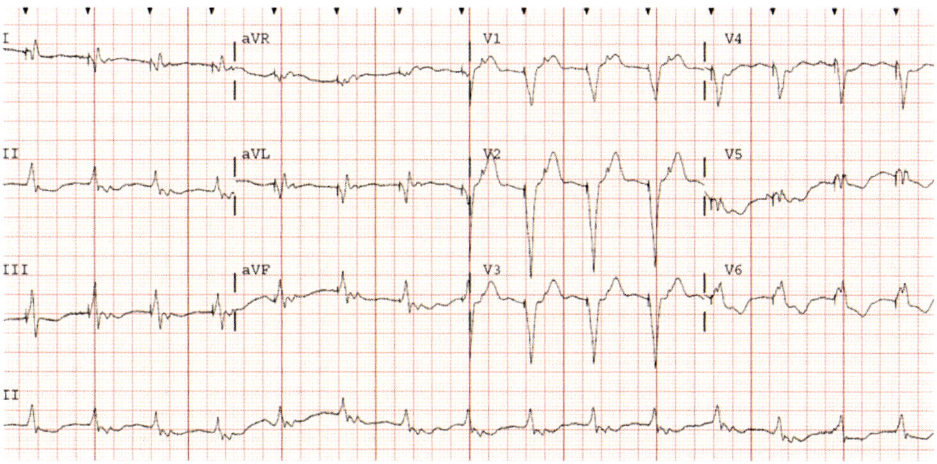

Figure 45. Retrograde conduction may be intermittent even during VVI pacing at constant rate – in this case, it starts after the 2nd beat and ends 3 beats before the recording ends.

4. Pacemaker or lead malfunction

Most common pacemaker and lead related malfunctions, that should be promptly identified and corrected, include oversensing, undersensing and ineffective stimulation. These may be related to inappropriate settings that may be easily corrected with a programmer, however, pacemaker lead related issues (dislocation, fracture, insulation failure) may present similarly and require hardware revision. If true pacemaker dysfunction cannot be ruled out with certainty based on ECG, device interrogation should be performed – this is especially important, if the patient was exposed to factors with potential device interaction, such as MRI, therapeutic irradiation, trauma, or drugs with known effect on pacing threshold (Goldschlager, 2001).

Pure undersensing may be identified by a pacing spike that comes early compared to the anticipated timing, with appropriate capture, if the paced chamber is not refractory. Transient arrhythmias, such as premature ventricular beats, may lead to intermittent undersensing, as their intracardiac signal amplitude may be low (Figure 46). Atrial fibrillation is often undersensed and elicits different behavior in AAI and DDD systems (Figures 47-48).

Loss of capture is easily recognized, however, post-pacing artifacts should not be misinterpreted as capture (Figure 49). Complete lead fracture usually leads to exit block with no visible spikes, while lead dislocation or insulation failure may manifest in various ways (Figures 50-54).

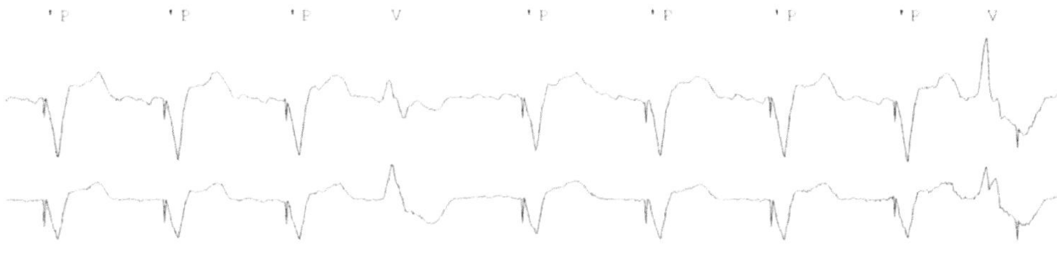

Figure 46. Ventricular undersensing in a patient with VVI pacemaker after AV node ablation for AF. The first PVC was detected and the pacing cycle was reset, however, the second PVC with a different morphology was not detected and inappropriate ventricular pacing occurred in the refractory period of the ventricles.

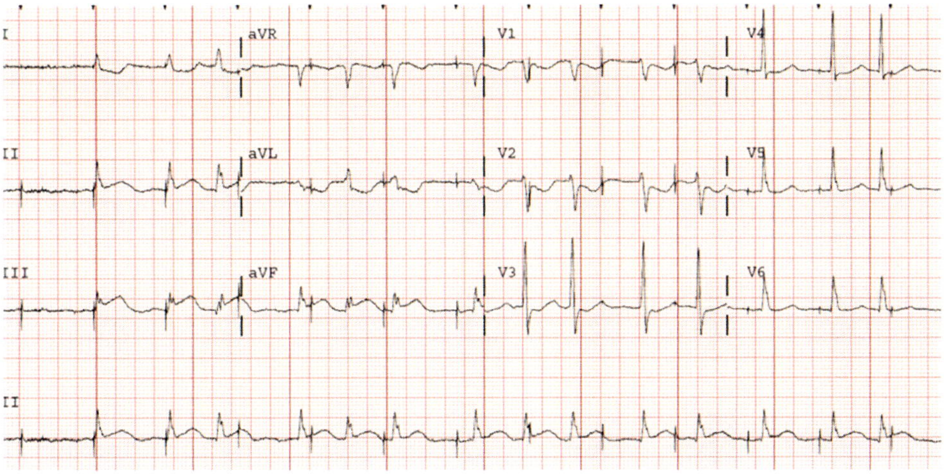

Figure 47. Undersensing of atrial fibrillation with an AAI pacemaker – there is asynchronous atrial pacing without capture. Pseudo pseudofusion beats are seen (2nd, 3rd). VVI pacing would give a similar picture in case of complete sensing failure and loss of capture.

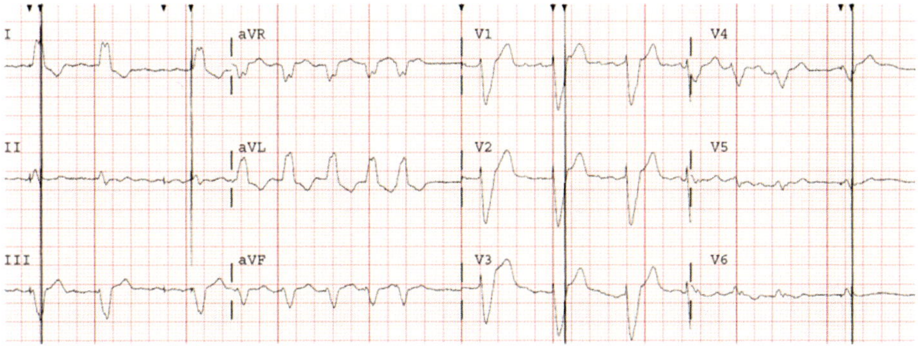

Figure 48. Undersensing of atrial fibrillation with a DDD pacemaker. When the ventricular rate during AF falls below the basic pacing rate, the PM delivers an atrial stimulus, which is not capturing as the patient is in AF. If conduction does not occur after the preset AV delay, a ventricular stimulus is delivered. If conduction occurs after the atrial spike within the ventricular safety period, a ventricular safety pace is delivered, which is not capturing as the ventricles are refractory.

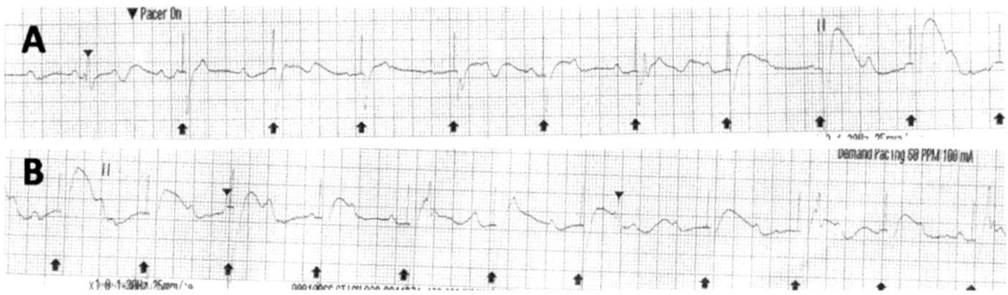

Figure 49. Pseudocapture during temporary external pacing. Transcutaneous pacing was initiated due to complete heart block (underlying rhythm is sinus tachycardia). An escape beat is seen (marked with a black triangle), then pacing is initiated and pacing energy is increased rapidly, causing progressively increasing post-pacing artifacts, which may be misinterpreted as capture (A). However, the slow escape rhythm is still visible between the spikes (best seen after the 6th spike). Later, dissociation between pacing and ventricular rhythm is even more evident despite marked post-pacing artifacts (B).

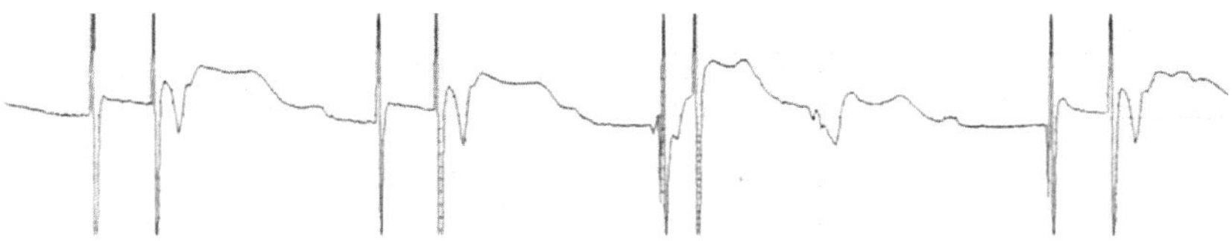

Figure 50. Atrial lead dislocation of a DDD pacemaker. The atrial activity is not sensed, which leads to asynchronous pacing without atrial capture, followed by ventricular pacing with capture. The 3rd beat is a sinus beat conducted with prolonged AV delay, which is sensed in the ventricular safety pacing interval, so a ventricular safety pace is delivered without capture – the ventricle is refractory at this time.

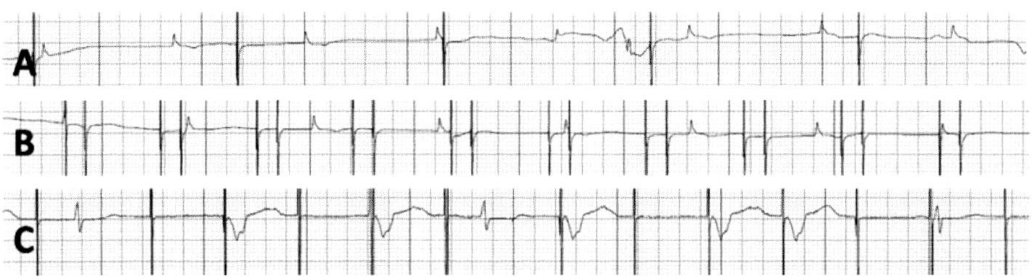

Figure 51. (A) Undersensing and ineffective pacing with a unipolar pacemaker. Both single chamber atrial and ventricular pacemakers would present similarly in case of lead dislocation. (B) Complete failure of sensing and pacing in a dual chamber pacemaker. There is asynchronous dual chamber pacing, without capture in either chamber. Unipolar pacing causes notable post-spike artifacts, which should not be confused with cardiac electrical activity. (C) Intermittent loss of capture with a ventricular pacemaker. Sensing appears to be normal as each spontaneous QRS resets the pacing cycle. The last spontaneous beat comes very early after the pacing stimulus and is likely not detected due to sensing in the blanking period.

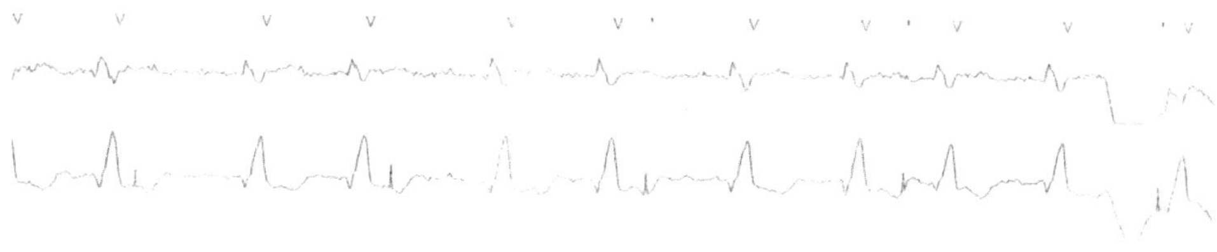

Figure 52. Lead dislocation in a recently implanted single chamber ICD. There is no ventricular sensing, so the pacing is at 40/min, asynchronous to the intrinsic rhythm. There is also lack of capture – attention should be paid when assessing capture as spikes 1-3 come very early when the ventricles may still be refractory. However, spike 5 should have lead to capture.

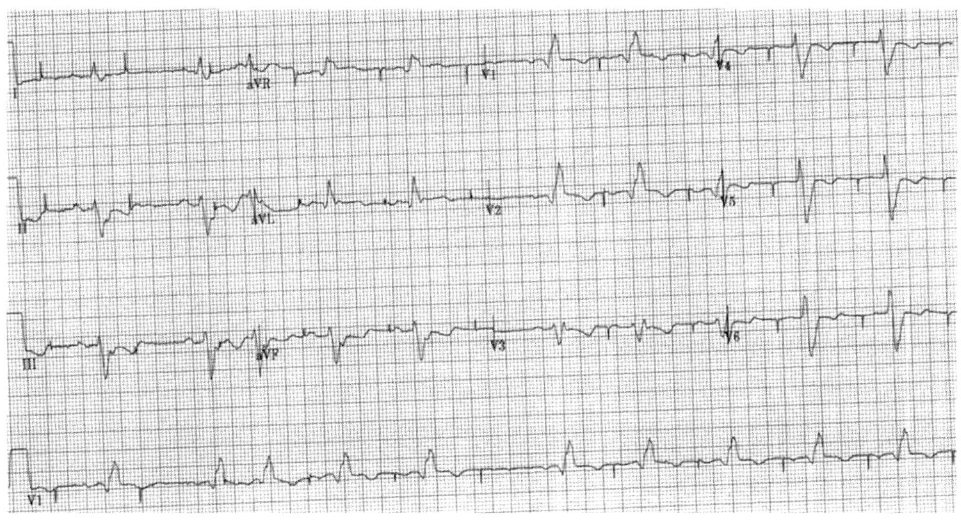

Figure 53. Intermittent loss of atrial capture during AAI stimulation. There is also intermittent undesensing - the atrial activation before the 3rd spike was not detected by the device. This scenario is suspicious for lead disclocation.

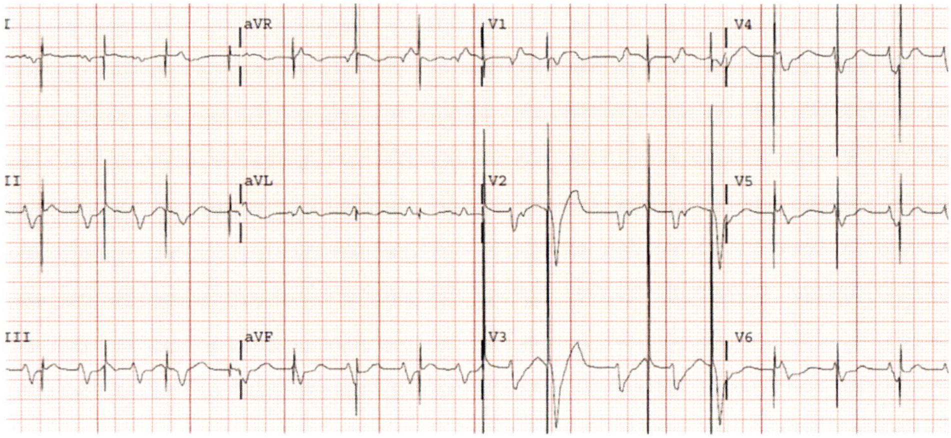

Figure 54. Loss of sensing with oversensing in a ventricular pacemaker. The first few beats may be misinterpreted as atrial pacing, however, the spike to QRS interval is not constant. Fusion and paced beats are seen when pacing occurs during an excitable period. Transient oversensing caused delayed pacing (3rd spike in V3). This scenario is suggestive of lead dislocation or failure.

6. Evaluation of ICD function

Implantable cardioverter defibrillators have multiple therapeutic zones (bradycardia, „physiological", ventricular tachycardia and fibrillation - VT, VF), that should be taken into account when interpreting ECG changes. While issues due to undersensing or ineffective capture usually manifest similarly to a pacemaker, oversensing may lead to inappropriate therapy due to false VT/VF detection.

As ICD therapies may cause severe patient distress or proarrhythmia, prompt device interrogation and expert consultation is required after such events, unless appropriate device behavior is evident (Figures 55-56). Even when appropriate therapies have been delivered, the patient has to be fully evaluated and appropriate measures should be taken to reduce the risk of arrhythmia recurrence (Mishkin, 2009). In cases when inappropriate therapy is suspected and the risk of recurrence is high (atrial fibrillation with rapid ventricular rate, oversensing), a magnet may be applied to temporarily inhibit tachyarrhythmia therapies, until the device may be interrogated and appropriately reprogrammed (Figure 57). Continuous monitoring is required in the meantime as the patient will not be protected from malignant tachyarrhythmias while in magnet effect.

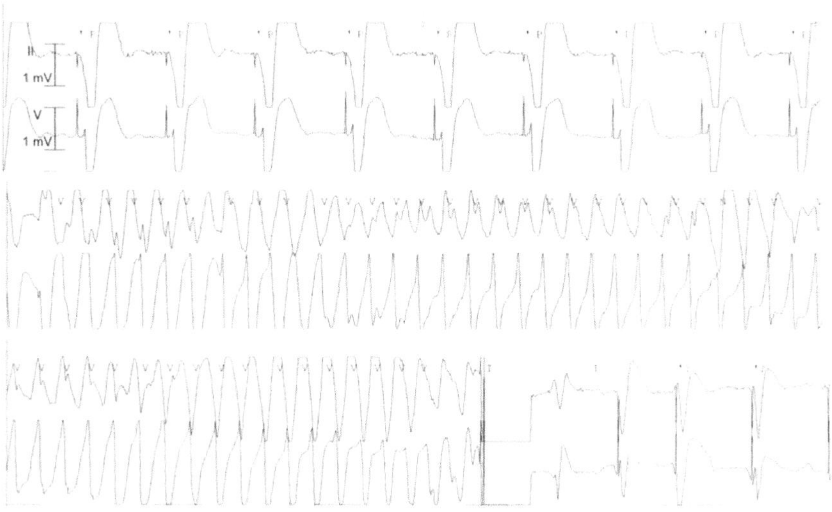

Figure 55. Appropriate ICD function recorded on telemetry. Following ventricular paced rhythm, rapid polymorphic ventricular tachycardia develops, which is terminated by a single endocardial shock after appropriate detection.

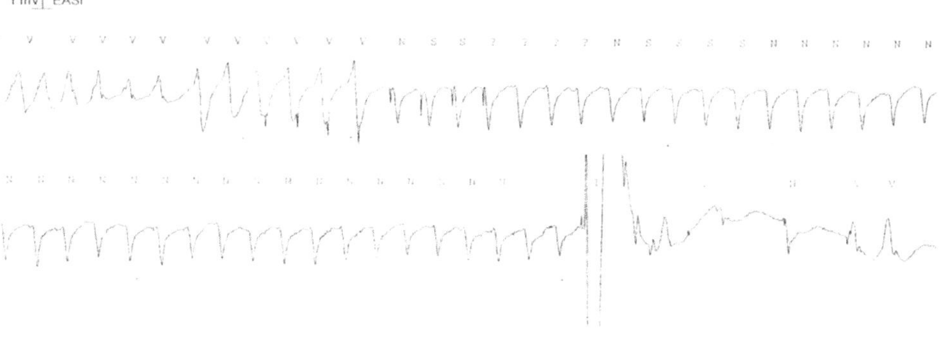

Figure 56. Appropriate ICD function recorded on telemetry. Following ventricular paced rhythm, rapid polymorphic ventricular tachycardia develops, then burst antitachycardia stimulation is attempted, however, fails to terminate the arrhythmia, although changes it to monomorphic VT. The tachyarrhythmia is terminated by an endocardial shock.

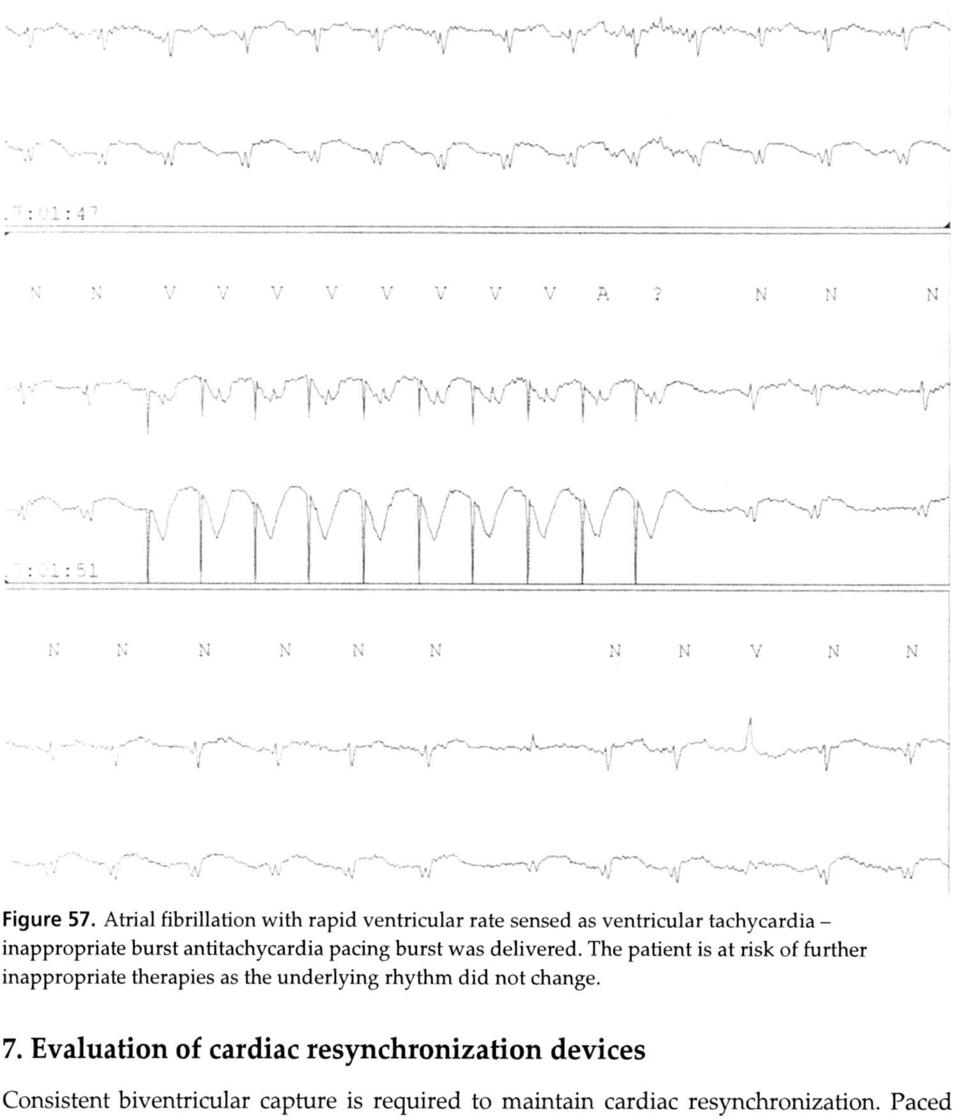

Figure 57. Atrial fibrillation with rapid ventricular rate sensed as ventricular tachycardia – inappropriate burst antitachycardia pacing burst was delivered. The patient is at risk of further inappropriate therapies as the underlying rhythm did not change.

7. Evaluation of cardiac resynchronization devices

Consistent biventricular capture is required to maintain cardiac resynchronization. Paced QRS morphology may vary based on underlying conduction abnormalities, lead location, interventricular delay and the amount of myocardium captured by each lead, relative to each other. Typically, right axis deviation and atypical RBBB pattern is present. If interventricular delay is set greater than 0 ms, usually two pacing spikes can be seen prior to the QRS (Figure 58). In rare cases, conventional RV pacing may mimic biventricular paced QRS morphology (Figure 59). QRS morphology may change due to variable fusion with conducted beats either from variable AV delay or atrial fibrillation (Figures 60-61).

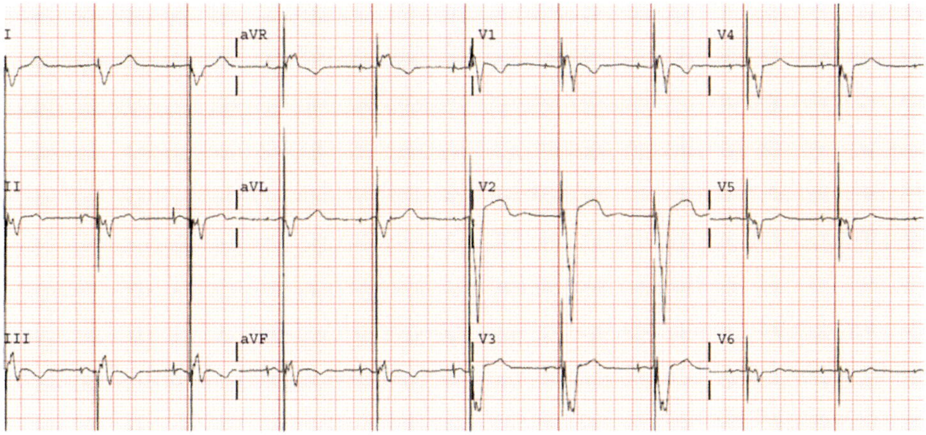

Figure 58. Typical atriobiventricular pacing. The paced QRS usually shows right axis deviation and an atypical RBBB pattern in V1. Two distinct pacing spikes, representing right and left ventricular stimulation with a delay around 20 ms, can be best seen in II and V3 on this tracing.

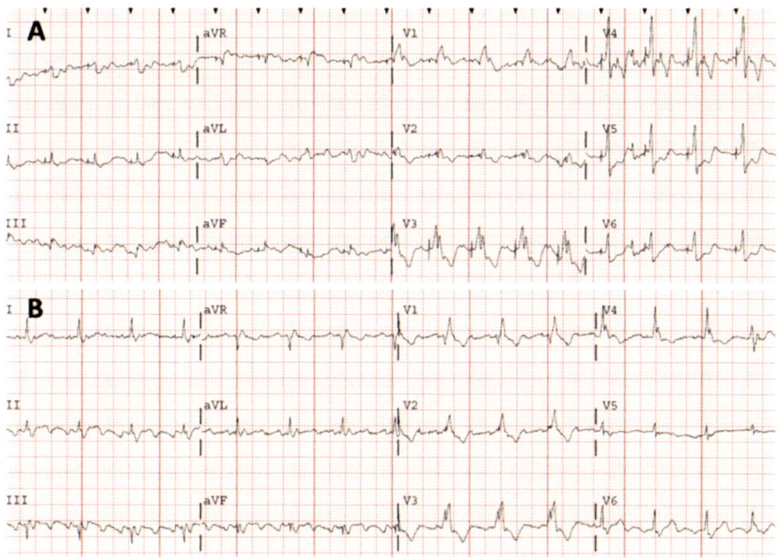

Figure 59. Although biventricular pacing may be recognized in most cases, underlying RBBB may mimic this QRS morphology during right ventricular pacing, especially, if fusion is present – this patient has a DDD pacemaker (A). His previous ECG showed atrial flutter with RBBB (B).

Sense response pacing is an algorithm that was designed to maintain the benefits of biventricular stimulation with premature beats or fast AV conduction – in case a ventricular event is sensed, a pacing stimulus is delivered simultaneously to decrease ventricular activation time. The resulting QRS morphology is affected by the origin of the premature beat and the amount of fusion (Figures 62-64).

Loss of left ventricular lead capture changes QRS morphology, so it becomes similar to RV pacing. A full 12-lead ECG should always be obtained during follow-up (Barold, 2011a and Barold, 2011b). Comparison with previous tracings is recommended as biventricular paced QRS morphology varies individually (Figure 65). Undersensing or oversensing may be more difficult to identify with resynchronization devices, than with conventional pacemakers, due to the algorithms designed to maintain biventricular pacing (Figure 66-67). In uncertain cases, device interrogation should be performed to prevent loss of resynchronization.

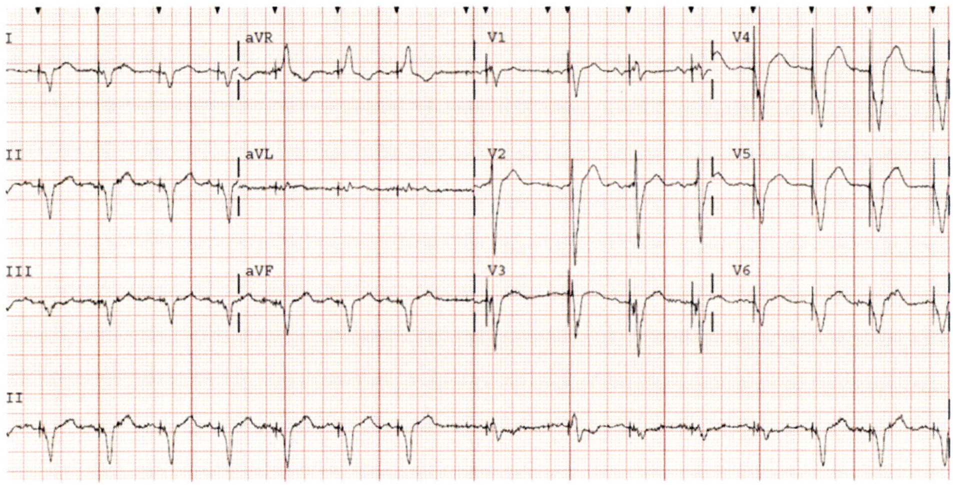

Figure 60. Variable fusion during biventricular pacing due changes in the atrial rate – the degree of ventricular fusion is different for atrial sensed and atrial paced beats, due to different atrioventricular delay, affecting how much of the ventricular myocardium can be activated through the native conduction system during biventricular pacing.

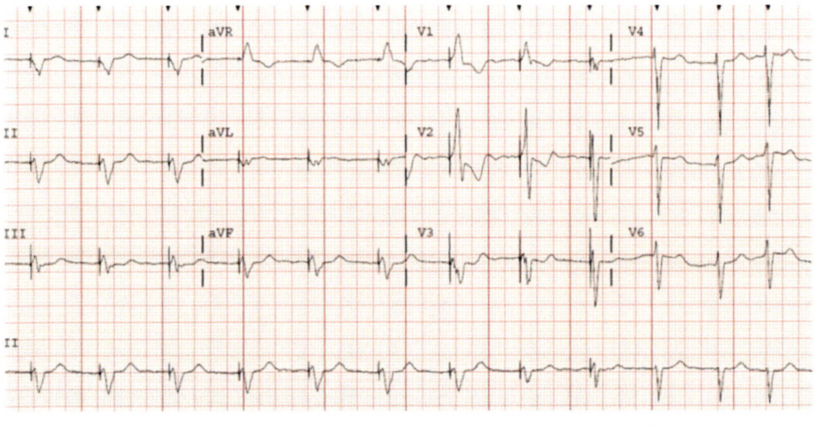

Figure 61. AF with biventricular pacing. When the ventricular rate increases, first it leads to more fusion, then to sense response pacing – appropriate response of the system.

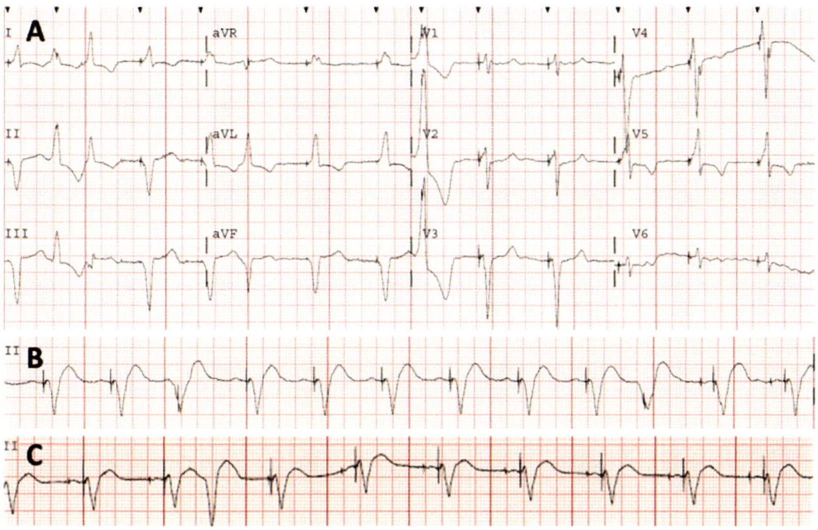

Figure 62. Sense response pacing during biventricular stimulation – each ventricular sensed event (PVC, rapidly conducted AF) leads to simultaneous pacing, aiming to maintain optimal hemodynamics of biventricular pacing. Due to the various origin of these early beats, the result can be fusion of even pseudofusion. Despite irregular rate and variable QRS morphology, this tracing shows appropriate biventricular pacemaker function (A). This function may be easier to evaluate when the underlying rhythm is regular, such as in sinus rhythm (B). There is an appropriate sense response pace for each premature beat. Depending on the coupling interval of the premature beat and the atrial rate, this may lead to post-event atrial pacing, if the compensatory pause exceeds the basic pacing rate. Very early PVCs do not trigger sense response pacing if that would exceed a maximal tracking rate (C).

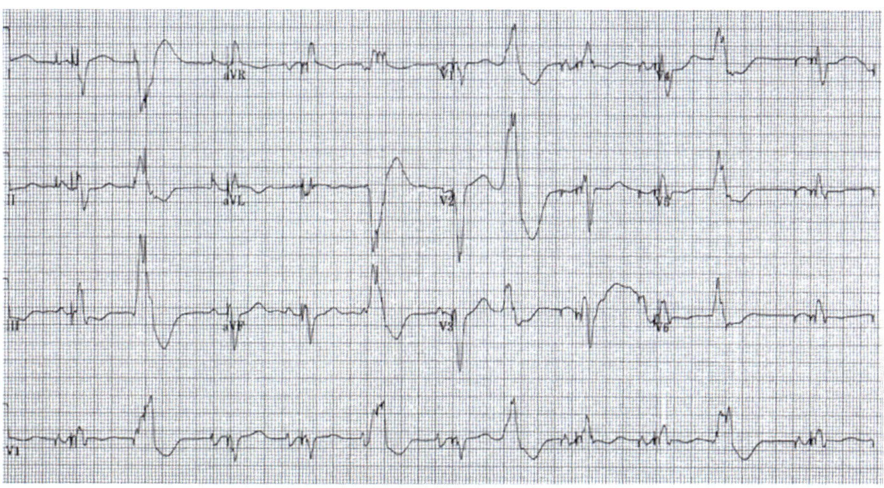

Figure 63. Atriobiventricular pacing with irregular ventricular rhythm due to frequent PVCs. Appropriate device behavior with sense response pacing during PVCs (best seen during the 1st PVC). There is notable interventricular delay between the right and left ventricular stimulation (60 ms).

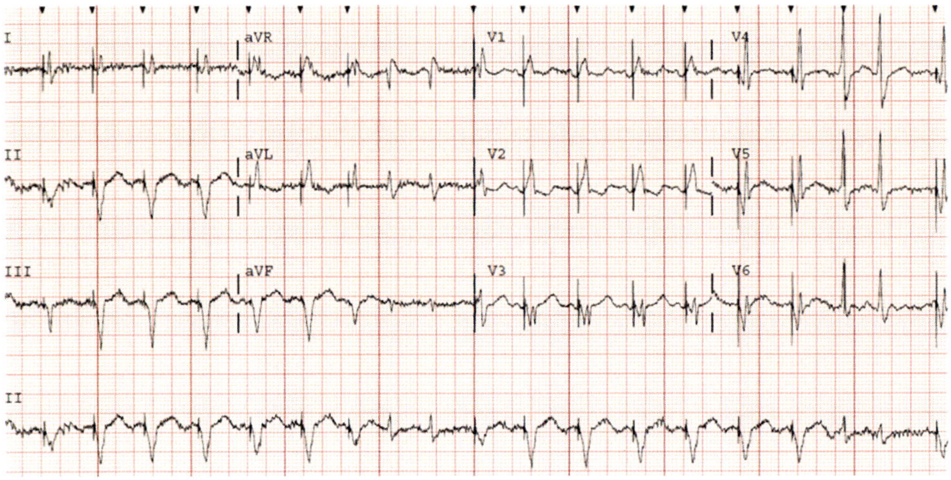

Figure 64. Biventricular (sense response) pacing ceases above the upper biventricular tracking rate – this is appropriate pacemaker function, however, may lead to rapid deterioration if the tachycardia persists.

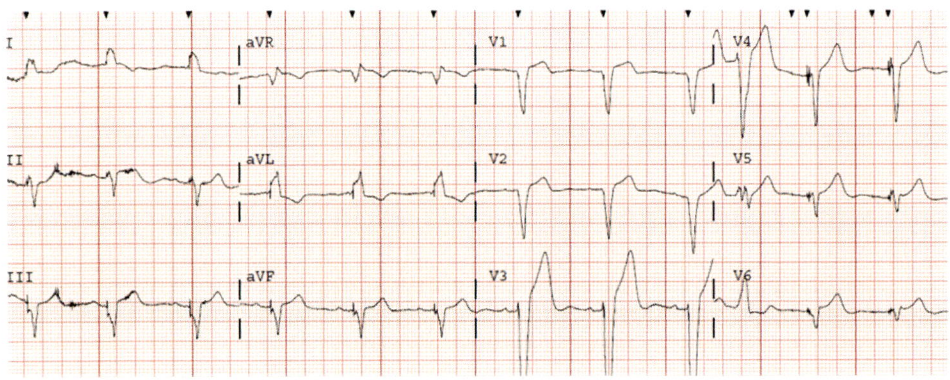

Figure 65. LBBB QRS morphology in a patient with a biventricular system should raise the suspicion of left ventricular non-capture. Other causes include suboptimal LV lead placement or too long RV-LV delay – these may diminish the amount of myocardium activated by the LV lead during biventricular pacing. In this case, biventricular pacing with 40 mm VV delay is apparent in V4.

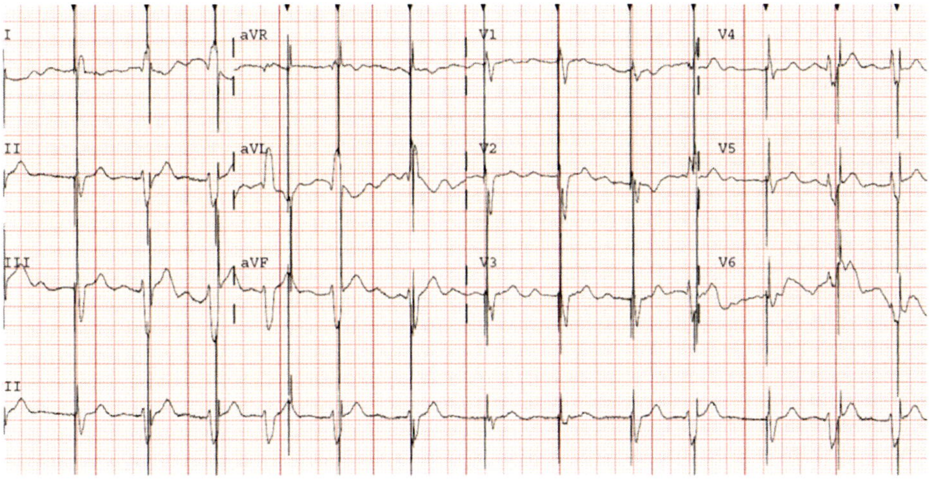

Figure 66. Intermittent ventricular undersensing in a biventricular system. Most ventricular beats are biventricular paced at 75/minute or sense response paced (occurring faster that 75/min). However, there are few spikes coming late (instead of a sense response pace), at 75/minute – the ventricular activation was not detected by the device. The undersensing is intermittent, as the sense response paced beats present on this tracing require a sensed event.

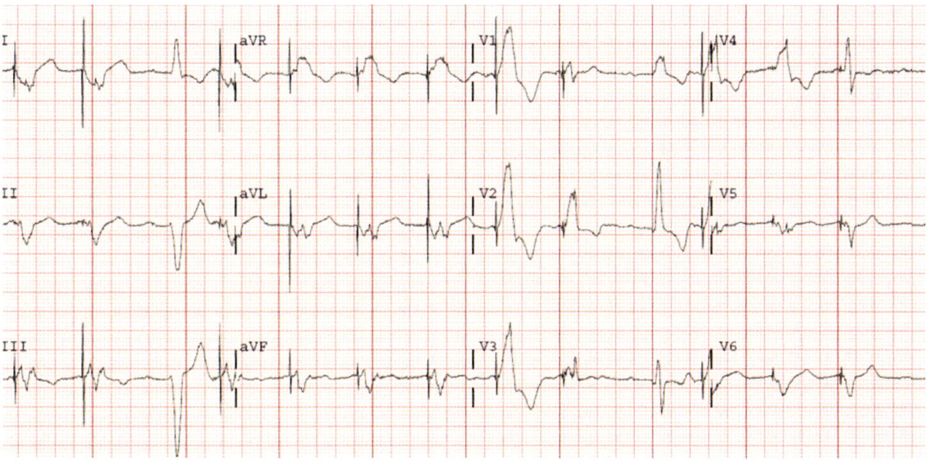

Figure 67. Pacing below the basic rate in an atriobiventricular system is always abnormal – algorithms are designed to maintain the ventricular rate, track premature beats and provide sense response pacing. This patient with a biventricular defibrillator had a fracture of the right ventricular sensing/pacing/shock ICD lead, leading to intermittent ventricular oversensing and multiple inappropriate shocks.

7. Conclusion

Conventional 12-lead ECG is an important tool to evaluate CIED function. A systematic approach is required to identify appropriate device function and to decide whether further investigation is necessary. As advanced devices, such as implantable cardioverter-defibrillators and cardiac resynchronization systems become more abundant, even common malfunctions and pseudo-malfunctions may be more difficult to identify, due to the presence of special pacing algorithms. In uncertain cases, review of prior patient data, device interrogation and expert consultation is required.

Author details

Attila Roka
Hospital of St. Raphael, New Haven, CT, USA

8. References

Balachander, J., et al., Pacemaker trouble shooting and follow up. Indian Heart J, 2011. 63(4): p. 356-370.

Barold, S.S., et al., Usefulness of the 12-lead electrocardiogram in the follow-up of patients with cardiac resynchronization devices. Part I. Cardiol J, 2011. 18(5): p. 476-486.

Barold, S.S., et al., Usefulness of the 12-lead electrocardiogram in the follow-up of patients with cardiac resynchronization devices. Part II. Cardiol J, 2011. 18(6): p. 610-624.

Goldschlager, N., et al., Environmental and drug effects on patients with pacemakers and implantable cardioverter/defibrillators: a practical guide to patient treatment. Arch Intern Med, 2001. 161(5): p. 649-655.

Ip, J.E., et al., Differentiating pacemaker-mediated tachycardia from tachycardia due to atrial tracking: Utility of V-A-A-V versus V-A-V response after postventricular atrial refractory period extension. Heart Rhythm, 2011. 8(8): p. 1185-1191.

Israel, C.W., Analysis of mode switching algorithms in dual chamber pacemakers. Pacing Clin Electrophysiol, 2002. 25(3): p. 380-393.

Jacob, S., et al., Cardiac rhythm device identification algorithm using X-Rays: CaRDIA-X. Heart Rhythm, 2012. 8(6): p. 915-922.

Lahiri, M.K., et al., Strategies for pacemaker programming in acute heart failure. Heart Fail Rev, 2011. 16(5): p. 441-448.

McPherson, C.A., et al., Permanent pacemakers and implantable defibrillators: considerations for intensivists. Am J Respir Crit Care Med, 2004. 170(9): p. 933-940.

Mishkin, J.D., et al., Appropriate evaluation and treatment of heart failure patients after implantable cardioverter-defibrillator discharge: time to go beyond the initial shock. J Am Coll Cardiol, 2009. 54(22): p. 1993-2000.

Wilkoff, B.L., et al., HRS/EHRA expert consensus on the monitoring of cardiovascular implantable electronic devices (CIEDs): description of techniques, indications, personnel, frequency and ethical considerations. Heart Rhythm, 2008. 5(6): p. 907-925.

Chapter 4

Strategies and Pacemaker Algorithms for Avoidance of Unnecessary Right Ventricular Stimulation

D. Bastian and K. Fessele

Additional information is available at the end of the chapter

http://dx.doi.org/10.5772/48747

1. Introduction

Since the first implantation of a pacemaker was done in 1958, this effective form of antibradycardia therapy has evolved in an amazing way. Besides ensuring the survival of patients with asystole or complete AV block who lack a sufficient intrinsic escape rhythm, today there is a wide range of further indications including advanced therapy strategies for pacing therapy. After it was shown that frequent right ventricular (RV) stimulation (especially in the RV apex (RVA)) can be associated with clinical deterioration in patients with implanted cardioverter-defibrillators (ICD) the avoidance of unnecessary RV pacing (RVP) has become one of the cornerstones of modern ICD- and PM-therapy.

2. Pathophysiology of RV-stimulation

With intact cardiac conduction, the physiological excitation of the ventricles occurs with high velocity (3-4m/s) over the His-Purkinje-system (HPS) nearly synchronously. This is the basis for an optimum hemodynamic contraction sequence in all heart chambers.

Similar to the excitation in a premature ventricular contraction (PVC) or following conduction through an antegrade conducting bypass tract, ectopic ventricular stimulation will result in a more or less non-physiologic activation and therefore non-physiologic contraction sequence of the ventricles. For example, the conduction after stimulation in the RV apex (RVA) will occur mostly in the working myocardium with a significantly lower velocity ≤1 m/s in an apico-basal direction from the RV via the interventricular septum to the left ventricle (LV). The exact individual sequence of excitation and contraction will be influenced by stimulus location, activation of parts of the specific conduction system and electroanatomical characteristics of the myocardium (fibrosis, scars). The dyssychronous contraction resulting from atypical excitation due to pacing can be compared to the situation in patients with conduction delay or block in the left Tawara-bundle (left bundle branch block (LBBB)).

At the start of systole (isovolumetric phase) the myocardial fibers near the RVA-pacing site will be the first ones to shorten, whereas the more remote left lateral ventricular areas will go into passive stretching, as they are lacking electrical excitation at this point. In the ejection phase the early activated areas will be able to contract only a little further, whereas the later activated areas will contract 1) delayed and 2) increased due to the previous stretching (Fig.1 and 4).

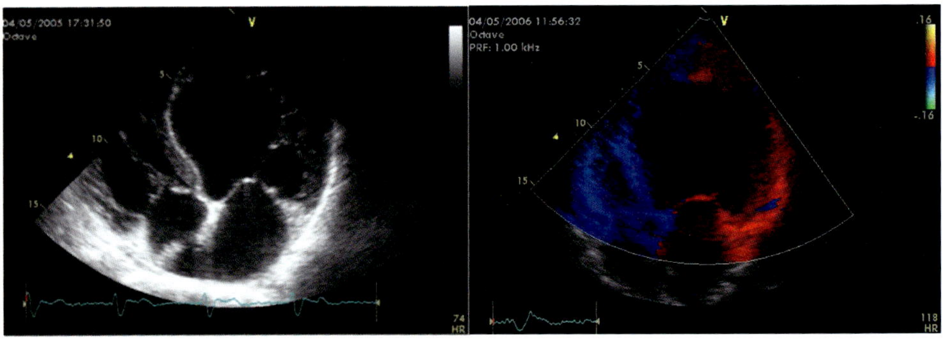

Figure 1. Transthoracic echocardiogram (TTE, apical 4-chamber view (A4CH)). There is preserved global systolic LV-function but longstanding left ventricular dyssynchrony (here resulting from LBBB) causes a typical hypertrophy of the left lateral wall compared to the interventricular septum. This is due to the delayed systolic LV lateral wall activation and the increased contraction after the preceding passive stretching.

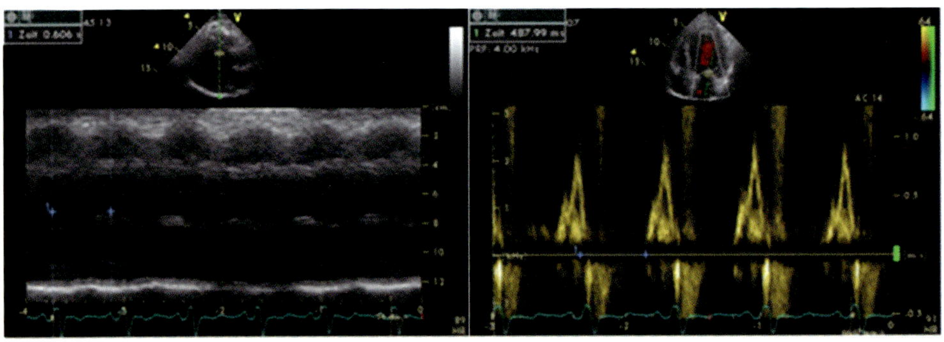

Figure 2. a. TTE, m-mode, parasternal long axis (PLAX); 2b. Doppler at mitral inflow, A4CH. Demonstration of systolic contraction of the left posterolateral ventricular wall (LV-PLW) while there is already left ventricular filling. The time interval Δt 1 from the beginning of the QRS complex to the end of anterior movement of the LV-PLW (fig. 2a) is longer than Δt 2: from the beginning of the QRS complex to the start of transmitral filling (figure 2b). Transmitral doppler shows fusion of E- and A-wave, representing an overlap of the passive and active LV-filling, which is therefore shortened and reduced.

The electromechanical dyssynchrony influences the diastole as well. Whereas the first activated areas of myocardium already enter the relaxation cycle, the delayed activated ones can still be in systolic contraction. This late systolic contraction delays the passive ventricular filling and thereby shortens the effective duration of diastole (Fig. 2) [1].

The delayed dyssynchronous activation of the ventricle with RV stimulation is visible in the ECG by a more or less deformed and widened QRS complex (Fig. 3).

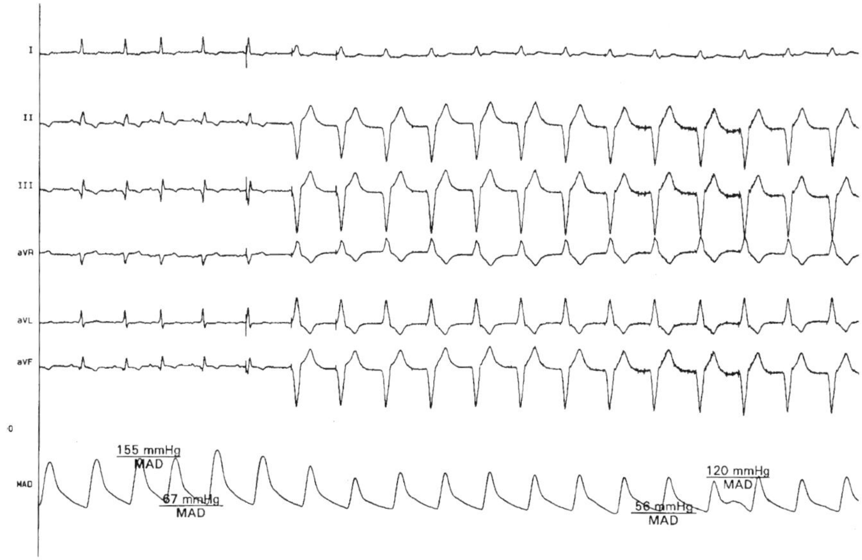

Figure 3. 12 Lead-ECG of VVI pacemaker stimulation in the right ventricular apex. The stimulated QRS complex is visibly widened, shows a negative deflection in the inferior leads (II, III, aVF) and LBBB-like deformation. Note the fall of aortic pressure with VVI stimulation here in a patient with sinus rhythm.

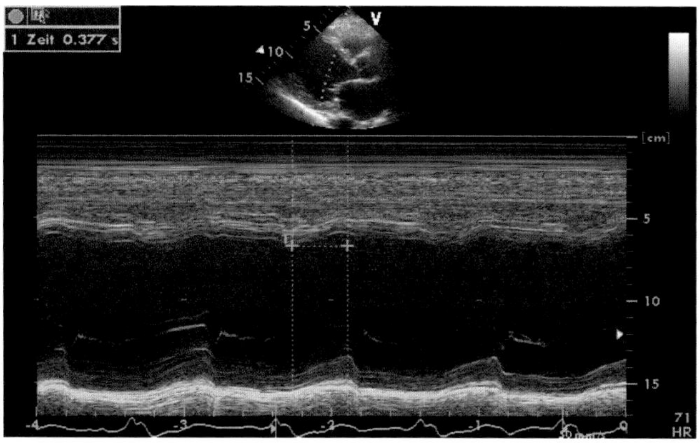

Figure 4. TTE, m-mode, PLAX. Demonstration of the different times for maximum systolic contraction of the interventricular septum and the LV posterolateral wall. The "septal to posterior wall motion delay" (SPWMD) is measured as 377 ms in this case. Values > 130 (140) ms are considered pathological.

Echocardiography allows excellent noninvasive estimation of global and regional electromechanical dyssynchrony and hemodynamic consequences. Examples are shown in Fig 1, 2 as well as 4 and 5). For more detailed information further specialized reading is recommended [2-5].

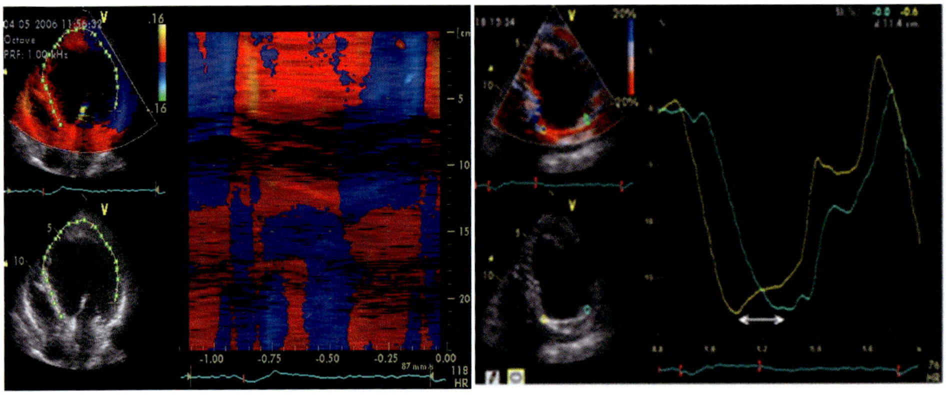

Figure 5. Visible shift of the contraction phases of interventricular septum and lateral LV wall, color-m-mode (5a) and tissue-doppler / strain (5b).

3. Clinical consequences of unnecessary right ventricular pacing

The first evidence for clinically relevant negative effects of a high percentage of RV pacing was found interestingly in studies that were originally intended to show benefits of "physiologic" AV sequential DDD stimulation compared to VVI stimulation.

The original intention of the DAVID trial (Dual Chamber and VVI Implantable Defibrillator) was to show a survival benefit of dual chamber ICD systems compared to single chamber ICDs. Patients with an ejection fraction <40% and chronic heart failure were enrolled, who didn´t have an indication for antibradycardia stimulation. The study was stopped early after enrollment of 506 patients: the patients with the supposedly "physiological" AV sequential DDD pacing (at least 70/min) had a 1.61 increased risk for mortality or hospitalization because of new onset or deteriorated heart failure compared to patients with VVI backup stimulation (40/min) only [1,6,7]. The proportion of ventricular stimulation was 55.7% in the DDD group compared to 2.9% in the VVI patients.

In a sub-study of the MOST trial (Mode selection Trial) it was shown that patients with DDD(R) stimulation for sick sinus syndrome / sinus node dysfunction (SSS / SND) and normal QRS duration (<120 ms) had a significant increase of their risk for heart failure hospitalization (HFH) associated with an increase of cumulative percentage RVP (cum%RVP) up to 40% [1,8].

Interestingly the correlation between the percentage of RV stimulation and the risk for HFH was different for patients with DDDR versus VVIR stimulation.

After detailed review it seemed that the risk for HFH stayed nearly constant for percentages of VP >40% in the DDDR mode. It was therefore speculated that the risk of HFH in the DDDR mode would not increase with further increases in cum%RVP above 40%, but a further risk reduction to about 2% could be achieved with minimization of unnecessary RV pacing (VP <10%).

Overall the relative risk for hospitalization due to heart failure was always higher for VVIR patients compared to DDDR patients who had a comparable percentage of cumulative right ventricular stimulation.

Furthermore a linear relationship, between RV pacing and the incidence of atrial fibrillation (AF), was found up to a right ventricular stimulation percentage of 85% [8].

This observation was confirmed in a prospective randomized study including 177 patients with SSS, by demonstrating that AAIR stimulation was associated with a significantly lower incidence of AF compared to DDD stimulation with a short (≤150 ms) or a long (300 ms) AV interval [9]. Furthermore no significant changes were observed for left atrial (LA) or left ventricular diameters in the AAI(R) population, whereas in both DDD(R) groups the LA diameter increased significantly.

A sub-analysis of the MADIT II study (Multicenter automatic defibrillator trial II) was also able to show a clear correlation between more frequent RV stimulation and increasing morbidity and mortality for the included collective of ICD patients [10]. With increased RV stimulation the percentage of VT episodes was higher. If there was a cum%RVP of ≥50% a significant increase of the risk for HFH was observed (p<0.001).

Gardiwal et al. showed that apart from an LV ejection fraction (EF) <40% a cum%RVP >2% is an independent predictor for the occurrence of ventricular tachyarrhythmias, mortality and episodes of heart failure in ICD patients (who had predominantly secondary prophylactic ICD indications) [11].

Since the implementation of specific algorithms for avoidance of unnecessary RV stimulation in modern PM and ICD systems several studies have shown the clinical relevance and necessity of this approach. The details of these studies will be shown in the following sections respectively.

4. Strategies and algorithms for avoiding unnecessary right ventricular stimulation

4.1. Single-chamber AAI(R) pacing

In patients with single SND and completely intact AV conduction, the implantation of an AAI(R) system theoretically appears to be the best form of pacemaker therapy especially considering the - here 100% - avoidance of RV stimulation [12]. It has to be emphasized, that this pacing modality is so far the only one with a prognostic benefit (overall and cardiovascular mortality of 225 PM patients with SND) that was proven in a study: in the

DANISH trial the AAI(R) stimulated patients had a higher survival rate, less deaths due to heart failure (HF) and other cardiac causes, less AF and fewer thromboembolic complications compared to the group with VVI(R) stimulation [7,12-14].

Indication:

In principle all AAI systems can be indicated in single SND without evidence of impaired AV conduction or concern over development of AV block in the future.

The following conditions have to be present:

- No AV block of any degree (including °1)
- Narrow QRS complex
- Antegrade 1:1 conduction / Wenckebach point >120 (130)/min
- No need for any medication causing conduction delay
- No carotid sinus syndrome
- No loss of consciousness as primary indication for pacing therapy.

Patients with carotid sinus syndrome or vasovagal syncope are not suitable for AAI systems, because apart from the inhibition of the sinus node intermittent AV block is encountered. [14].

Whereas the overall percentage of AAI(R) pacemaker systems is about 9-10% in Scandinavian countries [1,7], atrial single-chamber pacemakers are only implanted in selected cases in other countries. The German PM register lists for the year 2009 a nearly constant low implantation rate of 0.5% AAI systems [15]. The reasoning behind it is, that relevant AV conduction disturbances are often not detectable or foreseeable at the time of implantation, however a later manifestation cannot be predicted or excluded for the individual patient. The incidence of new onset AV block is overall low and is reported to be approximately between 0.65% and 1.8% per year [1,12,16]. In studies on atrial pacing for SND a median annual incidence of third-degree AV block of 0.6% (0%-4.5%) with a total prevalence of 2.1% (0-11.9%) was revealed. Potential clinical manifestations include

- Clinical symptoms due to AV block associated bradycardia, pauses or asystole, if there is no sufficient intrinsic escape rhythm. The incidence of syncope or near-syncope is high within the group of patients with onset of higher degree AV block.
- AAI pacemaker syndrome with non-physiologic long intrinsic, hemodynamically unfavorable AV delay (Fig. 6)

The fixation of the atrial lead in the appendage usually provides a stable position and good results for sensing and pacing threshold. Relevant ventricular far field signals should be ruled out carefully. Alternatively septal atrial (active) lead placement in the area of Bachmann´s bundle (Fig. 7) can provide a more synchronous atrial activation resulting in a shorter P wave duration. There is some evidence that septal atrial pacing might have preventive effects on the incidence and progression of atrial fibrillation [51,52].

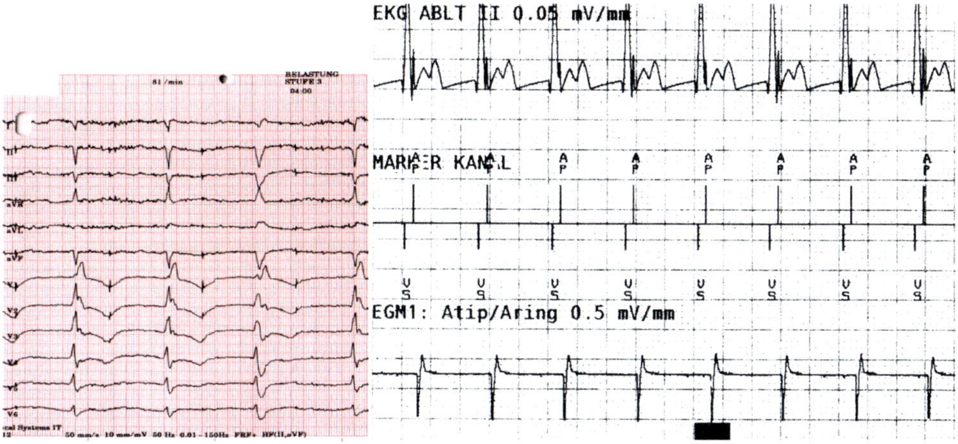

Figure 6. a. 12-lead stress test ECG: Unlike the normal physiologic response there can be a lack of shortening or even an increase of the intrinsic AV conduction delay during AAI stimulation with exercising in some patients with SND: the atrial stimulation can appear in extreme cases within the preceding systole (atrial stimulus shortly after or even within the QRS complex), the (nearly) simultaneous contraction of atria and ventricles can be the consequence, resulting in an AAI PM syndrome (6b).

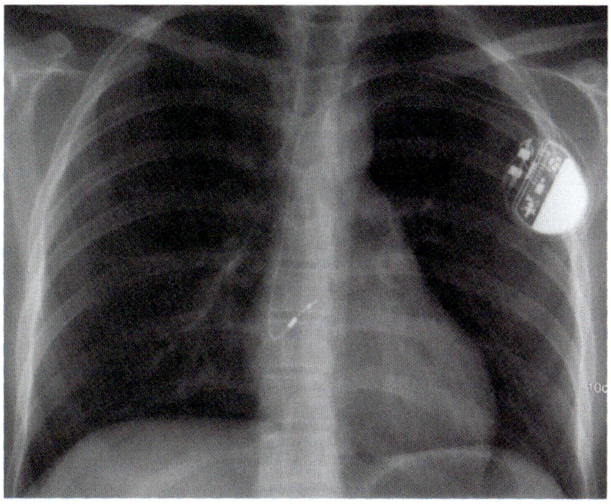

Figure 7. Chest x ray. Single-chamber AAI PM implanted on the right side in a young female patient with symptomatic idiopathic sinus bradycardia. The active atrial electrode is placed at the septum, resulting in a narrow P wave indicating better synchronized activation of the atria.

If there is impaired AV conduction, a dual- or triple-chamber pacemaker system should be implanted. This should be considered in patients with advanced cardiac disease as well [14].

The indication for implantation of single-chamber AAI PM in patients with SND is currently questioned even more after the results of the DANPACE trial (The Danish multicenter randomised trial on AAIR versus DDDR pacing in sick sinus syndrome) [Nielsen, ESC Congress 2010]. The aim of this study was to compare AAIR with DDDR stimulation (lower rate 60/min, upper rate 130/min, paced/sensed AV-interval ≤220 / ≤200 ms). As main finding there was no survival difference for the 1415 patients in the two groups after follow up over 5.4±2.6 years. The mortality of all causes was 29.6% in the AAIR group versus 27.3% in the DDDR group (p=0.53.). There was a doubling of reoperation risk with AAIR pacing. After correction for baseline variables, the patients in the AAIR group had a 27% risk increase for the development of atrial fibrillation. This contradicts the results of previous studies and therefore was not expected. However there was no monitoring regarding atrial fibrillation before enrollment, which means that a preexisting difference between the groups in AF prevalence already at baseline cannot be excluded. Additionally, monitoring in the follow up was not very sensitive for recognizing of AF episodes. The conclusion of the DANPACE authors was, that single-chamber (AAIR) pacing should be avoided in patients with SND and that DDDR stimulation using an AV interval ≤220 ms should be the pacing modality of choice for SND.

In his guest editorial for PACE in 2001 S. Barold concluded that permanent single-chamber atrial pacing is *obsolete*: "Proponents of AAI(R) pacing claim it is safe but dual-chamber pacing is *safer* than AAI(R) pacing and more suitable for the overall care of SSS patients." [17].

4.2. VVI stimulation with low intervention rate („VVI backup")

The guidelines of the German society of cardiology state that VVI stimulation with a low intervention rate (e.g. <45/min) can be indicated, if there is rare disturbance of AV conduction (occurrence <5%) [indication class I B]. [14,18,19].

Fröhlig justifies the indication for implantation of a simple „VVI backup"-PM system in patients with recurrent syncope due to paroxysmal AV block, BBB and normal HV interval [1]. These patients have a high risk for further syncopal episodes. If there is no need for antibradycardia pacing apart from the short phases of paroxysmal AV block, this subgroup can be fitted adequately with a sole VVI „backup" stimulation of 40/min.

Compared to pacemaker patients the situation looks different in patients with an ICD indication only, without need for antibradycardia pacing. The above mentioned DAVID study showed superiority of single chamber ICD systems with a programming of VVI 40/min to a dual-chamber mode [1,6,7].

In 2007 the INTRINSIC RV trial enrolling 988 ICD patients showed that the group with DDD pacing (60-130/min) with AV search hysteresis (AVSH, Boston Scientific) was not inferior to the VVI backup pacing group (40/min) in terms of all-cause mortality and heart failure hospitalization after 10 months follow up [20]. In the DDDR AVSH group the mean cum%RVP was 10% compared to 3% in the VVI pacing group. It has to be emphasized however, that prior to randomization only patients that had <20% ventricular stimulation in the first week after implantation in DDDR AV search hysteresis mode were selected and therefore would be regarded as likely "responders" to AVSH.

The MVP trial was a prospective, multicenter, randomized, single-blind, parallel, controlled clinical trial which didn`t succeed in showing that atrial-based dual-chamber managed ventricular pacing mode (MVP™) is equivalent or superior to backup only ventricular pacing (VVI 40/min) with regard to time to death, heart failure hospitalization and heart failure–related urgent care in patients with standard indication for ICD therapy and no indication for antibradycardia pacing. The overall HF event rate was found to be slightly higher during AAI pacing and mainly seen in patients with a PR interval ≥230 ms in the MVP-60 group compared to VVI-40. There were no differences between the two compared ICD pacing modes for atrial fibrillation, ventricular tachyarrhythmias, quality of life, or echocardiographic measurements. [21].

There is an ongoing discussion with regard to a possible improvement of discrimination between supraventricular and ventricular tachyarrhythmias due to additional atrial information in dual-chamber ICD compared to VVI systems as this could avoid inadequate therapy deliveries by the ICD.

The DATAS trial found a reduction of clinically significant adverse events (CSAE) in dual-chamber ICD versus single-chamber devices or simulated single-chamber mode in implanted dual-chamber systems [22]. It was possible to reduce the occurrence of inadequate ICD shocks for atrial fibrillation in dual-chamber ICDs. Procedure related complications were more frequent with dual-chamber devices.

A meta-analysis from 2008 (748 patients) found less inappropriate treated episodes with dual-chamber discrimination but the number of patients experiencing inadequate therapies was not reduced [23]. It has to be known that the programmed criteria for differentiation of supraventricular and ventricular tachyarrythmias in the VVI ICD in this study were most commonly "onset" and "stability". Modern single-chamber ICDs offer markedly improved discrimination algorithms as standard today.

In summary the majority of patients with ICD indication only, i.e. lacking foreseeable demand for antibradycardia pacing or indication for CRT at the time of implantation, can be fitted adequately with a modern VVI ICD system and a backup-rate of 30-40/min. Advantages include avoidance of unnecessary RV stimulation, less expensive and less complex systems, less complications at implantation and in the long term course by using just a single lead. Most of the time in current single-chamber ICDs using modern algorithms there isn´t worse SVT/VT discrimination compared to dual-chamber ICDs.

The disadvantage of this strategy is: If the need for regular pacing arises in the clinical course of patients with single-chamber ICDs the upgrade to a dual-chamber or CRT system is often a more complex procedure.

Therefore, dual-chamber ICD systems should be preferred (of course unnecessary RVP should still be avoided when possible):

- Conventional PM indication (especially SND; with permanent AV block II º or IIIº consider CRT-system)
- Long-QT-Syndrome

- History of (frequent) atrial tachyarrhythmias.

4.3. DDD stimulation with fixed long AV delay

Programming of a fixed long atrioventricular delay (AVD) supports intrinsic conduction in patients with largely intact or only mildly impaired atrial and atrioventricular conduction and thereby avoids unnecessary RV stimulation.

However, even in patients with isolated disease of the sinus node and a programmed fixed AVD of 300 ms, a percentage of >10% RV stimulation is found in about every third patient [1,24]. It has to be kept in mind that the IEGM determined AVD of the PM is not identical with the PQ interval measured in the surface ECG. The relevant AV interval for the timing of the PM in atrial stimulation consists of: conduction time from the stimulus to the atrium, intra- and interatrial conduction times, AV conduction and the time to the expected actual detection of ventricular activation, which sometimes can be markedly delayed up to the S wave of the chamber complex [25].

In clinical practice the following problems have to be considered with fixed long AVD programming [25]:

- A prolonged AVD results in an extension of the total atrial refractory period (TARP, fig. 8). Depending on the programmed postventricular atrial refractory period (PVARP) a limitation of the upper rate behavior can be the consequence, i.e. respectively lower limitation of the upper 1:1 AV conduction rate (upper tracking rate, 2:1-block rate), which can lead to problems with higher degree AV block on exercising.

  Example: with an AVD of 300 ms plus a PVARP of 300 ms, the PM is not able to detect atrial rates above 100/min 1:1 anymore and if there is a higher degree AV block to track AV sequentially 1:1.

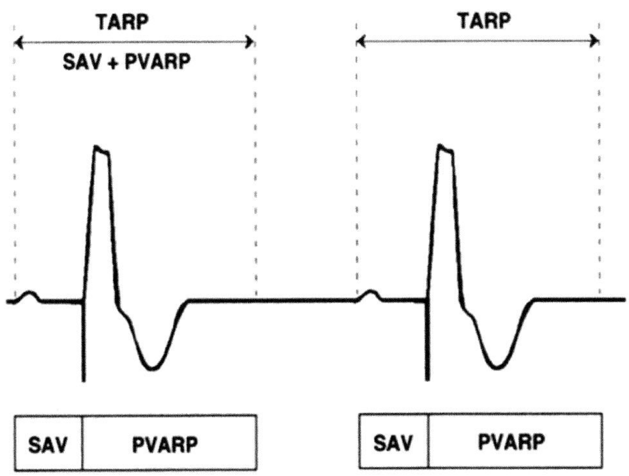

Figure 8. TARP = AV Delay + PVARP

- If as compensation the PVARP is programmed shorter in patients with preserved VA conduction, the occurrence of pacemaker mediated tachycardias (PMT) is facilitated.
- With an extremely long AVD the frame for detection of intrinsic atrial activities is limited, which sometimes - depending on the postventricular atrial blanking period (PVAB) - can possibly lead to an impairment of the mode switch reaction in atrial tachyarryhthmias [26].
- In case of higher degree AV block with resulting need of ventricular stimulation the (ultra-) long fixed AVD may result in a less favorable hemodynamic situation.
- If there is intermittent atrial undersensing (typically in atrial fibrillation) a very long AVD may favor proarryhthmogenic pacemaker-induced R-on T-stimulation. To avoid this a short postatrial ventricular blanking period should be programmed and the ventricular safety stimulation (safety window pacing) should be activated [25].

With SND and preserved AV conduction DDIR mode is recommended if a long AV delay is programmed [25,27]. Unfortunately this is not really an option in patients with intermittent AV block, as intrinsic P waves (AS-events) can't trigger AV sequential response then.

In summary the programming of fixed long AVD is associated with numerous problems. Nielsen et al. entitled a publication in 1999: "Programming a fixed long atrioventricular delay is not effective in preventing ventricular pacing in patients with sick sinus syndrome" [24]. For the effective avoidance of unnecessary RV stimulation the following modern algorithms should be preferred, if the implanted DDD PM offers these options.

4.4. AV hysteresis

To escape the problems associated with long fixed AVD the AV hysteresis was developed. The term "hysteresis" originates from the Greek *hysteros* = thereafter, later.

The algorithm distinguishes intact versus impaired / non-physiologically prolonged intrinsic AV conduction. A longer intrinsic AV conduction time is permitted ensuring stimulation with an optimized AV interval in case of a higher degree AV block.

Basically there are 2 sets of sensed or paced (AV / PV) atrioventricular intervals:

- The shorter AV-/PV delay becomes active, if the conducted intrinsic ventricular sensed (VS) event is missing.
- The longer (hysteresis) AVD will be switched to after VS events or when there is a search for intrinsic conduction [28].

The AV sequential cycle is mandatory for every beat.

- If *AV hysteresis* is activated the stimulated or sensed (short base) AV time will be extended by a programmable amount of time after a spontaneous VS event. This now long AV interval remains unchanged, as long as there is intrinsic AV conduction within this interval (VS). After ventricular stimulation (VP) the shorter AV interval becomes active. (fig. 9).

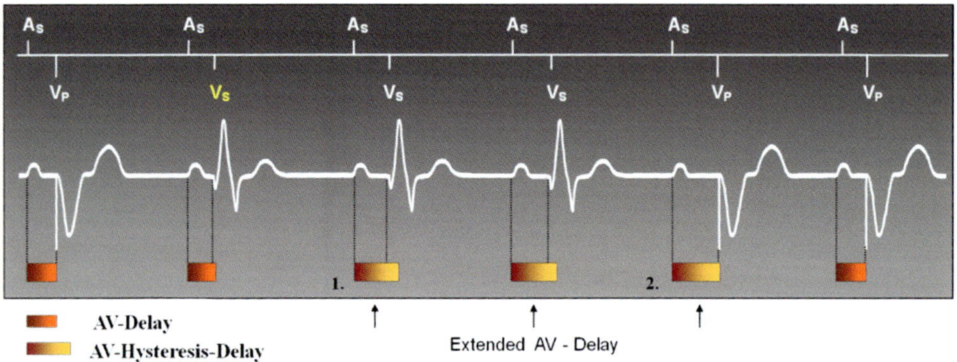

Figure 9. AV hysteresis: 1. After ventricular sensing (VS) the short AVD is extended by the programmed hysteresis interval. 2. A ventricular stimulation (VP) after the active long AVD deactivates the hysteresis and stimulation continues with the programmed short AV/PV delay.

- If an *AV repetitive hysteresis* is activated, a single VP event will not immediately result in switching to the short base AV interval, but the long AV hysteresis interval will remain for a programmed number of cycles. The set back to the short AVD will come if there is no intrinsic conduction during these cycles.
- The *AV search hysteresis* looks actively for preserved intrinsic conduction: In determined intervals the short base AV interval will be prolonged actively by the hysteresis duration for a set number of cycles (fig. 10).

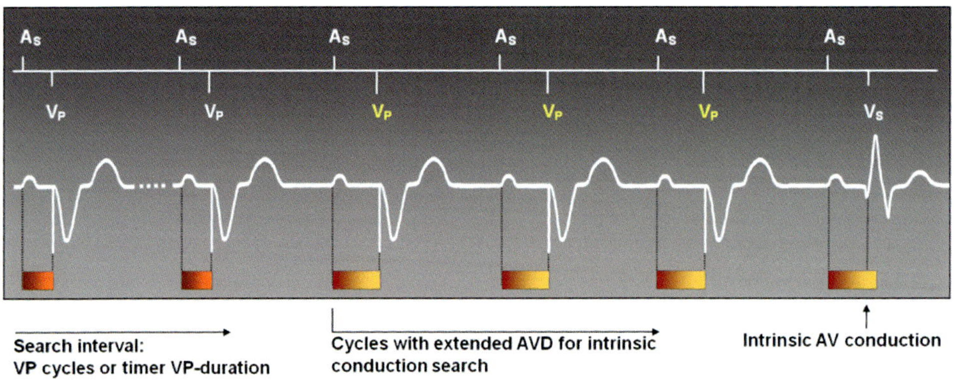

Figure 10. AV search and repetitive hysteresis.

Generally in modern devices these 3 algorithms can be activated combined in 1 function. The exact criteria that can be programmed (maximum AV time extension, search intervals) vary between the device manufacturers and models.

As examples available algorithms of 4 manufacturers are explained:

a. AV search hysteresis (AVSH (+)), Boston Scientific

- Example devices: INSIGNIA®, ALTRUA®, ADVANTIO™, INGENIO™
- Programming options (depending on the model):
  - AV delay 10 (30) up to 300 respectively 400 ms in 10 ms steps (device dependent)
  - Dynamic AVD
  - Minimum (10 to 290 ms) and maximum AVD (20 to 300 respectively 400 ms; device dependent)
  - AV search interval (off, 32, 64, 128, 256, 512, 1024 cycles)
  - AV increase (proportional increase of AVD extension during one search cycle; 10% to 100%)
- The AV delay will be extended periodically fixed or dynamical for up to 8 cycles to look for intrinsic conduction.
  - If the search was successful (ventricular sensing: VS), the extension will be continued, as long as there is intrinsic conduction (fig. 11). A switch back to the programmed AV / PVD is done after the first ventricular stimulus with long hysteresis AVD.
  - If the search is not successful, the stimulation continues with the programmed short AVD and a new AV search interval starts.

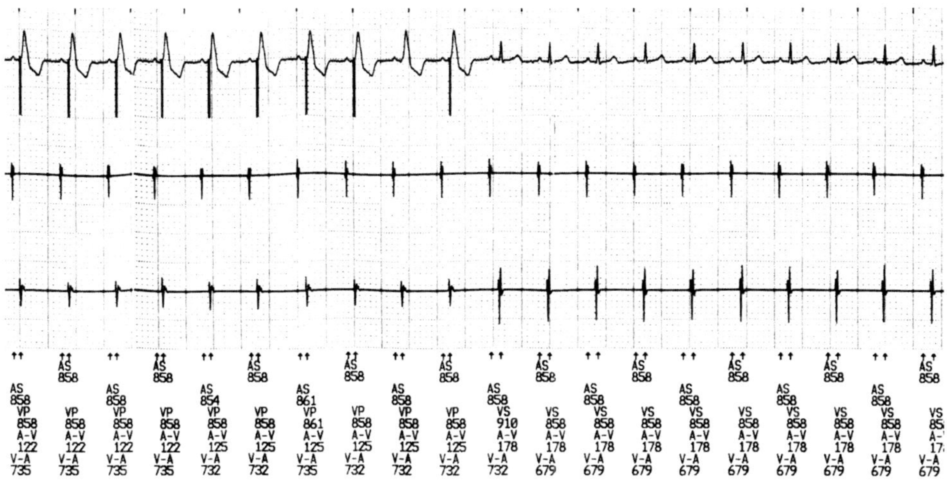

Figure 11. AVSH, BSCI. The tracing begins with AV sequential ventricular stimulation (AS/VP) with a programmed AVD of 125 ms. The extension of the AVD by the AV search hysteresis results in intrinsic conduction: AS/VS with an intrinsic AV interval of 178 ms.

b. AutoIntrinsic Conduction Search™ (AICS), St. Jude Medical

- Example device: INTEGRITY™ [53]
- With ventricular stimulation the function extends the AV / PVD every 5 minutes with a programmable hysteresis time (in ms) to search for intrinsic conduction.
  - On ventricular sensing the extension of the AV / PVD is set, a switch back is done after the first ventricular stimulus.
- The maximum AVD is 350 ms.

- The function becomes inactive in the following situations:
  - DDD(R) or VDD(R) mode + base rate ≥90/min + active rate dependent AVD
  - Intrinsic atrial rate or sensor rate ≥90/min
  - During rate search hysteresis.

c. Intrinsic Rhythm Support (IRSplus), Biotronik

- Example device: Philos II DR.
- When the IRSplus is activated, the following features are set:
  - AV hysteresis is at a fixed length of 300 ms. The long AV interval stays active if an intrinsic ventricular signal is sensed (VS).
  - In AV repetitive hysteresis there are five cycles with the prolonged AV /PV interval after a VS event has occurred. The AV hysteresis remains active, if intrinsic ventricular activity is sensed during one of these five cycles. However after five repetitive cycles without spontaneous AV conduction the device changes back to the short AV / PV interval.
  - In AV scan hysteresis there is extension of the AV delay for five cycles after 180 consecutive ventricular paced cycles. If in these five cycles a spontaneous AV conduction is detected, the AV hysteresis stays active. If no ventricular event has been detected within these five cycles the device switches back to the short AV delay interval and the cycles end with ventricular stimulation. The cycle counter is reset and commences counting the consecutive paced cycles.

d. Search AV™/Search AV™+, Medtronic

- Example devices: Kappa 700 DR, EnPulse™
- The PM will try to detect intrinsic conducted events in an "AV delay window" that precedes scheduled VP events by -55 to -15 ms.
- If the device classifies 8 out of 16 AV conduction sequences as too long /"late" (≤15 ms before scheduled VP), it prolongs the operating SAV and PAV intervals by 31 / 62 ms for the next 16 pacing cycles to facilitate intrinsic conduction until the maximum AVD. If the previous 8/16 AV intervals are defined as too short (>55 ms before scheduled VP), the device will shorten the operating SAV and PAV intervals by 8 ms for the next 16 pacing cycles.
- In the case of inadequate AV conduction (8/16 VP with maximum AVD) the search will be repeated after 15 and 30 minutes and then after 1, 2 … 16 hours. The algorithm is deactivated after 10 unsuccessful searching attempts / 16 hours until the next device interrogation.
- With the help of this algorithm intrinsic conduction is promoted even in cases with slightly changing AV conduction times and unnecessary long AV delay intervals are avoided.
- The maximum AVD is 350 (*Search AV™*) respectively 600 ms (*Search AV™+*).

Melzer et al. compared the above mentioned algorithms Search AV™ (max. AVD sensed 230 / paced 260 ms) versus Search AV+™ (max. AVD 300 / 360 ms) in a randomized study with 30 PM patients [29]. It could be shown that prolonging the AV interval above 300 ms results in an additional significant reduction of the percentage of ventricular stimulation (19±28% versus 70±40%, p<0.001).

A larger prospective non randomized multi-centre study enrolling 197 patients with a dual-chamber PM (EnPulse) demonstrated a Reduction of cum%RVP from 97.2% without AV interval extension to 23.1% with Search AV+™ [30]. There were no adverse events reported under Search AV+™ .

4.5. AAI(R)⇔DDD(R) mode switch

This strategy is currently considered the most effective form of reducing unnecessary RV stimulation. A dual-chamber system (PM or ICD) is implanted in the usual way with conventional atrial and ventricular leads. The programming follows a special AAI(R) mode, by which the device controls AV conduction with every beat. If intrinsic conduction is preserved, the stimulation will be in a functional AAI(R) mode. However, as the algorithm still maintains ventricular sensing to assess AV conduction, it acts technically like ADI(R) mode. In contrast to conventional dual-chamber systems with e.g. AV hysteresis these devices are allowed to accept even single non conducted p waves, e.g. as in second-degree AV block type Wenckebach (fig. 12).

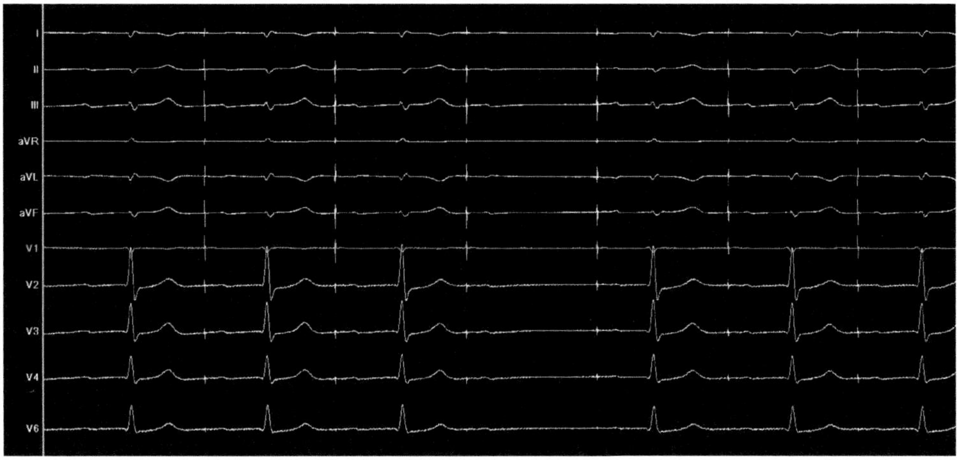

Figure 12. A dual-chamber PM with AAI⇔DDD mode switch (Reply DR, *AAISafeR2*™) accepts a single non conducted p wave in second-degree AV block type Wenckebach.

If a higher degree AV block occurs the device switches automatically to a dual-chamber mode according to defined criteria and keeps this up until improvement of intrinsic conduction.

This strategy thereby is thought to combine the advantages of the AAI(R) mode in avoiding unnecessary RV stimulation with the safety of DDD(R) backup.

To show examples 4 currently available systems will be explained.

a. AAISafeR™, AAISafeR2™, ELA Medical, Sorin Group
- Example devices: Symphony™ DR, Reply™ DR.

- AAISafeR™: loss of sufficient intrinsic AV conduction:

The switch to dual-chamber mode occurs following a defined pattern, by which the AV conduction is classified:

- 7 consecutive AV / PV intervals, that are too long (programmable for rest and exercise "first-degree AV block" criterion, fig. 13)
- 3 AS / AP events without VS within the last 12 atrial cycles ("second-degree AV block" criterion, fig. 14,15)
- 2 consecutive AS / AP without VS ("high degree AV block" criterion, fig. 16)
- Ventricular pause >2 up to 4 sec. (length of pause programmable, fig. 20)

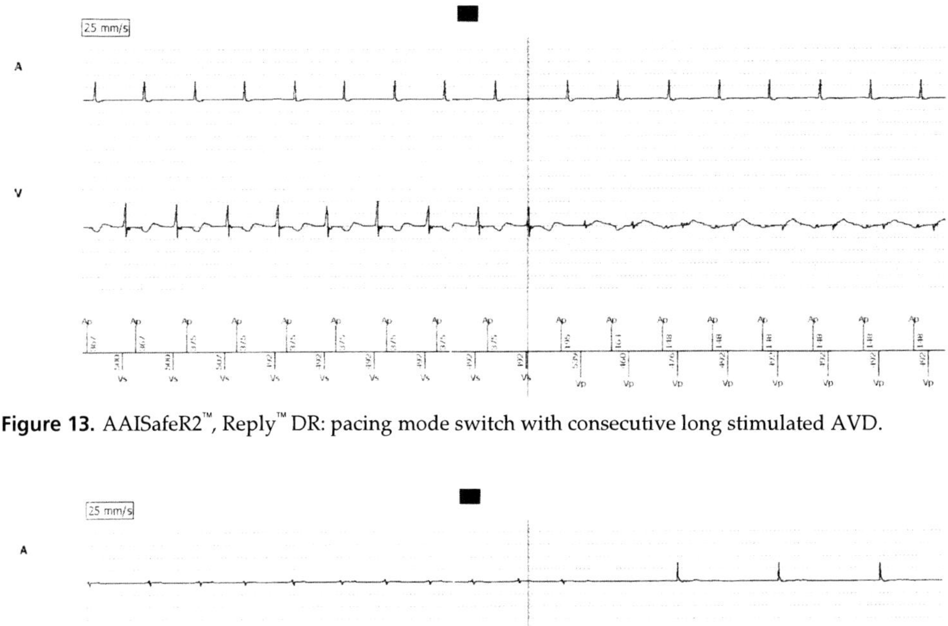

Figure 13. AAISafeR2™, Reply™ DR: pacing mode switch with consecutive long stimulated AVD.

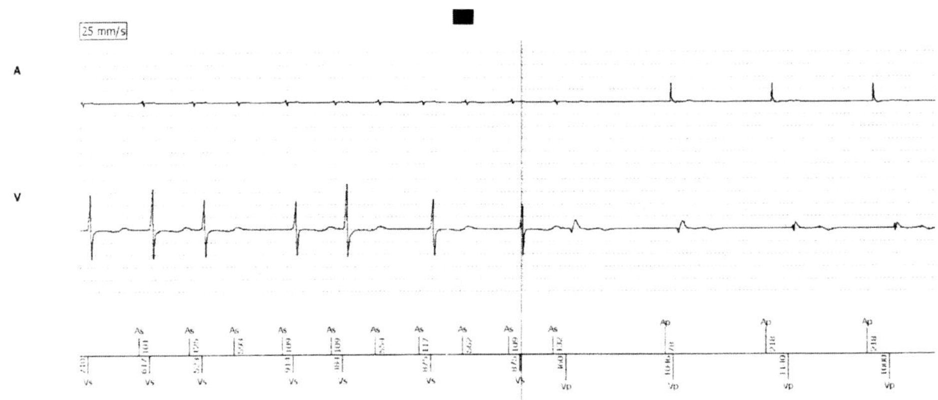

Figure 14. AAISafeR2™, Reply™ DR: mode switch after 3 of 12 consecutive sensed or stimulated atrial events without VS. (In this particular case the pacing mode switch is triggered by a frequency-dependent AV block caused by a short run of an atrial tachycardia, atrial CL about 450 ms).

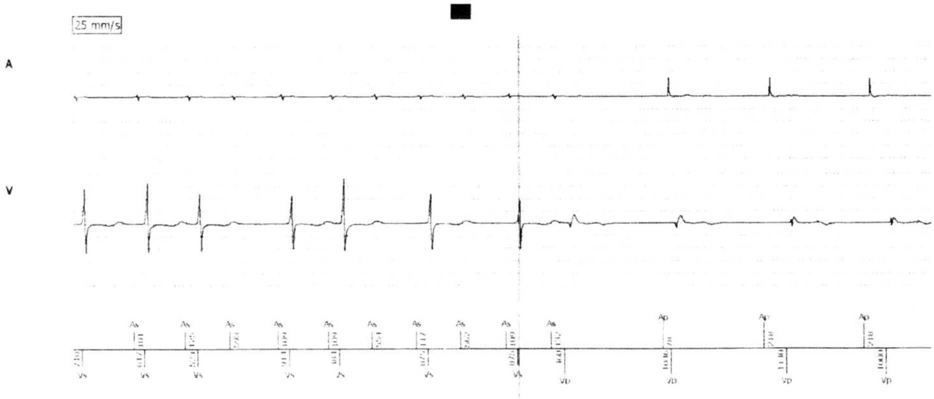

Figure 15. AAISafeR2™, Reply DR, Holter-monitoring: switch from AAI(R) to DDD(R) after 3 (in this case stimulated) atrial events without intrinsic conduction within the last 12 AA intervals.

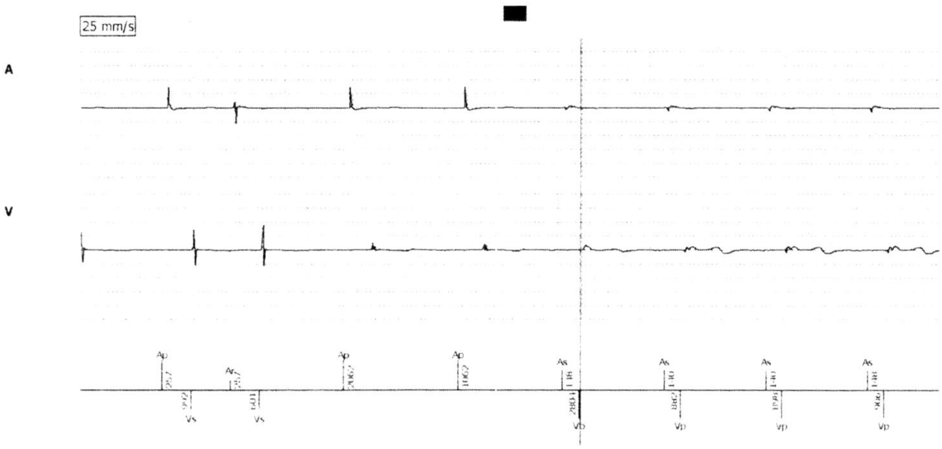

Figure 16. AAISafeR2™, Reply™ DR: paroxysmal AV block, possibly phase 4 block caused by critical prolongation of the PP interval after a conducted atrial premature beat ("Ar"). Switch from AAI to DDD after 2 consecutive atrial stimulated events (AP) without intrinsic conduction.

- AAISafeR™: Recurrence of sufficient intrinsic AV conduction

After 100 ventricular stimulations (VP) the device checks intrinsic AV conduction (fig. 17, 18, 20). A switch back from DDD(R) to AAI(R) takes place after 12 cycles of spontaneous conduction.

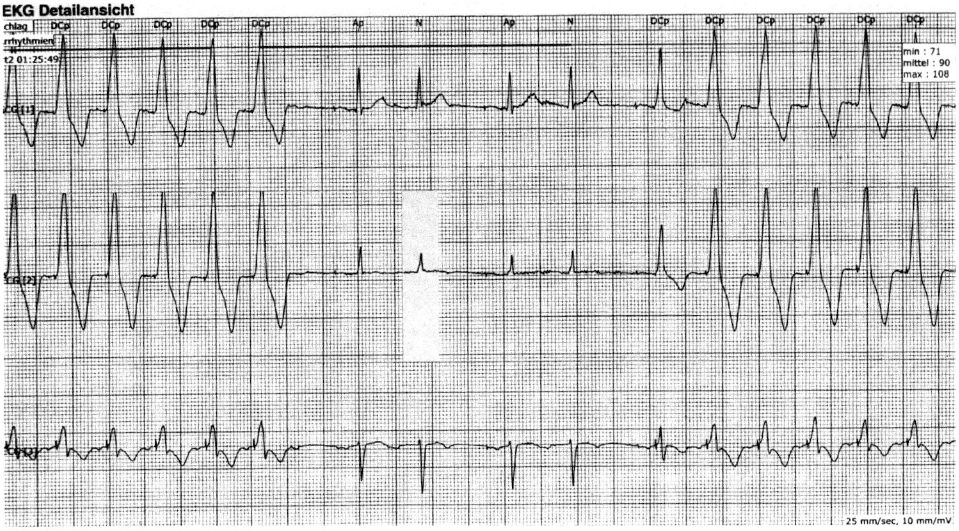

Figure 17. AAISafeR2™: After unsuccessful search for sufficient intrinsic conduction DDD(R) stimulation is continued.

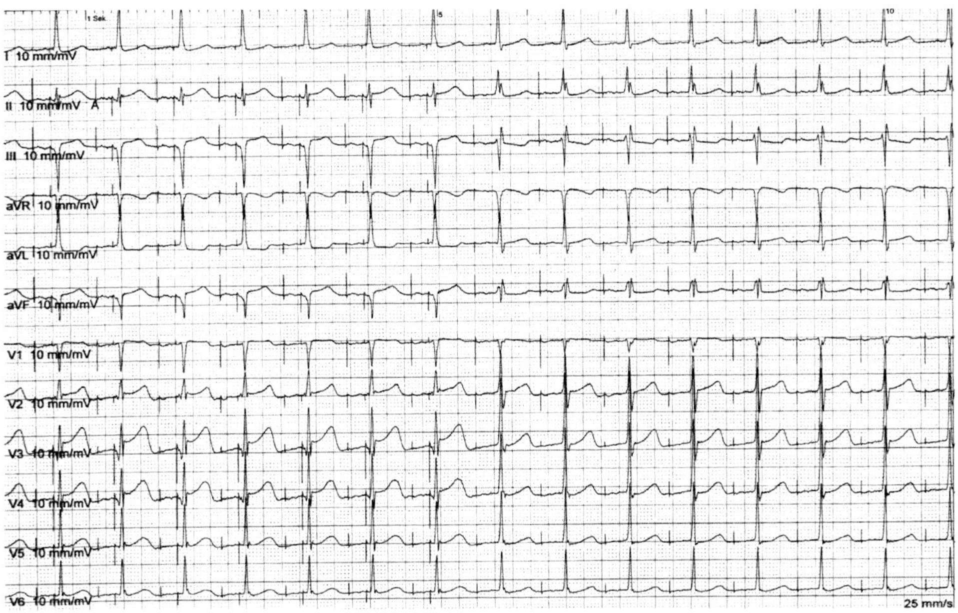

Figure 18. AAISafeR2™, Symphony™ DR: Successful mode switch from AV sequential DDD pacing with ventricular fusion to AAI mode resulting in intrinsic AV conduction (APace/VSense).

In contrast to MVP® the AAISafeR™ is programmed for a permanent switch to DDD(R) mode in case of persisting AV conduction disturbance:

- If there are ≥15 mode switches within 24 hours
- If there are >5 mode switches per day on 3 consecutive days

A specific feature is the pacing mode switch when there is sensing of a ventricular event within the committed window (ventricle, 94 ms after atrial stimulation, Vr). Whereas in the DDD mode after the Vr event a ventricular safety stimulation occurs, the SafeR mode is not counting a sensed Vr as conducted in this committed interval. This can lead to a switch from AAI(R) to DDD(R) (fig. 19)

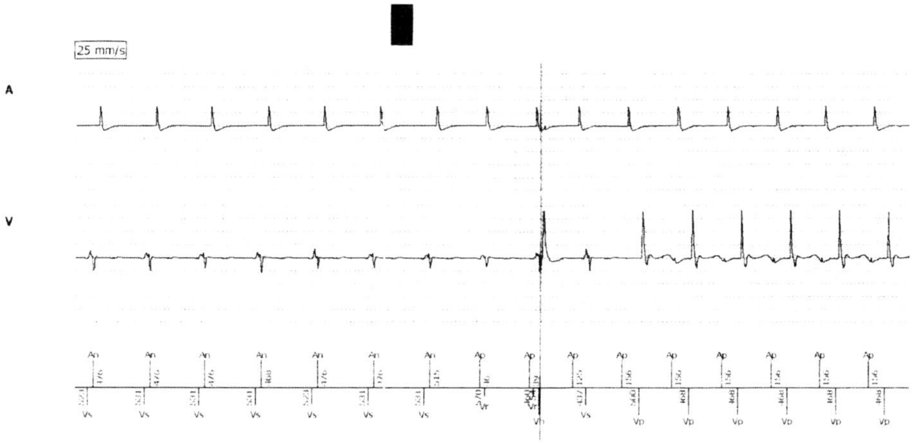

Figure 19. AAISafeR2™, Reply™ DR: With AAISafeR mode the occurrence of 2 consecutive ventricular events within the committed interval (Vr) results in mode switch to DDD. Once in DDD mode a safety stimulus is delivered here (Vn).

The efficiency of the AAISafeR™ algorithm was shown in an approval study enrolling 43 patients with SSS and intermittent AV block: after 1 month 65% of the patients remained in AAI(R) mode with a ventricular stimulation percentage of only 0.2±0.4%, in 35% of the patients the device automatically changed to permanent DDD(R) mode due to frequent mode switches (73±23% VP) [1,7,31,32].

AAISafeR2™ offers the following modifications [33]:

- The amount of time with stimulation in dual-chamber mode (>50%) is used as a criterion for a persisting impairment of AV conduction.
- If there is AV block with an exercise induced heart rate >100 this is not used as criterion for "persisting AV conduction impairment".
- The switch criterion "too long consecutive AV intervals" can be inactivated for resting.
- Even after switch to DDD(R) with persisting AV block the device runs a search for intrinsic conduction every morning (fig. 20).

Fröhlig et al. investigated the algorithm in 123 PM patients with SND, paroxysmal AV block or Bradycardia Tachycardia Syndrome (BTS). In 97/123 patients an adequate switch to DDD was seen, with 69 patients (56%) this wasn´t persisting, the average %VP was 0.2±0.5 [33].

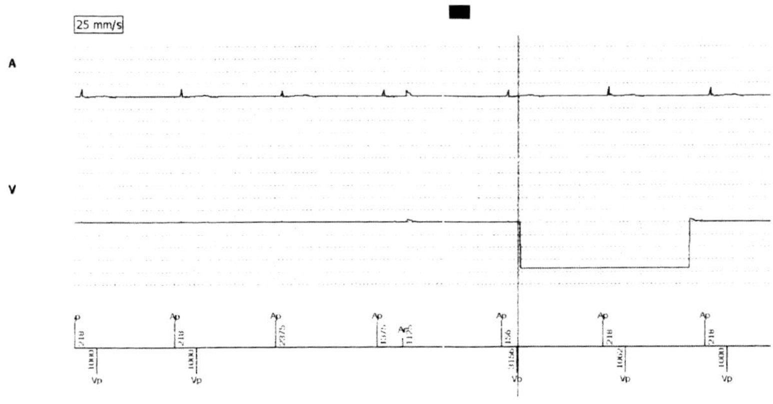

Figure 20. AAISafeR2™, Reply: Unsuccessful search for intrinsic conduction in a patient with third-degree AV block, resulting in a long pause > 3 sec. DDD mode is maintained.

The majority of publications about AAISafeR2™ didn´t report any adverse events [32-35].

Thibault et al. observed 2 SafeR related adverse events among 208 PM patients:

1 patient with SND and second-degree AV block complained of dizziness. 24-hour electrocardiogram revealed ventricular pauses as cause, another patient with SND and first-degree AV block presented with unexplained syncope. In both of these cases the device was reprogrammed to DDD [36].

b. Ventricular pace suppression (Vp Suppression), Biotronik.
- Example devices: Evia / Entovis.

Depending on evaluation of intrinsic AV conduction the device works either in DDD(R) or ADI(R) mode. Independent of that the system offers a mode switch to DDI(R) for atrial tachyarrhythmias (fig. 21).

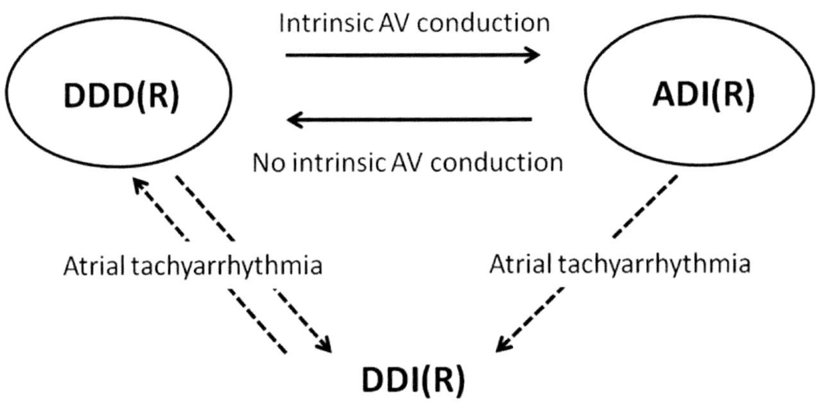

Figure 21. Stimulation forms of the Vp Suppression algorithm, Biotronik

- Vp Suppression: DDD(R) mode

With Vp Suppression activated the system stimulates first in the DDD(R)-mode with a programmed AVD. A VS search is started after a VS event or if there is no intrinsic conduction within 0.5 min. AVD is then extended to 450 ms to search over 8 cycles for intrinsic conduction. The device switches to ADI(R), if the programmable criterion "x consecutive VS" is met. It is possible to program 1, 2…8 consecutive VS events in individual steps, default 6. If the criterion isn´t met within the VS search period, the device continues to work in the DDD(R) mode with the programmed AVD and the searching interval is doubled up to maximum of 128 min. Thereafter the next search is initiated every 20 h, as long as Vp Suppression is activated.

- Vp Suppression: ADI(R) mode

A cycle without intrinsic conduction / VS within 450 ms triggers an observation period of 8 repetitive cycles, to make the decision about switching back to DDD(R) mode according to the following criteria:

- x/8 cycles without VS (programmable)
- 2 consecutive cycles without VS
- No VS for at least 2 sec.

c. RYTHMIQ™, Boston Scientific

- Example devices: ADVANTIO™, INGENIO™, ENERGEN™, INCEPTA™

The algorithm is automatically activated, if the indication-based programming (IBP) is used.

- RYTHMIQ™: Intact intrinsic AV conduction

If there is preserved intrinsic AV conduction, the system works in the AAI(R) mode at the lower rate limit (LRL) or sensor rate (SIR) with backup VVI stimulation at a rate which is 15/min below the programmed LRL [37]. The VVI backup can be provided between a rate not slower than 30/min but not faster than 60/min. During AAI(R) mode the device continuously checks AV synchrony.

- RYTHMIQ™: Loss of sufficient intrinsic AV conduction

The device automatically switches to DDD(R) mode, if three blocked or "slow ventricular beats" are documented within a rolling detection window of 11 beats. RYTHMIQ™ defines a "slow ventricular beat" as a ventricular event (VS or VP) occurring at least 150 ms slower than the atrial pacing rate (LRL of SIR) [37].

- RYTHMIQ™: Reoccurrence of sufficient intrinsic AV conduction

From DDD(R) mode a regular search for intrinsic conduction is carried out by using the AV Search+ algorithm. The pacing mode is switched back to AAI(R) with VVI backup, if AV Search+ 1) can remain in AV hysteresis for a minimum of 25 intervals and 2) less than two out of the last ten cycles are VP events [37].

- RYTHMIQ™: Mode switch for atrial tachyarrhythmias

The algorithm is able to detect atrial tachyarrhythmias from either AAI(R) with VVI backup or DDD(R). In the case of detection of atrial tachyarrhythmias the system immediately changes to the ATR mode switch.

d. Managed Ventricular Pacing® (MVP®), Medtronic
- Example devices: Adapta L ADDRL, Ensura DR MRI™, Protecta DR.
- MVP®: Intact intrinsic AV conduction [38]

The device works in the AAI(R) mode with programming and timing for atrial single-chamber stimulation. At the same time there is active surveillance of AV conduction.

The atrial refractory period (ARP) cannot be programmed. It is set to 600 ms for rates <75/min respectively 75% of ventricular cycle length (CL) for rates ≥75/min. This dynamic ARP is intended to stop unnecessary switch episodes with singular non conducted atrial extra beats (PAC) or R wave far-field sensing.

If there are fast intrinsic ventricular events (e.g. PVC, VT) the atrial stimulation is inhibited. This is done to avoid unnecessary atrial stimulation, if the intrinsic ventricular rate is higher than the stimulation rate. Additionally the recognition of tachyarrhythmias is facilitated, if there is no interference by the blanking periods after atrial stimulation.

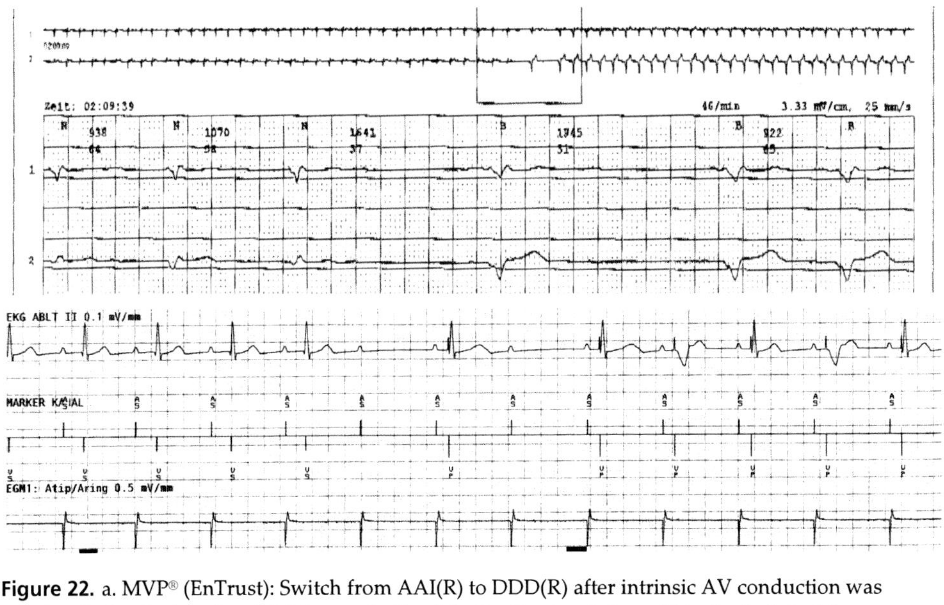

Figure 22. a. MVP® (EnTrust): Switch from AAI(R) to DDD(R) after intrinsic AV conduction was missing during 2 of the last 4 AA intervals. Special attention has to be paid to the fact, that the ventricular backup stimulation fires 80 ms after the intended (actually given or inhibited!) atrial stimulus after each AA interval without ventricular sensing (VS). (This ECG was sent to us per emergency fax as suspected ICD dysfunction: the specifics of AAI ⇔DDD mode switch can lead to substantial uncertainties).
b. MVP® (Protecta DR): Switch from AAI(R) to DDD(R) due to sudden second-degree AV block with 2:1 AV conduction.

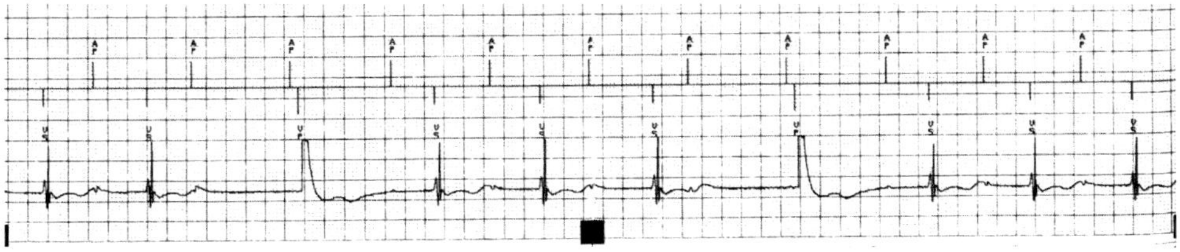

Figure 23. MVP® (Adapta DR): Action of the algorithm in a patient with second-degree AV block type Wenckebach. After there is a consecutive prolongation of the intrinsic AV conduction time (AP/VS) a singular AV conduction is missing and after the next stimulated atrial beat a ventricular stimulus is given.

The AAI(R) mode is maintained as long as intrinsic AV conduction is present. The criterion of intact intrinsic AV conduction is considered to be met, if there is a sensed ventricular event detected before the next atrial sensed event (AS) or atrial stimulation (AP).

The programmed AVD (PAV / SAV) is not relevant in this mode and will be only active after switch to DDD(R) mode.

- MVP®: loss of sufficient intrinsic AV conduction

The device switches automatically to a temporary DDD(R) mode, if there was no intrinsic ventricular event (VS) during 2 of the last 4 atrial intervals. After a missing VS event, there will be a ventricular backup stimulation following the next atrial action (fig. 22). If the following atrial event is not conducted either, the device switches to DDD(R) mode. Thereby singular missing VS events are tolerated (fig. 23). Two consecutive missing ventricular events however are not permitted. This behavior can cause pauses with duration of twice the cycle length of the intervention rate before switch to DDD(R), if there is a sudden loss of intrinsic AV conduction (fig. 24).

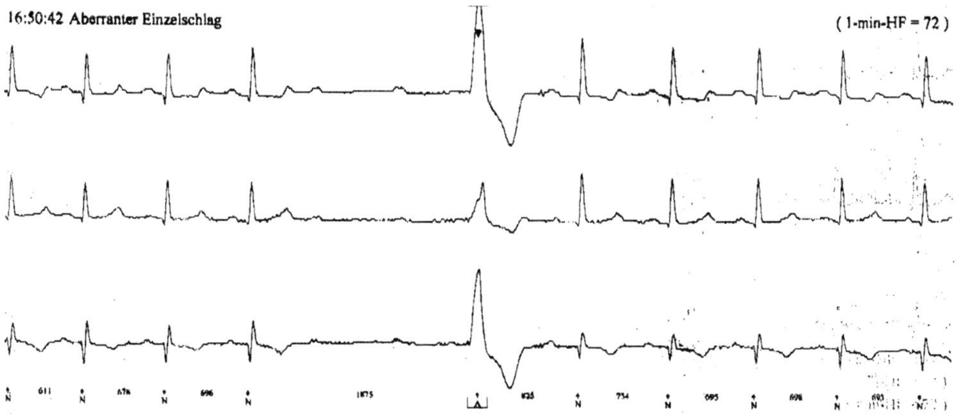

Figure 24. MVP® (Adapta DR): basic rate 50/min (1200 ms). When AV conduction is lost, a ventricular backup stimulus is given, but not with the normal AV time after the 2nd blocked P wave, but 80 ms after the next intended (here inhibited!) atrial stimulus. The "pause" between the first blocked P wave and

the ventricular backup-stimulus is here 1280 ms. Because the following intrinsic AV conduction was intact again, the device stayed in the AAI(R) mode.

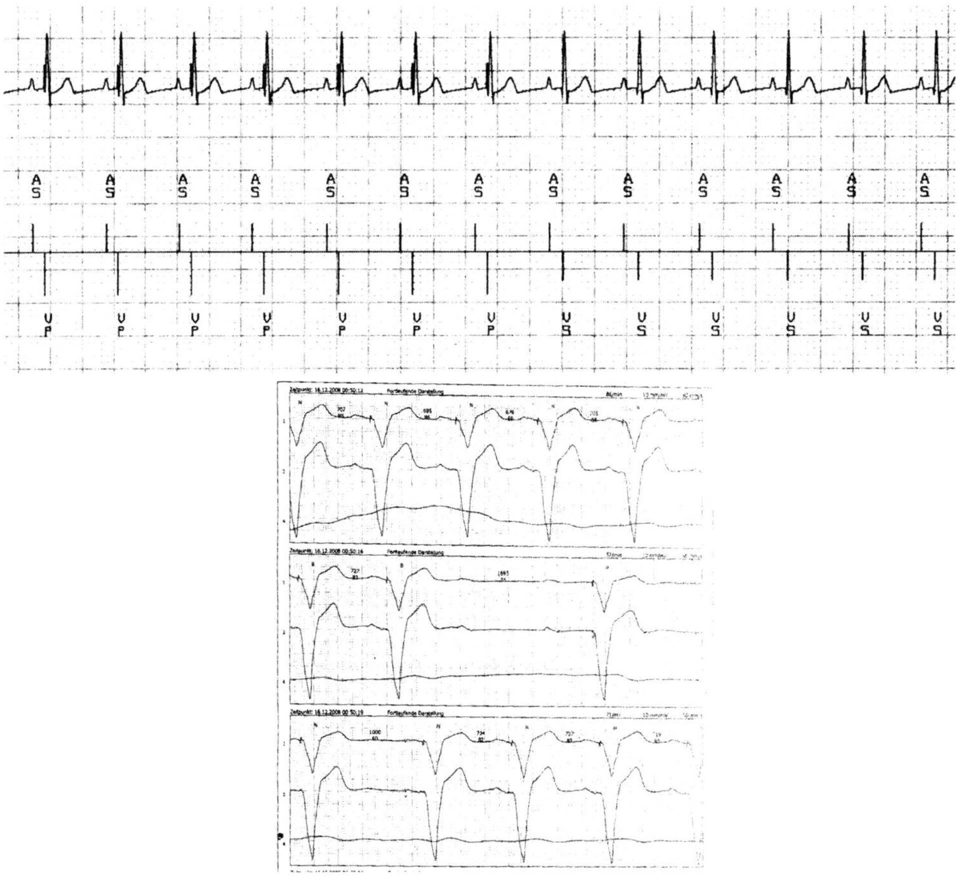

Figure 25. a. MVP® (Protecta DR): Successful test for intrinsic AV conduction, switch from DDD (AS/VP, ventricular fusion) to AAI (AS/VS).
b. MVP®: Negative test for intrinsic AV conduction in a patient with third-degree AV block.

There is no automatic switch over to a permanent DDD(R) mode.

- MVP®: Reoccurrence of sufficient intrinsic AV conduction

After switching to DDD(R), the device checks the intrinsic conduction in regular intervals and thereby checks the possibility for return to AAI(R). This starts already one minute after change to DDD(R) with a switch to AAI(R) for one cycle.

- If there is a VS event following the next AA interval, the device remains in AAI(R) (fig 25a).
- If there is no VS event following the next AA interval, the conduction test was negative and the device remains in DDD(R) (fig. 25b).

After each negative test the time interval doubles to the next control (1 => 2 => 4 => 8 =>…min). The maximum time interval is 16 hours.

As a consequence of this periodic check, patients with permanent complete AV block will have a single missing ventricular beat every 16 hours.

- MVP®: Mode switch for atrial tachyarrhythmias

The device switches to DDIR both from AAI(R) and DDD(R) on the onset of an atrial tachyarryhtmia to avoid fast atrial 1:1 triggering. The mode switch to DDIR for atrial tachyarrhythmias is given a higher priority than MVP®. Once the termination of the atrial tachyarrhyhtmia is recognized, there is a change to DDD(R) no matter which mode was active before that episode. Then an AV conduction test (1 beat) is performed and the device returns to functional AAI(R), if AV conduction is verified. If not, the DDD(R) mode is maintained and regular conduction tests are carried out (1, 2, 4, 8 min … 16 h), as described above.

The MVP® algorithm is a highly effective in avoiding unnecessary RV stimulation.

In a randomized pilot study including 30 patients with dual-chamber ICDs without history of AV block MVP® "dramatically" reduced cum%RVP from 80.6±33.8% to 3.79±16.3% ($p<0.0001$) [39]. 15% of AV intervals under MVP® were longer than 300 ms. There were no relevant symptoms or adverse effects with MVP®.

In 181 ICD patients, that were randomized in a prospective manner, a 99% relative reduction of the cumulative ventricular pacing percentage (cum%VP 4.1±16.3 vs. 73.8±32.5, $p<0.0001$) by application of the MVP®-algorithm versus DDD(R) was found, again without adverse events [40].

In principle it is possible to reduce cum%RVP in all patients with SND and intermittent impairment of AV conduction. According to an investigation by Gillis et al. the reduction of ventricular stimulation percentage is higher in PM patients with SND than in patients with AV block (median relative reduction 99.1% vs. 60.1%) [41]. In a mixed PM population it was possible to reduce cum%VP to ≤40% with the MVP® algorithm in 72% of patients [42]. Compared to AV search hysteresis Search AV+™ there was a significantly lower median percent VP by application of MVP® with the exception of the patients with persisting third-degree AV block [43]. Of the 322 PM patients in this study the best VP reduction was found in mildly impaired AV conduction.

The safe and effective use of MVP® was shown for pediatric patients and grown up patients with congenital heart disease as well [44]. In this study it was necessary to change the programming to DDD in one case of symptomatic intermittent AV block.

The (hemodynamically) optimal form of stimulation for patients with a long AV conduction time ("long AV-block °1") remains still unclear and has to be tested in the individual patient. Especially for these patients one has to consider that MVP® depending on the intervention rate will tolerate any length of AV conduction time, as long as there is a ventricular sensed event (VS) before the next atrial sensing (AS) or atrial stimulation (AP).

This can lead to hemodynamically unfavorable (ultra-) long intrinsic AV times (Fig. 6). In this clinical scenario permanent DDD(R) stimulation with a fixed AV delay optimized e.g. by echocardiography may be more favorable [45].

As already mentioned before, the effective ventricular rate can drop to half of the intervention rate before switch to DDD(R), if there is a sudden loss of intrinsic conduction. Therefore it is recommended to program the basic rate of patients with sinus bradycardia or frequent AV block to a minimum of 50/min.

When the available literature is reviewed, only few cases concerning clinical problems with MVP® are to be found. Mostly the algorithm worked as specified; the most common findings were:

- Atrial events, in which functional undersensing occurred due to the long atrial refractory period (fig. 26)
- Ventricular events, in which functional undersensing occurred during the ventricular blanking time following the next atrial stimulation
- Major variations in AV delays
- Ultra long AV delays being accepted with the result of short VA intervals
- Long atrial pauses
- Occurrence of unnecessary RV pacing because of "linking", i.e. repetitive retrograde invasion of ventricular depolarization into the AV junction resulting in non-conducted P waves

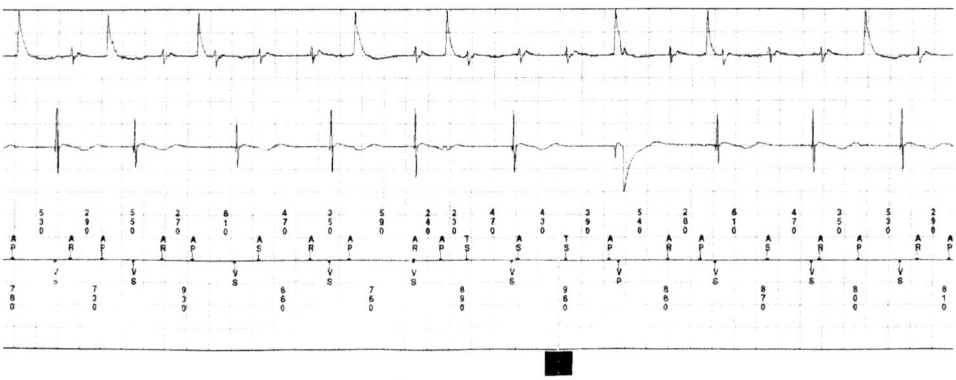

Figure 26. MVP®, EnRhythm DR: Functional undersensing of atrial events due to the long atrial refractory period in a patient with a fast atrial rhythm (sinus or atrial tachycardia), CL about 480 ms.

Murakami et al. reported 2 out of 127 Patients suffering from chest discomfort and one case with mild dizziness due to 2nd or 3rd degree AV block with frequent non-conducted atrial events in MVP mode [46]

A serious potentially proarrhythmogenic effect of MVP was observed by van Mechelen and Schoonderwoerd. In a patient with implanted PM for complete AV block a polymorphic VT degenerated to ventricular fibrillation which successfully was terminated by external defibrillation. Pacemaker interrogation showed correct device function in AAI mode (MVP) before the VT episode with irregular ventricular events (slow escape rhythm with frequent PVCs) and no AV synchronicity. The slow ventricular escape rhythm together with short coupled PVCs constituted proarrhythmogenic short-long-short cycles. Combined with documented hypokalemia, this caused the VT. As a consequence the MVP algorithm was switched off [47].

Clinical Benefit of Ventricular Pacing Reduction by AAI(R)⇔DDD(R) mode switch

Meanwhile, first study results became available showing the clinical benefit of reducing unnecessary RV-stimulation by AAI(R)⇔DDD(R) mode switch algorithms.

In the SAVE PACe trial patients with symptomatic bradycardia due to sinus node disease were evaluated for the primary endpoint "time to persistent atrial fibrillation" [48]. Excluded were patients with persistent atrial fibrillation or cardioversion for atrial fibrillation in the preceding 6 months, second- or third-degree AV block and wide QRS complex. The 1065 enrolled pacemaker patients were randomized to either DDD(R) pacing mode (AVD 120 to 180 ms) or to a dual-chamber pacing mode with a minimal ventricular pacing algorithm (MVP or SAV+). The study was stopped when in the interims analysis the pre-specified efficacy boundary ($P=0.007$) for difference in persistent atrial fibrillation between the two groups was reached (after 1.7 ± 1.0 years). The difference in the median cum%RVP was substantial: 99 % in the DDD group vs. 9.1 % in the MVP group ($P<0.001$). The reduction of the risk for development of persistent atrial fibrillation was significant: 40% relative risk reduction ($P=0.009$) and 4.8% absolute risk reduction in the SAV+/MVP group. As clinical outcome there was a trend towards more strokes in patients who developed persistent atrial fibrillation, compared to those who did not (n.s., $P=0.18$). There was no significant difference for mortality between the two groups. The conclusion of the authors was that in their examined group of patients with SND dual-chamber pacing with the use of a minimal ventricular pacing feature (MVP or SAV+) prevents ventricular desynchronization and is of advantage in reducing risk of persistent atrial fibrillation.

A single center randomized clinical trial done by Xue-Jun et al. compared follow up results after 3 months of pacing in DDD mode (AV delay 250 ms with 30 ms extension) with AAISafeR mode. 30 patients with sick sinus syndrome were randomized to one of the two modes for 3 months and then switched over to the other mode for another 3 months. After 3 months in DDD mode echocardiographic analysis showed that left atrial diameter, left ventricular end-diastolic diameter and left ventricular end-systolic diameter had increased significantly and left ventricular ejection fraction had decreased. However after 3 months of pacing in the AAISafeR mode no obvious changes were noted. In the AAISafeR mode cum%RVP was significantly reduced compared to the DDD mode. The authors of this randomized trial using echocardiographic follow up concluded that AAISafeR mode is not only effective in reducing the amount of unnecessary RV pacing in sick sinus syndrome substantially, but also prevents harmful effects on cardiac performance [49].

5. Conclusion

Recently the importance of reducing unnecessary RV stimulation has been recognized widely. This is reflected in the ACC/AHA/HRS 2008 Guidelines for Device-Based Therapy of Cardiac Rhythm Abnormalities, which for the first time includes a separate chapter regarding this topic ("Importance of Minimizing Unnecessary Ventricular Pacing") [50].

Today we have several options available for this task. Which one to use has to be considered individually for each patient with an indication for a device, at the time of implantation and during follow-up.

The use of atrial single-chamber systems will stay limited to singular cases even in patients with SND, because of the missing ventricular backup if impairment of AV conduction occurs. Apart from the indication for bradycardia in permanent atrial fibrillation, single-chamber VVI PM systems as "backup" can be used as an option for patients with rare paroxysmal AV block. The other major application of single-chamber VVI backup devices with low intervention rate is in ICD therapy, if there is no need for concomitant antibradycardia pacing.

In dual-chamber systems the programming of a fixed long AVD offers a "makeshift-programming", if there is no other specific algorithm available. AV search hysteresis permits markedly longer intrinsic AV conduction times with stimulation with optimized AV interval in the event of higher degree AV block. An effective reduction of unnecessary RV stimulation is possible with the new AAI⇔DDD mode switch algorithms. The clinical effects of wider use of these new functions need to be further evaluated in ongoing trials.

Author details

D. Bastian and K. Fessele
Klinikum Nürnberg Süd, Nuremberg, Germany

6. References

[1] Fröhlig G. [Why, when and how should right ventricular pacing be avoided?] Herzschr Elektrophys 2004; 15:165-176.
[2] Pitzalis MV, Iacoviello M, Romito R et al. Cardiac Resynchronisation Therapy Tailored by Echocardiographic Evaluation of Ventricular Asynchrony. J Am Coll Cardiol 2002; 40:1615-1622.
[3] Bax JJ, Ansalone G, Breithardt OA et al. Echocardiographic evaluation of cardiac resynchronisation therapy: ready for routine clinical use? J Am Coll Cardiol 2004; 44: 1-9.
[4] Søgaard P, Egeblad H, Kim WY et al. Tissue Doppler Imaging Predicts Improved Systolic Performance and Reversed Left Ventricular Remodeling During Long-Term Cardiac Resynchronisation Therapy. J Am Coll Cardiol 2002; 40: 723-730.

[5] Breithardt OA, Sinha AM. Improved identification of suitable patients for cardiac resynchronisation therapy by transthoracic echocardiography. Herzschr Elektrophys 2005; 16:10-19.
[6] Wilkoff BL, Cook JR, Epstein AE et al. Dual-Chamber Pacing or Ventricular Backup Pacing in Patients With an Implantable Defibrillator: The Dual Chamber and VVI Implantable Defibrillator (DAVID) Trial. JAMA 2002; 288:3115-3123.
[7] Anelli-Monti M, Mächler H, Anelli-Monti B et al. [Avoiding Unnecessary Ventricular Stimulation in Sinus Node Disease. New strategies in bradycardia pacing.] J Kardiol 2005; 12:238-242.
[8] Sweeney M, Hellkamp A, Ellenbogen K, et al, for the MOde Selection Trial (MOST) Investigators. Adverse effect of ventricular pacing on heart failure and atrial fibrillation among patients with normal baseline QRS duration in a clinical trial of pacemaker therapy for sinus node dysfunction. *Circulation* 2003; 107:2932-2937.
[9] Nielsen JC, Kristensen L, Andersen HR et al. A randomized comparison of atrial and dual-chamber pacing in 177 consecutive patients with sick sinus syndrome: echocardiographic and clinical outcome. J Am Coll Cardiol 2003; 42(4): 614-623.
[10] Steinberg JS et al. The clinical implications of cumulative right ventricular pacing in the multicenter automatic defibrillator trial II. J Cardiovasc Electrophysiol 2005; 16(4):359-65.
[11] Gardiwal A, Yu H, Oswald H et al. Right ventricular pacing is an independent predictor for ventricular tachycardia/ventricular fibrillation occurrence and heart failure events in patients with an implantable cardioverter-defibrillator. Europace 2008; 10:358-363.
[12] Andersen HR, Thuesen L, Bagger JP, Vesterlund T, Thomsen PEB. Prospective randomised trial of atrial versus ventricular pacing in sick-sinus syndrome. Lancet 1994; 344:1523-1528.
[13] Andersen HR, Nielsen JC, Thomsen PEB, et al. Long-term follow-up of patientsfrom a randomised trial of atrial versus ventricular pacing for sick-sinus syndrome. Lancet 1997;350:1210-1216.
[14] Deutsche Gesellschaft für Kardiologie (DGK) [German Cardiac Society]. Lemke B, Nowak B, Pfeiffer D (Hrsg). Leitlinien zur Herzschrittmacher-Therapie [Guidelines for pacemaker therapy]. Z Kardiol 2005; 94:704-720.
[15] Markewitz A. Jahresbericht 2009 des Deutschen Herzschrittmacher-Registers. Herzschr Elektrophys 2011; 22:259-280.
[16] Rosenqvist M, Brandt J, Schüller H. Long-term pacing in sinus node disease: effects of stimulation mode on cardiovascular morbidity and mortality. Am Heart J 1988; 116:16-22.
[17] Barold SS. Permanent Single Chamber Atrial Pacing Is Obsolete. Pacing Clin Electrophysiol 2001; 24:271-275.
[18] Connolly SJ, Kerr CR, Gent M, et al. Effects of physiologic pacing versus ventricular pacing on the risk of stroke and death due to cardiovascular causes. N Engl J Med 2000; 342:1385-1391.

[19] Tang ASL, Roberts RS, Kerr C, et al. Relationship between pacemaker dependency and the effect of pacing mode on cardiovascular outcomes. Circulation 2001; 103:3081-3085.
[20] Olshansky B, Day JD, Moore S et al. Is dual-chamber programming inferior to single-chamber programming in an implantable cardioverter-defibrillator? Results of the INTRINSIC RV (Inhibition of Unnecessary RV Pacing With AVSH in ICDs) study. Circulation 2007; 115(1):9-16.
[21] Sweeney MO, Ellenbogen KA, Tang AS et al. Atrial pacing or ventricular backup–only pacing in implantable cardioverter-defibrillator patients. Heart Rhythm 2010; 7:1552–1560.
[22] Almendral J, Arribas F, Wolpert Ch et al. Dual-chamber defibrillators reduce clinically significan adverse events compared with single-chamber devices: results from the DATAS (Dual chamber and Atrial Tachyarrhythmias Adverse events Study) trial. Europace 2008; 10:528-535.
[23] Theuns DA, Rivero-Ayerza M, Boersma E, Jordaens L. Prevention of inappropriate therapy in implantable defibrillators: A meta-analysis of clinical trials comparing single-chamber and dual-chamber arrhythmia discrimination algorithms. Int J Cardiol 2008; 125(3): 352-357.
[24] Nielsen JC, Pedersen AK, Mortensen PT et al. Programming a fixed long atrioventricular delay is not effective in preventing ventricular pacing in patients with sick sinus syndrome. Europace 1999; 1:113-120.
[25] Wiegand UKH. Avoidance of ventricular pacing in patients with sinus node disease or intermittend AV block. Herzschr Elektrophys 2008; 19:3-10.
[26] Israel CW. Analysis of mode switching algorithms in dual chamber pacemakers. Pacing Clin Electrophysiol 2002; 25:380-393.
[27] Nitardy A, Langreck H, Dietz R, Stockburger M. Reduction of right ventricular pacing in patients with sinus node dysfunction through programming a long atrioventricular delay along with the DDIR mode. Clin Res Cardiol 2009; 98(1):25-32.
[28] Fröhlig G, Koglek W. Schrittmacherfunktion: Algorithmen zum Erhalt der intrinsischen AV-Überleitung. In: Herzschrittmacher- und Defibrillator-Therapie. Thieme 2006: 200-204.
[29] Melzer C, Sowelam S, Sheldon T, et al. Reduction of right ventricular pacing in patients with sinus node dysfunction using an enhanced search AV algorithm. Pacing Clin Electrophysiol. 2005; 28(6):521-527
[30] Milasinovic G, Sperzel J, Smith TW et al. Reduction of RV Pacing by Continuous Optimization of the AV Interval. Pacing Clin Electrophysiol 2006; 29:406–412.
[31] Savoure A, Anselme F, Galley D et al. A new dual-chamber pacing mode to prevent ventricular pacing. Europace 2003; 4(Suppl B):B175.
[32] Savoure A, Fröhlig G, Galley D, Defaye P, Reuter S, Mabo P, Sadoul N, Amblard A, Limousin M, Anselme F. A new dual-chamber pacing mode to minimize ventricular pacing. Pacing Clin Electrophysiol 2005; 28 (1):43-46.
[33] Fröhlig G, Gras D, Victor J, Mabo P, Galley D, Savoure A, Jauvert G, Defaye P, Ducloux P, Amblard A. Use of a new cardiac pacing mode designed to eliminate unnecessary ventricular pacing. Europace 2006; 8 (2):96-10.

[34] Pioger G, Leny G, Nitzsche R, Ripart A. AAIsafeR limits ventricular pacing in unselected patients. Pacing Clin Electrophysiol 2007; 30 (1):66-70.

[35] Stockburger M, Trautmann F, Nitardy A, Teetzmann MJ, Schade S, Celebi O, Krebs A, Dietz R. Pacemaker-Based Analysis of AtrioventricularConduction and Atrial Tachyarrhythmias in Patients with Primary Sinus Node Dysfunction. Pacing Clin Electrophysiol 2009; 32:604–613.

[36] Thibault B, Simpson C, Gagné CE. Blier L, Senaratne M, McNicoll S, Stuglin C, Williams R, Pinter A, Khaykin Y, Nitzsche R. Impact of AV Conduction Disorders on SafeR Mode Performance Pacing Clin Electrophysiol 2009; 32:S231–S235.

[37] INCEPTA ICD Manual, Boston Scientific, 358431-001 EN Europe 05/10, E 0086, 4-27.

[38] Medtronic, Inc. ENSURA DR MRI™ SURESCAN™ ENDR01. [Handbuch für Ärzte und Klinikpersonal]. Medtronic, Inc. Minneapolis, MN; 2010.

[39] Sweeney MO, Shea JB, Fox V et al. Randomized pilot study of a new atrial-based minimal ventricular pacing mode in dual-chamber implantable cardioverter-defibrillators. Heart Rhythm 2004; 1:160-167.

[40] Sweeney MO, Ellenbogen KA, Kasavant D et al. Multicenter, Prospective, Randomized Safety and Efficacy Study of a New Atrial-Based Managed Ventricular Pacing Mode (MVP) in Dual Chamber ICDs. J Cardiovasc Electrophysiol 2005; 16:811-817.

[41] Gillis AM, Pürerfellner H, Israel CW et al. Reducing Unnecessary Right Ventricular Pacing with the Managed Ventricular Pacing Mode in Patients with Sinus Node Disease and AV Block. Pacing Clin Electrophysiol 2006; 29:697–705.

[42] Milasinovic G, Tscheliessnigg K, Boehmer A et al. Percent ventricular pacing with managed ventricular pacing mode in standard pacemaker population. Europace 2008; 10:151–155.

[43] Pürerfellner H, Brandt J, Israel CW et al. Comparison of Two Strategies to Reduce Ventricular Pacing in Pacemaker Patients. Pacing Clin Electrophysiol 2008; 31:167–176.

[44] Kaltman JR, Ro PS, Zimmerman F, Moak JP, Epstein M, Zeltser IJ, Shah MJ, Buck K, Vetter VL, Tanel RE. Managed Ventricular Pacing in Pediatric Patients and Patients With Congenital Heart Disease. Am J Cardiol 2008; 102:875-878.

[45] Bastian D. Präsynkope unter physiologischer Schrittmacherstimlation [Pre-syncope under physiologic pacemaker stimulation]. 31th Autumn Meeting German Cardiac Society, Cologne 2007. Abstract L174. Oral Presentation. [German]

[46] Murakami Y, Tsuboi N, Inden Y, Yoshida Y, Murohara T, Ihara Z, Takami M. Difference in percentage of ventricular pacing between two algorithms for minimizing ventricular pacing: results of the IDEAL RVP (Identify the Best Algorithm for Reducing Unnecessary Right Ventricular Pacing) study. Europace 2010; 12:96-102.

[47] van Mechelen MR, Schoonderwoerd R. Risk of managed ventricular pacing in a patient with heart block. Heart Rhythm 2006; 3 (11):1384-1385.

[48] Sweeney MO, Bank AJ, Nash E, et al, for the Search AV Extension and Managed Ventricular Pacing for Promoting Atrioventricular Conduction (SAVE PACe) Trial. N Engl J Med. 2007; 357(10):1000-1008.

[49] Xue-Jun R, Zhihong H, Ye W et al. A clinical comparison between a new dual-chamber pacing mode-AAI safeR and DDD mode. Am J Med Sci 2010; 339(2):145-147.

[50] ACC/AHA/HRS 2008 Guidelines for Device-Based Therapy of Cardiac Rhythm Abnormalities.
[51] Epstein AE, DiMarco JP, Ellenbogen KA, et al [published correction appears in JACC. 2009;53:147]. JACC 2008;51(21):e1-62.
[52] Bailin SJ, Adler S, Giudici M. Prevention of chronic atrial fibrillation by pacing in the region of Bachmann's bundle: Results of a multicenter randomized trial. J Cardiovasc Electrophysiol 2001; 12:912-917.
[53] Israel CW. [Alternative Stimulationsorte zur Prävention von Vorhofflimmern.] Herzschr Elektrophys 2002; 13:30-43.
[54] INTEGRITY™ AFx DR Modell 5346. User's Manual. St. Jude Medical, Inc. 2000:28-29.

Chapter 5

Implanted Devices and Atrial Fibrillation

Federico Guerra, Michela Brambatti,
Maria Vittoria Matassini and Alessandro Capucci

Additional information is available at the end of the chapter

http://dx.doi.org/10.5772/47449

1. Introduction

Atrial fibrillation (AF) is a supraventricular tachyarrhythmia characterized by uncoordinated atrial activation with consequent deterioration of atrial mechanical function. On the electrocardiogram (ECG), AF is characterized by the replacement of consistent P waves with rapid oscillations or fibrillatory waves associated with an irregular ventricular response. AF is the most common arrhythmia in clinical practice: its prevalence varies from 0.4% to 1% in the general population and increases with age, reaching 8% in patients older than 80 years [1]. AF may occur in a temporary causing condition setting, such as acute myocardial infarction, cardiac surgery, pericarditis, myocarditis, hyperthyroidism and pulmonary embolism, or in association with underlying cardiac disease such as valvular disease, coronary artery disease, hypertensive cardiomyopathy and others cardiomyopathies, especially those associated with left ventricular dysfunction and heart failure (HF). AF may also occur in younger patients without underlying cardiovascular disease and it is often referred to as "lone AF". AF may develop in isolation or in association with other tachyarrhythmias, most commonly atrial flutter or atrial tachycardia, or bradyarrhtythmias especially due to sinus node dysfunction [1].

Atrial fibrillation is very common in pacemaker recipients because of the wide range of conditions that could require device implantation and promote AF development.

1.1. Patients implanted with dual chamber pacemaker

Paced patients could develop AF for several reasons. On average, half of patients with dual chamber pacemaker have sinus node disease (SND) that is in turn associated with the development of AF in 20-50% of patients, defining the clinical picture of bradycardia-tachycardia (brady-tachy) syndrome [2,3]. Moreover, nearly one third of all patients with complete atrioventricular (AV) block also shows tachy-brady syndrome. Right ventricular (RV) pacing has been demonstrated to increase the risk of developing AF in patients with permanent pacemaker implantation for both SND or AV block [4,5], because of its association with a number of pathophysiological changes which reduce left ventricular function and may promote AF. These changes include: an abnormal activation sequence (intraventricular and interventricular dyssynchrony), depressed left ventricular ejection fraction (EF), diastolic abnormalities and reduced myocardial perfusion [6]. As in general population, in paced patients aging is associated with a higher prevalence of AF, irrespectively of the pacing mode.

1.2. Patients implanted with Implantable Cardioverter Defibrillator (ICDs)

AF is particularly common in patients with left ventricular dysfunction and its prevalence depends on the severity of the underlying pathology. Prevalence is usually 10%-20% in mild to moderate HF, and up to 50% in patients with more advanced disease [7]. Therefore, AF is frequent in ICD recipients, the vast majority of whom have structural heart disease. Approximately 25% of patients who receive an ICD have documented atrial tachyarrhythmias before implantation. Furthermore, a large proportion of patients without prior history of atrial tachyarrhythmias will develop AF after ICD implantation. AF occurs in about 25% of the patients with secondary prevention indication while its prevalence in patients with primary prevention indication is more difficult to define. Prevalence seems to be higher in patients with left ventricular dysfunction due to non-ischemic etiology (ranging from 15% to 25%), and lower in patients with ischemic cardiomyopathy (about 5-10%). Management of atrial tachyarrhythmias in patients with ICDs is important because of the increased morbidity and mortality and the increased cost of medical care.

1.3. Patients implanted with Cardiac Resynchronization Therapy

Cardiac resynchronization therapy (CRT) has emerged as an important and established therapy for patients with end-stage drug refractory HF due to systolic dysfunction and cardiac dyssynchrony. Several clinical trials have demonstrated the efficacy of CRT; however, the vast majority of patients included in all major trials were in sinus rhythm (SR) [8,93]. The low prevalence of AF patients in these trials is justified for several reasons. First, patients with AF are usually patients with more comorbidities and therefore less likely to be included in a clinical trial. On the other hand, in the absence of atrioventricular node ablation, AF reduces the likelihood of obtaining adequate pacing percentage and introduces a reasonable element of confusion when interpreting study results. Daily clinical practice is however quite different: approximately one-fifth of all patients receiving CRT in Europe has permanent AF, as reported in a recent ESC survey [9]. Patients suffering from AF are typically older, more likely to receive a CRT with pacemaker function (CRT-P), and have higher morbidity and mortality rates than patients in SR.

2. International recommendations for pacemaker and defibrillator implants in AF patients

Implantable devices are being commonly used for patients with AF. First of all, AF can occur in patients with SND. In SND, a wide range of cardiac arrhythmias such as sinus bradycardia, sinus arrest, sinoatrial block and junctional rhythm, often coexist with concomitant episodes of supraventricular tachyarrhythmias, generally AF. This peculiar clinical entity is also called brady–tachy syndrome. AF is often triggered by sudden deceleration in heart rate, sinus arrest and, in other cases, by long-short cycle sequence induced by extrasystoles. Sometimes a prolonged sinus arrest or severe bradycardia may follow the end of AF and this phenomenon is probably due to the prolonged suppression of sinus node induced by tachyarrhythmia. Patients with SND may be symptomatic for both bradyarrhythmias (fatigue, exercise intolerance, dizziness, syncope or pre-syncope) and tachyarrhythmia (palpitations, dyspnea, angina, heart failure). In these clinical situations, the implantation of a pacemaker may be necessary in order to prevent AF recurrence and control the symptoms related to bradyarrhythmia. Cardiac pacing can also facilitate the use of optimal dosages of antiarrhythmic drugs, thus preventing the bradycardia induced by the drugs themselves. Moreover, the activation of rate-responsive and dedicated algorithms can increase the benefits of antiarrhythmic atrial stimulation especially during exercise.

Permanent AF with low ventricular rate is another important clinical condition requiring pacemaker implantation. The degenerating process culminating into long-standing AF may be associated to a spontaneous disturbance of the atrio-ventricular conduction or it could be due to a scarce adherence to therapy. In this instance, the implantation of a single-chamber rate-responsive PM is indicated in presence of symptoms, such as fatigue, dizziness, presyncope, syncope or heart failure.

In patients with permanent or paroxysmal AF, in which adequate control of ventricular rate cannot be achieved with drug therapy, device implantation may be also beneficial. Patients with symptoms related to rapid ventricular rates during AF require prompt medical management, and cardioversion should be considered if symptomatic hypotension, angina, or HF occurs. A sustained, uncontrolled tachycardia may lead to deterioration of ventricular function, the so-called tachycardia-induced cardiomyopathy, which tends to resolve within 6 months of rate or rhythm control. When tachycardia recurs, LV ejection fraction declines faster and HF develops over a shorter period. In this case, when pharmacologic antiarrhythmic treatment fails, atrioventricular junction ablation and pace-maker implantation and substrate catheter ablation are reasonable non-pharmacologic alternatives. A meta-analysis of 21 studies published between 1989 and 1998 that included a total of 1181 patients concluded that AV nodal ablation and permanent pacemaker implantation significantly improved cardiac symptoms, quality of life, and healthcare utilization for patients with symptomatic AF refractory to medical treatment [10].

The last issue concerns AF patients eligible to CRT. The European Society of Cardiology guidelines were the first to include patients with AF between the candidates for CRT in 2007 [11], and were recently revised and updated [12]. Nowadays, it is reasonable to implant a CRT-P in patients with LVEF≤35%, QRS duration≥130 ms and NYHA III-IV despite optimal pharmacological treatment with level of evidence B for patients dependent on ventricular pacing and C for those with slow ventricular response who are expected to achieve an adequate percentage of biventricular pacing.

3. Pacemakers and ICDs in detecting AF

3.1. Definition, prevalence and prognosis of asymptomatic AF

AF can manifest itself through symptoms or it can be silent and consequently subclinical. The true prevalence of AF is dependent upon the method used for the diagnosis of this arrhythmia [13]: in general, current data showed an increased AF detection rate with longer monitoring durations. Twelve leads electrocardiogram controls are not very sensitive, detecting less than 30% of all AF episodes [14], whereas more AF paroxysms can be unmasked by using Holter recordings, telemedicine techinques, and loop recorders. Implanted devices, whether pacemakers or ICDs, further enhance the diagnostic yield of asymptomatic atrial arrhythmias by providing continuous rhythm monitoring.

In a study of patients with paroxysmal AF and conventional indication for permanent pacemakers, Israel et al. found that more than one third of all device documented AF of at least 48 hours duration were asymptomatic [15]. A multicenter study on pacemaker diagnostics also reported a high incidence of atrial arrhythmia in the pacemaker population, with atrial high rate episodes (AHRE) documented in 89% and 46% of patients with and without prior history of atrial tachyarrhythmia by 24 months of follow-up, respectively [16]. This study demonstrated that patients with prior history of atrial arrhythmia had higher arrhythmia burden and, again, most device-detected AHRE were asymptomatic.

However, silent AF and symptomatic AF share exactly the same risk for cardiovascular death and cardiovascular events [1]. A major concern with the onset of AF that progresses without any symptoms is the risk of cerebral embolism, with acute stroke its first manifestation. In about 25% of patients who have ischemic strokes, no etiologic factor is identified but subclinical AF is often suspected to be the cause. In the AFFIRM trial, which tested rate control versus rhythm control, stroke occurred in both groups, particularly in patients among whom anticoagulants were discontinued on the assumption that sinus rhythm was successfully maintained [17]. Recently, the ASSERT study found that pacemaker patients who have no history of atrial tachycardia AT or AF, but do have device-detected arrhythmias, are approximately 2.5 times more likely to have a stroke than patients who do not have device-detected arrhythmias [18]. Nevertheless, it is currently unknown if treatment of asymptomatic episodes detected by the device should be the similar to what already recommended for symptomatic AF.

Another relevant aspect related to the absence of symptoms is the development of atrial remodeling. Intermittent asymptomatic AF episodes can cause changes in the electrophysiological and histological matrix of the atria, thereby facilitating the creation of appropriate conditions for degenerating AF into permanent type.

3.2. Usefulness of implanted device in AF detection – New diagnosis, relapse monitoring, event recording, fibrillation burden and rate-control

All implanted devices (pacemakers, ICDs and CRTs) including loop recorders are capable of identification, recording and transmission of electrocardiographic data. Among all the data available, a modern device can store total number of episodes, time of onset and duration of each episode, the overall burden of arrhythmia and the ventricular electrocardiogram morphology (VEGM) associated with each detected episode. These continuous monitoring modalities have improved knowledge into the characteristics of AF.

As previously underlined, implanted devices are useful to detect new episodes of AF. Ricci et al. detected AF in 42 of 166 patients using implanted pacemakers or ICD over a period of 18 months. Interestingly enough, AF was not known before device implantation in more than half of these patients [19].

In patients without a definitive device implant indication implantable leadless loop recorders may be useful in order to detect AF and quantify its burden. The XPECT trial tested an AF detection algorithm incorporated into an implantable leadless loop recorder against traditional monitoring through 48-h ECG Holter [20]. The results of this study indicated a higher sensitivity of loop recorder for detecting AF. However, specificity was limited by falsely stored AF episodes in 15% of the patients. In addition, continuous monitoring can contribute to better therapy management, through better rate control therapy or monitoring of rhythm control especially after catheter ablation. In the latter case, continuous assessment of freedom from tachyarrhythmia recurrences may lead to discontinuation of oral anticoagulation after a successful procedure in selected patients.

3.3. Supraventricular tachycardia or ventricular tachycardia? Discriminating algorithms in modern devices

The MADIT-II, SCD-HeFT, and MUSTT trials indicate that ICD therapy improves survival with a significant reduction in mortality [21-23]. However, nearly half of all shocks experienced by ICD patients are inappropriate, an outcome resulting in poorer quality of life, pain, psychological distress, shorter battery life and device-induced arrhythmias. To reduce inappropriate therapy of supraventricular tachycardia (SVT), ICDs include algorithms engineered to discriminate ventricular tachycardia (VT) from SVT. Programming of discrimination algorithms varies from single chamber to dual chamber ICDs, and should be tailored according to the patient's specific needs, comorbidity and previous history of SVT such as paroxysmal AF.

3.3.1. Single-Chamber SVT-VT discriminators

Most single chamber devices currently include four elements into detection algorithms: RR onset, RR stability, VEGM and sustained rate duration. RR onset is based on the evidence of abrupt onset present in most VT, in contrast to the gradual onset of sinus tachycardia. It has high specificity for rejecting sinus tachycardia but may prevent detection of VT that originates during SVT and VT that starts abruptly with an initial rate below the VT detection rate.

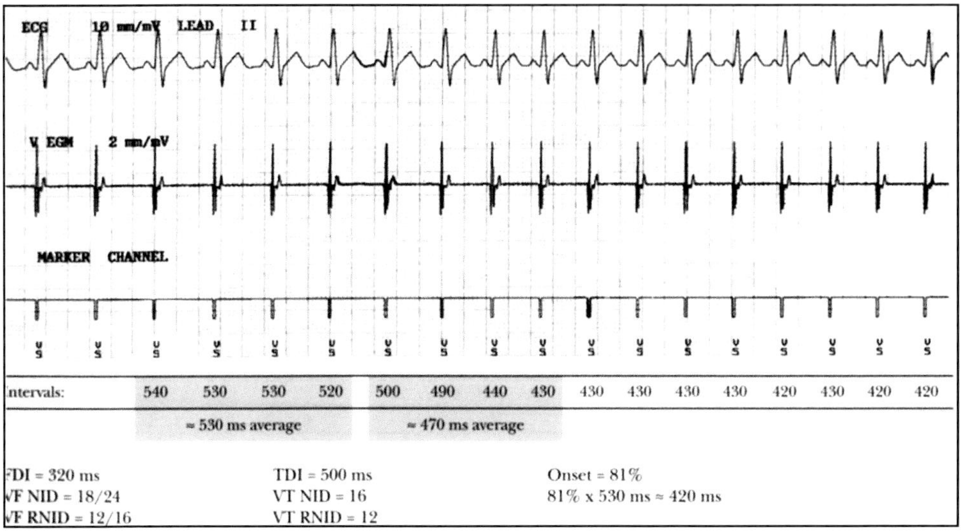

Figure 1. This particular RR onset algorithm analyses eight beats and compares mean ventricular rate of last four beats to mean ventricular rate of first four beats. If the ratio is over a pre-specified cut-off then the device recognises the tachycardia as VT.

RR stability discriminates monomorphic VT from AF based on regularity of the RR interval. The criterion depends on the analysis of cycle length variations and is continuously active during an episode; hence, when programmed "on", the stability algorithm withholds therapy despite ventricular rates in the tachycardia zone if the cycle length intervals are irregular. For most VT, the measured stability or the variation between RR intervals is<21 ms, as opposed to AF, where typically varies by 35–50 ms. Unlike onset, which is determined only once, stability algorithm continuously reevaluates the rhythm diagnosis during tachycardia. Nevertheless, it may misclassify a supraventricular arrhythmia with 2:1

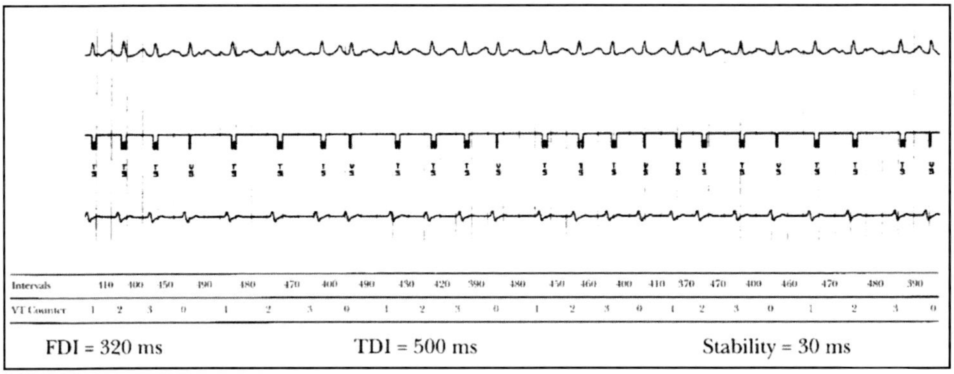

Figure 2. RR stability. Each RR interval is compared to the previous three. If the differences between the RR interval and each of the previous three are under a pre-specified stability cut-off then the arrhythmia is considered as VT.

conduction block, such as atrial flutter or a rapidly conducted AF with a pseudoregular ventricular pattern. Antiarrhythmic drugs may also affect the algorithm's performance. Use of amiodarone or Class IC antiarrhythmic drugs (e.g., flecainide or propafenone) may cause monomorphic VT to become irregular or polymorphic VT to slow down, leading to rhythm misclassification. For this reason, stability should not be programmed "on" unless AF with a rapid ventricular response has been documented.

Morphology discriminates VT from SVT on the basis of morphology-based algorithms that compare the differences between ventricular EGM in a previously stored template of a normally conducted beat with VT EGMs during a tachycardia episode. Common elements present in all morphology algorithms include: creation of a template by mathematically extracting electrocardiogram features and storing them; recording of electrocardiograms during an unknown tachycardia; time aligning templates and tachycardia electrocardiograms; classifying each tachycardia electrocardiogram as a match or non-match based on its comparison with the template; classifying the tachycardia as SVT or VT based on the number of electrocardiograms that match the template. Morphology analysis goes on until insufficient normal beats are recognized (and VT detection occurs) or until the heart rate slows out of the detection zone. Various morphology algorithms differ in their electrocardiogram source, methods of quantitative representation and alignment. In single-chamber ICDs, morphology algorithms are the only discriminators that distinguish regular SVT, such as atrial flutter or atrioventricular nodal reentrant tachycardia (AVNRT), from VT.

Nevertheless, morphology may detect VT inappropriately because of patient-related or algorithm-related factors. Patient-related factors include rate-dependent bundle branch block during SVT and exercise-induced myopotentials in sinus tachycardia [24]. Algorithm-related factors include misalignment of the sinus template with the tachycardia electrocardiogram, clipping of high-amplitude electrocardiograms, electrocardiogram changes during lead maturation, and shock-induced electrocardiogram changes [25]. In case of a possible sustained VT, a useful discriminator is the sustained-duration which overrides inhibition and starts therapy if the fast rate is persistent. It delivers therapy if a tachycardia

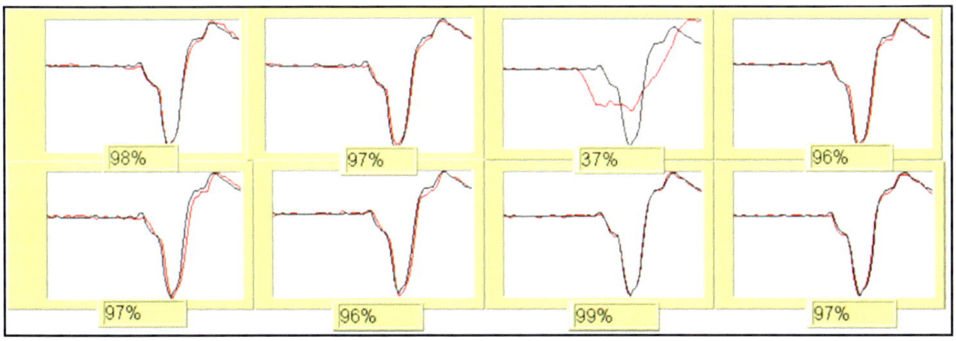

Figure 3. In this case morphology algorithm successfully discriminates a sinus tachycardia by matching tachycardia ventricular morphology with another morphology previously stored during sinus rhythm.

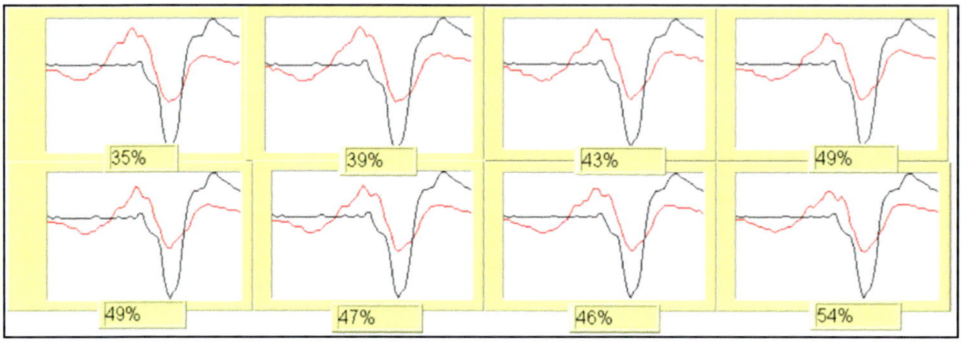

Figure 4. Ventricular morphology recorded during a tachycardia episode is recognized as different by morphology algohirthm, which in turn starts VT counter.

satisfies the VT rate criterion for a programmed duration, even if the discriminator indicates SVT. Since many cardiac patients are unable to maintain prolonged sinus tachycardia, the presumption is that sustained regular tachycardia lasting more than 3 min reflects VT. Thus, this feature ensures appropriate therapy of sustained VT at the price of decreased specificity for rejecting SVT. Indeed, inappropriate therapy is delivered for those SVT that remain above the rate boundary at the end of the programmed period.

3.3.2. Dual-Chamber SVT-VT Discriminators

Dual-chamber discriminators include analysis of atrial and ventricular rates and AV relationship, since dual chamber defibrillators acquire information simultaneously from the atrial and the ventricular leads. VT therapy is delivered immediately if ventricular rate is greater than atrial rate for a set number of beats. This occurs in more than 90% of detected arrhythmias which fall in the VT zone of dual-chamber ICD and in this case, no other data are necessary for therapy delivery. Therefore additional criteria for device diagnosis may be required only in less than 10% of VT. For instance, patients with AF may develop a slow VT, an atrial/ventricular counting algorithm would classify the situation as SVT because the atrial rate exceeds the ventricular rate, and other SVT discriminators may be necessary for a proper diagnosis. The best additional discriminator is morphology or stability.

Measures of AV association analyze the stability of the PR/RP interval and provide an implicit comparison of atrial and ventricular rates. Stable 2:1 AV association is what distinguishes atrial flutter from VT. Although 1:1 AV association does not discriminate between SVT and VT with 1:1 VA conduction, VT with 1:1 VA conduction begins often with transient AV dissociation.

P:R pattern identifies consistent timing relationships between atrial and ventricular electrocardiograms that occur during specific SVT, such as sinus tachycardia and atrial flutter. It identifies complex timing relationships, such as those present during variable AV block, and is insensitive to many transient perturbations. Yet, it is highly sensitive to sustained VT during SVT. The last discriminator, chamber of origin, is applied only to tachycardias with 1:1 AV association. It discriminates sinus or atrial tachycardia with 1:1 AV conduction from VT with 1:1 VA conduction. Atrial tachycardia begins with a short PP interval, whereas VT begins with a short RR interval. Chamber of origin depends on accurate sensing of all atrial and ventricular events at the onset of tachycardia. Thus, it is susceptible to errors based on a single oversensed or undersensed event. In summary, data have demonstrated that dual-chamber discriminators are able to diagnose 60–95% of SVT episodes correctly without significantly missing true VTs. Above all, they may be useful in selected patients, as those with a VT zone with rates < 200 bpm and patients with no permanent AF and no AV block.

3.4. Remote monitoring of AF through implanted devices

Remote monitoring, especially wireless monitoring, offers multiple advantages over traditional office-based device follow-up. For instance it is useful for diagnosing technical issues such as lead fracture, device malfunction, early detection of tachyarrhythmias and heart failure progression, permitting a prompt clinical reaction [26]. The main potential advantage of remote control application in AF management is represented by early detection and early reaction to the arrhythmia occurrences. The current device diagnostics are very sophisticated and may give the physician full information about arrhythmia episodes, their number and duration, date and time of occurrence, onset mechanism, arrhythmia burden, effects of antitachycardia therapies and heart rate during the arrhythmia. The remote transmission of all these data allows a quicker identification of asymptomatic episodes, anticoagulation treatment and cardioversion decisions in a timely manner while the risk of thrombus formation is limited. Currently, the exact impact of the remote control as a clinical tool is still unknown. Moreover, it is still a matter of debate if device detection of AF with remote monitoring could be useful in selecting anticoagulation strategies, as well as the critical threshold of AF burden warranting anticoagulant therapy [27]. Despite the fact that anticoagulation has been shown to significantly improve the outcome in patients with AF, it is also associated with potentially life-threatening side effects and is therefore not well tolerated by patients. Automatic AF detection could make anticoagulation approach easier, allowing a swift therapeutic intervention. This technology seems particularly promising in patients with ICDs. Despite improvements in discrimination algorithms, SVTs continue to be the most common cause of inappropriate shocks. In these cases, the quick identification of the arrhythmia underlying an inappropriate shock may help physician in order to avoid further episodes. In table 1, advantages of remote monitoring in supraventricular tachycardia management are resumed.

• Early detection of symptomatic and asymptomatic supraventricular tachycardia
• Electrical cardioversion within 48 hours of the onset of AF
• Evaluation of the effectiveness of antiarrhythmic therapy
• Modification of the previous antiarrhythmic therapy or anticoagulation
• Rapid reprogramming of ICD in case of inappropriate shocks
• Decrease of number of to traditional office-based device follow-up

Table 1. Main advantages of remote monitoring in SVT detection.

4. Cardioversion in patients with implanted pacemakers and defibrillators

Large-scale randomized trials have questioned the benefits of restoring normal sinus rhythm in patients with AF [17,28].However, the presence of AF in patients with implanted devices could lead to increased morbidity and mortality through adverse device-related complications, such as inappropriate shock deliveries or pacemaker mediated tachycardia with associated tachycardia induced cardiomyopathy. Therefore, AF termination could become necessary and, when appropriate precautions are taken, cardioversion becomes safe and effective in patients with implanted devices.

4.1. Internal cardioversion

Internal cardioversion (ICV) is a defibrillation technique performed through intracardiac electrodes which allows successful CV with very low energy levels. Low-energy ICV does not interfere with pacemaker function in patients with electrodes positioned in the RA, coronary sinus, or left pulmonary artery. ICV has been shown to be superior to conventional external cardioversion (ECV) in term of primary success rate, energy requirements and need of sedation instead of general anaesthesia [29]. However, there are some disadvantages related to the procedure such as the need for an electrophysiology laboratory and of specific technical competence for lead positioning that greatly hamper widespread use in clinical practice. Oesophageal cardioversion is another method to perform CV. This technique is quite simple, very fast and provides several advantages. The most important is a low energy requirement thanks to proximity of the oesophagus to the left atrium which warrants a lower energy dispersion and a lower defibrillation impedance. For this reason its safety has been demonstrated in patients with implantable devices [30]. In patients with ICDs, a programmed ventricular ICD discharge could be another option for a quick and safe cardioversion.

4.2. External cardioversion: how-to and precautions

ECV has long been a cause of concern regarding the potential adverse effects on the generator and on the leads induced by the electrical shocks. First of all, electricity conducted along an implanted electrode may cause endocardial injury and bring to a temporary or permanent increase in stimulation threshold, resulting in acute or chronic loss of ventricular capture. Moreover, other ECV related problems include physical dysfunction of the device, spurious programming or electrical reset induced by the shock and changes in sensing function or pacing impedance [31,32].

	Monophasic	Biphasic	p-value
AF duration before CV	18 (1–394) days	27 (1–1359) days	0.65
CV success	20/21 (95%)	22/23 (96%)	1.0
Success with initial shock	15/21 (71%)	17/23 (74%)	1.0
Cumulative shock energy	200 (200–1220) J	100 (100–650) J	0.001

Table 2. Comparison between AF cardioversion in patients with implanted rhythm devices treated with monophasic or biphasic shocks. For AF duration and cumulative shock energy, the median values and range are provided. Adapted from [31].

Devices assembled in last decades are considerably more sophisticated and better protected against sudden external discharges, even if data loss due to current surges is still possible. Voltage regulators protect the pacemaker circuitry by shunting the current away from the device through the lead to the electrode tip. However, this may result in concentration of the energy at the lead tip, causing burns and electrical trauma at the electrode-myocardial interface. This is the pathophysiological basis of the aforementioned pacing threshold and sensing changes.

Some precautions when performing ECV could be useful to ensure appropriate device function. First of all, the implanted device should be interrogated and, if necessary, reprogrammed before and after cardioversion. Prior to ECV, it is recommended to check pacemaker and leads function. Further precautions are necessary in pacemaker dependent patients such as programming higher voltage output in order to avoid loss of capture and switching to asynchronous mode (VOO or AOO). Current guidelines [33] do not set any interrogation timetable to follow after ECV. However, after the current discharge, it is safe to reassess device function immediately, at hospital discharge and 4-6 weeks later. Additional tests are needed in case of device malfunctioning.

Devices are typically implanted just under the collarbone, so the paddles used for ECV should be positioned as distantly as possible from the device. The positioning of paddles at least 8 cm away from pulse generator [31] did not produce changes in pacing thresholds or sensing measurements, preferably in the anterior-posterior configuration, as specified in AHA Guidelines [33]. The best paddles configuration is the anterior-posterior one. The antero-lateral orientation of cardioversion electrodes creates an electrical field parallel to the course of the leads thus maximizing current shunting through leads. The use of an antero-posterior orientation aims to prevent this 'antenna effect' since it creates an electrical field typically perpendicular to the main lead orientation. Furthermore, the anterior-posterior configuration needs, on average, lower energy requirements for termination of AF [31-33]. Different studies have demonstrated that biphasic shocks are superior to monophasic shocks for cardioversion because of the higher percentage of SR restoration, the fewer shocks needed and the lower energy delivered. However, few studies have focused the attention on patients with implanted devices. From the comparison of monophasic and biphasic shock energy application, it seems that there are no significant differences in terms of safety and efficacy. However, energy requirements are significantly lower for biphasic shocks when compared with monophasic shock waveforms.American and European guidelines do not specify the time between two consecutive shocks in patients with implanted devices. However, safe common practice might be a waiting time of at least 1 minute between shocks, as recommended for patients with AF without intracardiac devices [33].

5. Atrial pacing for AF prevention

Sustained AF depends on a complex electrophysiological substrate which has not been fully elucidated yet. Nonetheless, some animal models demonstrated that specific triggers, such as premature atrial beats, are needed for AF initiation and multiple atrial refractoriness patterns facilitate AF persistency. Some device strategies have been developed in order to prevent AF onset.

5.1. Trigger suppression algorithms

Suppression of AF triggers strategy is mainly based on suppression of premature atrial beats, either by elevating the lower rate or by dynamic overdrive. Both these options, although cheap and easy to perform in an out-of-hospital setting, are not very effective. Re-programming a lower rate 10 bpm faster than 24 hours mean heart rate prevented AF recurrence in approximately 60% of patients over a 30-day follow up [34]. In another study, while atrial pacing vastly reduced total premature atrial beats from 3.8 per hour to 0.5 per hour, no difference was found in AF recurrence prevalence or time to first recurrence between paced and not paced patients [35]. At one year, 43% of all patients developed permanent AF, suggesting that atrial pacing does not prevent the natural progression of AF.

This strategy has also the drawback or requiring specific programming whenever mean heart rate changes, a quite common occurrence in AF patients. To address these issues, dynamic overdrive algorithms has been introduced. These algorithms work by increasing the paced rate upon detection of a premature atrial complex. The increased lower rate is then decreased again in steps until spontaneous atrial rate appears or a new premature atrial beat is detected. Premature beats can also increase dispersion of atrial refractoriness through the long-short cycle which is caused by the extrasystolic pause. In this setting, overdrive suppression algorithms are optimized to deliver either a series of paced beats or a higher pacing rate for a prespecified duration.

The advantage of these algorithms is to reduce atrial pauses following a premature beat while avoiding a fixed high heart rate, possibly leading to palpitations and tachycardiomyopathy. In general, mean heart rate is not significantly increased when these algorithms are working, and are well tolerated by the patients [36].

Efficacy of these algorithms in preventing AF is still a matter of debate. In one of the first prospective studies, AF suppression algorithm (St. Jude Medical, Sylmar, CA) was associated with a 35% reduction of AF burden in patients already implanted with a DDDR device [37]. Moreover, some effects on atrial remodeling, although little in magnitude, have been demonstrated. Other algorithms, such as the Atrial Preference Pacing algorithm (Medtronic, Minneapolis, MN) failed to show any reduction in the number of mode-switching episodes and symptomatic episodes despite a reduction of premature atrial beats [38].

Multicenter trials specifically designed to test efficacy and safety of these algorithms failed to demonstrate a net benefit over traditional pacing. The ATTEST trial evaluated three different algorithms for AF prevention (Atrial Preference Pacing, Atrial Rate Stabilization and Post Mode Switching Overdrive), and showed no difference in total number of AF episodes or median AF burden between patients with either the algorithms switched "on" or "off" [39]. The PIPAF trial had similar results, showing no difference in number of AF paroxysms per week in a crossover population during a 3 months follow up [40]. Post Mode Switching Overdrive algorithm (Medtronic, Minneapolis, MN) provided no reduction of AF episodes at 120 bpm and was actually arrhythmogenic when programmed at 80 bpm.

5.2. Alternative site and multi-site pacing for AF prevention

Paroxysmal AF is usually related to an important inter-atrial and intra-atrial delay, which further increases atrial refractoriness dispersion and helps sustain AF. Unconventional atrial pacing techniques have been proposed in order to synchronize atrial activation and reduce dispersion of refractoriness. Alternative site pacing and dual-site pacing have been the most extensively studied strategies.

Alternative site atrial pacing attempts to reduce atrial activation time by selective pacing right atria at preferential conduction sites. The most common of these sites is probably the Bachmann's bundle, a band of fibrous tissue that travels from the superior part of the right atrium near the ostium of the vena cava superior to the upper part of the left atria appendage. Pacing at the Bachmann's bundle has been shown to reduce AF recurrence [41]. The incidence of AF recurrences at 1 year has been lowered with Bachmann's bundle pacing compared to traditional right atrial appendage pacing, and in those patients P-wave duration was actually shorter, providing an indirect evidence of a better inter-atrial and intra-atrial activation [42]. Another alternative site for atrial pacing is the low interatrial septum near the triangle of Koch, where most of the connections between right and left atria have been discovered. Pacing at the low interatrial septum has been associated with a reduced AF burden and again, with shorter P-wave duration [43]. These alternative pacing sites obviously require active-fixation leads, but appear to be as stable and safe as conventional, passive-fixation, atrial appendage leads.

Multi-site pacing is another promising strategy which has been quite successful in reducing atrial refractoriness dispersion. This approach is characterized by the use of two atrial leads. The first one is placed in the atrial appendage or actively fixated into the interatrial septum. The second one can be either placed into the distal coronary sinus or near its ostium. In the former case, specifically designed leads are necessary in order to avoid dislodgement whereas in the latter case an active-fixation lead is required.

Only a single multicenter trial has currently been performed in order to test feasibility and efficacy of multi-site pacing in AF prevention [44]. This study randomized 118 patients to multi-site pacing, overdrive atrial pacing or simple support pacing at a lower rate of 50 bpm. The study showed a reduction in AF recurrences and mean dose of antiarrhythmic drugs taken in both multi-site pacing and overdrive pacing, with no significant difference between these two groups.

To conclude, patients with paroxysmal AF and a P duration ≥90 ms may benefit from dual-site pacing as well as alternative site pacing. Hybrid therapy, using both alternative site pacing and suppression algorithms, could represent a future approach to AF prevention, though multicenter trials are still needed in order to gather enough evidence.

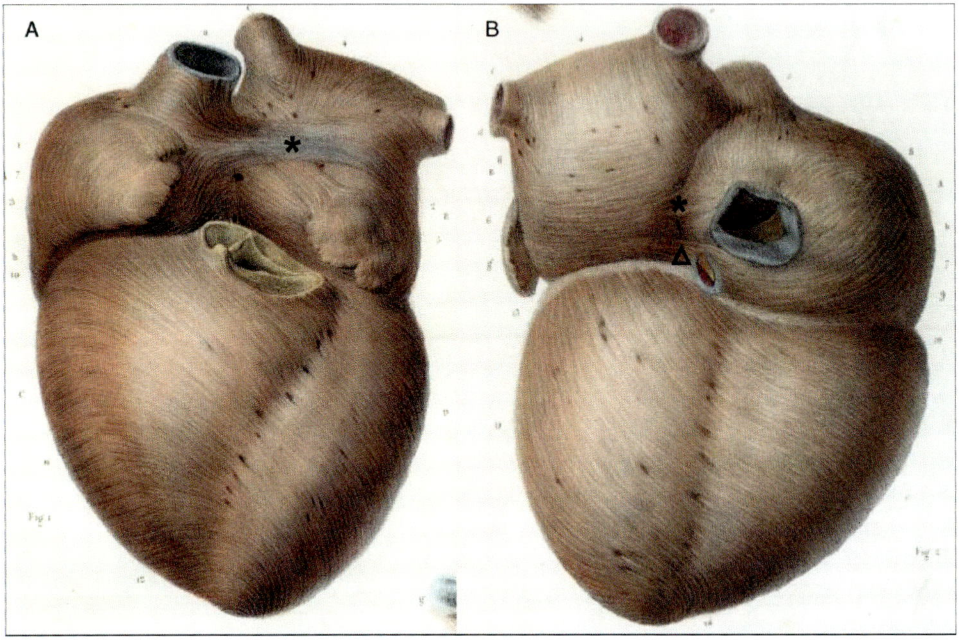

Figure 5. Superior (A) and inferior (B) view of the human heart. (A) Bachmann's bundle travels from the superior part of the right atrium near the ostium of the vena cava superior to the upper part of the left atrium (*). (B) components of the inferior interatrial route: asterisk denotes muscular bundles between the right atrium near the orifice of the vena cava inferior and the inferior surface of the left atrium; Arrowhead denotes interatrial bundles in the vicinity of the coronary sinus orifice (coronary sinus is removed). Reproduced from [41].

6. Atrial pacing for AF termination

Antitachycardia pacing (ATP) is a reliable method of suppressing ventricular arrhythmias, and is currently widespread as a standard ICDs therapy. More recently, its usefulness has been demonstrated also in terminating atrial tachyarrhythmias with a wide excitable gap such as atrial tachycardia or atrial flutter. Unfortunately, AF lacks a wide excitable gap, and its multiple reentrant wavelets do account for its resistance to ATP termination. Atrial ATP is now available in all modern implantable devices. Many different types of atrial ATP are available, as they differ from each producing company. The most common are: atrial burst (steady rate pacing), atrial ramp (auto-decremental pacing), atrial burst plus (steady rate pacing followed by two extrastimuli) and 50-Hz burst pacing for 3 seconds, none of which proved to be more effective than the others in terminating AF.

Efficacy of atrial ATP is low, mainly because of the aforementioned mechanisms, and it varies from 30 to 54% [39]. However, several variables must be taken into account. First of all, ATP success in terminating AF greatly depends on the cycle length of the arrhythmia:

being as low as 29% if the cycle length is ≤ 190 ms and as high as 65% when the cycle length is > 320 ms [45]. Also, atrial ATP is more effective if delivered in recent-onset AF paroxysms. Another possible use of atrial ATP depends on the common pathophysiology between AF and atrial flutter. In patients in whom those two arrhythmias coexist, ATP delivery while the patient is in atrial flutter may prevent further degeneration of atrial flutter into AF.

7. Ablate and pace

7.1. Rationale and indications for ablate and pace

Atrioventricular junction (AVJ) ablation and subsequent pacing, also called "ablate and pace" may be considered whenever it is not possible to achieve adequate rate control despite optimal pharmacological therapy or after unsuccessful AF ablation. Complete AV block is achieved by selective catheter-mediated destruction of the AV node or His bundle, with radiofrequency current serving as the predominant source energy. AVJ ablation is usually performed by a right-sided approach, which offers lower prevalence of complications and is related to shorter hospitalizations. When the right-sided approach fails, left-sided ablation can be performed during the same session or at another session. Left-sided ablation is usually faster, as requires fewer radiofrequency applications, but is associated with a significantly higher risk of bleeding [46,47]. An expert electrophysiologist can usually produce an effective AV block in more than 98% of cases. Regression of AV block late after ablation is rare, and occurs in less than 5% of total procedures [48].

Current European [1] and American [33] guidelines list ablate and pace as a palliative treatment. Indeed, in contrast to other ablative procedures in which the ablation erases the electrophysiologic substrate of the disease, ablate and pace only works indirectly, changing an irregular and fast ventricular rate into a regular, pacemaker-dependent, normofrequent rate. It could also be said that ablate and pace replaces one disease (uncontrolled AF) with another (iatrogenic complete AV block) [49]. Moreover, the procedure is completed by a pacemaker implant, with all the short- and long-term complications associated with a device implant procedure.

Nonetheless, ablate and pace improves symptoms and quality of life compared to medical therapy, and improves survival making it similar to survival rates in the general population [1,33]. Usually, patients who benefit the most of ablate and pace strategy are those patients with tachycardia-mediated cardiomyopathy, as symptoms are usually related to a fast ventricular response.

A meta-analysis, including less than 1200 patients affected by symptomatic permanent AF, demonstrated that AVJ ablation and pacemaker implantation significantly improved quality of life, reducing symptoms and hospitalizations [10]. Similar results have been shown for patients with paroxysmal or persistent AF refractory to any form of pharmacological rate control [50]. Ablate and pace seems also beneficial in restoring an adequate cardiac function: in the Ablate and Pace Trial (APT) 156 patients undergoing AV node ablation and pacemaker implant experienced an improvement of cardiac systolic function along with clinical status and quality of life [51]. Moreover, in a small study recruiting 56 patients with EF less than 40%, ablate and pace strategy was associated with an improvement of mean EF from 0.26 to 0.34, with one fourth of the patients actually achieving the goal of a normal (≥55%) EF.

The outcome of an ablate and pace strategy could be further improved by alternative sites pacing, such as the right ventricular outflow tract, the interventricular septum and the His bundle, although no clear evidence is currently available.

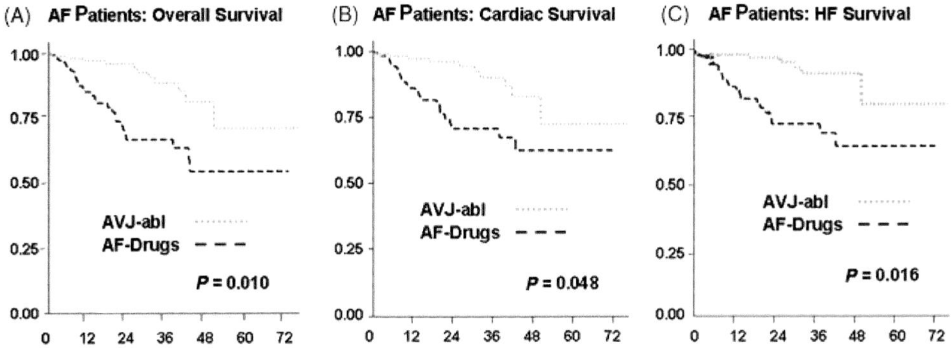

Figure 6. Comparison of Kaplan–Meier estimates of overall (A), cardiac (B), and heart failure (C) survival between AF patients who underwent AVJ ablation and AF patients treated only with anti-arrhythmic drugs. The p-values presented derive from the adjusted hazards ratio analysis stratified according to the corresponding cause of death. Reproduced from [51].

7.2. Which device in which patient? Recommendations for different types of devices in "ablate-and-pace" strategy

Selection of the appropriate device (pacemaker or ICD) and the optimal stimulation modality (VVI, DDD, or CRT) must be based on a number of clinical variables. First of all, type of AF (paroxysmal, persistent or permanent) is of the utmost importance to determine the correct strategy. In patients with paroxysmal AF, dual-chamber pacemakers are obviously preferred in an effort to maintain AV synchrony during sinus rhythm following ablation. Automatic mode switching capability of modern dual-chamber devices prevents rapid ventricular rate when AF occurs and, as already said, provides a major diagnostic tool in detecting AF episodes. The device can be easily reprogrammed to VVIR modality when AF becomes persistent or permanent.

Associated ischemic or valvular heart disease, systolic and diastolic function and the presence and severity of heart failure symptoms should also be taken into account. Current recommendations for cardiac resynchronization are still valid in this subtype of patients. In fact, it has been demonstrated that AF patients undergoing AVJ ablation before CRT implant have a better survival rate when compared with AF patients under a pharmacological rate control strategy [52]. Upgrading to a biventricular device should be considered for patients with HF and a right ventricular pacing system when AV node ablation is performed. It is not currently established whether biventricular pacing could be useful in patients without left ventricular dysfunction, although some recent evidences are in favor of a possible role in reducing AF-related symptoms [53]. In severely symptomatic patients with permanent AF, CRT significantly prevents hospitalization and worsening of clinical conditions during a 2-years follow-up [53].

7.3. Safety of ablate and pace therapy

As said before, ablation of the AV node produces a new illness (the iatrogenic AV complete block) out of an old one. Complications related to ablate and pace strategy include those commonly associated with device implant, thromboembolism associated with anticoagulation withhold and progression from paroxysmal to permanent AF. AVJ ablation procedure creates a temporary proarrhythmic state, which in turn can rarely lead to polymorphic VT and cardiac arrest. In fact, the 1-year mortality rate after ablate and pace is approximately 6.3%, which include a 2% risk of sudden cardiac death [54]. Although this issue has raised some criticisms, programming a higher lower rate of about 80-90 beats per minute for the first 1-2 months seems a viable option for reducing the risk of sudden death [55]. Nonetheless, mortality associated with ablate and pace is still low, reaching 10.5% in 5 years [56], with no significant difference in mortality between ablation and pharmacological control rate.

8. Two birds with one stone: Usefulness of implanted devices in AF associated with other cardiac diseases

8.1. Bradycardia and syncope: Recommended type of devices and optimal settings in low-response AF

VVIR is the mode of choice for patients with permanent AF and a slow ventricular response, in whom pacing is necessary. On the contrary, for most patients with brady–tachy syndrome, a dual chamber pacemaker is indicated. As most patients with symptomatic bradycardia often have associated chronotropic incompetence or at least the potential for this to occur, a dual-chamber pacemaker with rate-adaptive capabilities (DDDR) is recommended. In patients with frequent AF relapses associated with slow ventricular rates, DDDR becomes essential. Rate responsiveness in patients with chronic AF depends on autonomic regulation of the AV node, which is usually poorly regulated in this population. the DDDR pacemaker could be reprogrammed to VVIR afterwards if AF degenerates over time into permanent type. A DDD pacemaker, which has no rate-adaptive capability, could be reprogrammed only to VVI, which could not be optimal for the patient.

8.2. Heart failure: Cardiac resynchronization therapy in AF

Latest ESC [12] and AHA/ACC/HRS Guidelines [57] have considered atrial fibrillation patients, who constitute an important subgroup of HF patients, as eligible to receive CRT.

Both ventricular conduction delay and AF are associated with poor prognosis in HF and CRT may be therefore indicated in these patients. Few randomized trials have been done in order to assess the efficacy of CRT in AF patients [58-60]. The MUSTIC trial showed good one-year results of biventricular pacing in patients with severe HF and major intraventricular conduction disturbances with either SR or AF [58]. Because of the high drop-out rate, the impact of these results were limited even though the results underlined the importance of an high percentage of biventricular pacing to achieve real CRT-related benefits in patients with AF. The PAVE study demonstrated that in patients undergoing AV node ablation for AF, biventricular pacing provided a significant improvement in the 6-minute walk test and ejection fraction compared to right ventricular pacing [59]. These beneficial effects of CRT were greater in patients with impaired systolic function or symptomatic HF [59]. An intrinsic, intermediate-to-high, irregularly spontaneous AF rhythm reduces the percentage of effectively biventricular paced captured beats. Even in a patient who has normofrequent AF, phases of effective biventricular capture alternate with phases of competing AF rhythm which translates into spontaneous, fusion, or pseudo-fusion beats. The presence of fusion and pseudo-fusion leads to inaccuracy and overestimation of the effective pacing capture. Furthermore, the global effective 'CRT-dose' may be markedly reduced compared with atrial synchronous rhythm with a short AV interval achieved during SR, since the number of effective biventricular captured beats are reduced. Moreover, in AF patients, spontaneous ventricular rate tends to overdrive biventricular pacing rates during exertion, determining a further reduction of paced beats precisely when patients are most in need of biventricular capture, and thus greatly limiting functional capacity [60,61]. Another problem is the possible negative impact on prognosis of negative chronotropic therapy in achieving adequate rate control. In fact, the SCD-HeFT study has shown that amiodarone therapy provided no benefit in patients in NYHA class II and decreased survival among patients in NYHA class III, as compared with those who received placebo [62].

To achieve a ventricular rate control delivery, devices-derived features have been developed in order to maximize ventricular pacing during potentially disruptive events. These features are ventricular rate regularization and in ventricular sense response pacing. The former consist in performing biventricular pacing, which 'overrides' intrinsic rhythm, through faster ventricular-paced depolarization, allowing to reduce short cycles through retrograde concealed penetration of the AV node. The other feature is characterized by the activation of LV pacing soon after a premature RV sensed event is detected. Another mechanism in the management of AF is the combination between CRT and atrial tachyarrhythmia prevention pacing algorithm. The ADOPT trial [37] has demonstrated the efficacy and safety of the AF suppression algorithm in reducing symptomatic AF burden in patients with permanent pacemaker with prior history of AF and with normal EF. A subsequent study, the MASCOT trial, has been designed to determine whether the addition of atrial overdrive pacing to CRT could reduce the incidence of permanent AF. The overall incidence of permanent AF was low and was similar for the two treatment groups underlying that probably the advanced atrial remodelling in the setting of HF and AF may preclude benefit from atrial algorithms in this altered milieu [63].

AVJ ablation and placement of a permanent pacemaker has been used in patients with fast, symptomatic and drug-refractory AF to confer symptomatic relief and improve exercise tolerance. In the setting of CRT and AF, the AVJ ablation is emerging as a useful tool to optimize CRT delivery because it allows a complete heart rate control through a constant biventricular pacing.

From the current evidences it emerges that the real benefits of CRT in AF population seem to be confined only to AF patients treated with AVJ ablation. The magnitude of reverse remodelling, of improving of the systolic function and of the decrease in NYHA functional class, the percentage of responders seems to be higher in AF patients treated with CRT and AVJ ablation [51,52]. AVJ ablation in addition to CRT appears also to improve long-term overall mortality and hospitalization compared with CRT alone, primarily by reducing HF death [53].

The outcomes of AF with AVJ ablation patients are similar to the outcomes of patients in SR. Several trials have concluded that AF patients display similar survival as sinus rhythm patients provided that AVJ ablation is performed. However, data from larger randomized clinical trials will be needed before utilizing this as a standard practice since this would create a large number of pacemaker- dependent HF patients with all stimulation dependency-related problems.

In patients with permanent AF who undergo CRT without AVJ ablation, a few studies have suggested that cardioversion and aggressive rhythm control result in better clinical outcomes [64]. Limited data showed that in patients with severely depressed left ventricular EF, left bundle branch block and permanent AF a more vigorous approach to restoring SR is justified prior to implantation of a CRT device or after, in case of recurrences conferring clinical and instrumental improvement. However, currently available antiarrhythmic drugs are only partially effective in maintaining sinus rhythm, and this is achieved at the cost of potential risk [17]. In contrast, catheter ablation may offer another approach for achieving sinus rhythm in these patients. Several clinical trials have demonstrated catheter ablation as a promising alternative compared to pharmacologic therapy, that significantly improved LV function, NYHA class and exercise capacity in patients with AF and symptomatic LV dysfunction [65-68]. The results of these nonrandomized series provide a potent rationale for a randomized clinical trial comparing ablation to pharmacologic therapy.

Author details

Federico Guerra*, Michela Brambatti, Maria Vittoria Matassini and Alessandro Capucci
Cardiology Clinic, Marche Polytechnic University, Ancona, Italy

9. References

[1] Camm AJ, Kirchhof P, Lip GY, Schotten U, Savelieva I, Ernst S, et al. (2010) Guidelines for the management of atrial fibrillation: the Task Force for the Management of Atrial Fibrillation of the European Society of Cardiology (ESC). European Heart Journal. 31:2369-2422.

* Corresponding Author

[2] De Sisti A, Attuel P, Manot S, Fiorello P, Halimi F, Leclercq JF. (2000) Electrophysiological determinants of atrial fibrillation in sinus node dysfunction despite atrial pacing. Europace. 2:304-311.

[3] Lamas GA, Lee KL, Sweeney MO, Silverman R, Leon A, Yee R, et al. (2002) Ventricular pacing or dual-chamber pacing for sinus node dysfunction. New England Journal of Medicine. 346:1854-1862.

[4] Veasey RA, Arya A, Silberbauer J, Sharma V, Lloyd GW, Patel NR, Sulke AN. (2011) The relationship between right ventricular pacing and atrial fibrillation burden and disease progression in patients with paroxysmal atrial fibrillation: the long-MinVPACE study. Europace. 13:815-820.

[5] Sweeney MO, Bank AJ, Nsah E, Koullick M, Zeng QC, Hettrick D, et al. (2007) Minimizing Ventricular Pacing to Reduce Atrial Fibrillation in Sinus-Node Disease. New England Journal of Medicine. 357:1000-1008.

[6] Silberbauer J, Veasey RA, Freemantle N, Arya A, Boodhoo L, Sulke N. (2009) The relationship between high-frequency right ventricular pacing and paroxysmal atrial fibrillation burden. Europace. 11:1456–1461.

[7] Savelieva I, Camm J. (2003) Atrial fibrillation and heart failure: natural history and pharmacological treatment. Europace. 5: S5-S19.

[8] Cleland JG, Daubert JC, Erdmann E, Freemantle N, Gras D, Kappenberger L, Tavazzi L, for the Cardiac Resynchronization—Heart Failure (CARE-HF) Study Investigators. (2005) The effect of cardiac resynchronization on morbidity and mortality in heart failure. New England Journal of Medicine. 352:1539–1549.

[9] Dickstein K, Bogale N, Priori S, Auricchio A, Cleland JG, Gitt A, et al. (2009) The European cardiac resynchronization therapy survey. European Heart Journal. 30:2450 –2460.

[10] Wood MA, Brown-Mahoney C, Kay GN, Ellenbogen KA. (2000) Clinical outcomes after ablation and pacing therapy for atrial fibrillation: a meta-analysis. Circulation. 101:1138–1144.

[11] Vardas PE, Auricchio A, Blanc JJ, Daubert JC, Drexler H, Ector H, et al. (2007) Guidelines for cardiac pacing and cardiac resynchronization therapy. European Heart Journal. 28:2256–2295.

[12] Dickstein K, Vardas PE, Auricchio A, Daubert JC, Linde C, McMurray J, et al. (2010) Focused update of the European Society of Cardiology guidelines on device therapy in heart failure. An update of the 2008 European Society of Cardiology guidelines for the diagnosis and treatment of acute and chronic heart failure and the 2007 European Society of Cardiology guidelines for cardiac and resynchronization therapy. European Heart Journal. 31:2677-2687.

[13] Brignole M, Vardas P, Hoffman E, Huikuri H, Moya A, Ricci R, et al. (2009) Indications for the use of diagnostic implantable and external ECG loop recorders. Europace. 11:671–687.

[14] Nieuwlaat R, Capucci A, Camm AJ, Olsson SB, Andresen D, Davies DW, et al. (2005) Atrial fibrillation management: a prospective survey in ESC member countries: the Euro Heart Survey on Atrial Fibrillation. European Heart Journal. 26:2422-2434.

[15] Israel CW, Grönefeld G, Ehrlich JR, Li YG, Hohnloser SH. (2004) Long-term risk of recurrent atrial fibrillation as documented by an implantable monitoring device: implications for optimal patient care. Journal of the American College of Cardiology. 43:47-52.

[16] Orlov MV, Ghali JK, Araghi-Niknam M, Sherfesee L, Sahr D, Hettrick DA. (2007) Asymptomatic atrial fibrillation in pacemaker recipients: incidence, progression, and determinants based on the atrial high rate trial. Pacing and Clinical Electrophysiology. 30:404-411.

[17] Wyse DG, Waldo AL, DiMarco JP, Domanski MJ, Rosenberg Y, Schron EB, et al. (2002). A comparison of rate control and rhythm control in patients with AF. New England Journal of Medicine. 347:1825–1833.

[18] Healey JS, Connolly SJ, Gold MR, Israel CW, Van Gelder IC, Capucci A, et al. (2012) Subclinical AF and the Risk of Stroke. New England Journal of Medicine. 366: 120-129.

[19] Ricci RP, Morichelli L, Santini M. (2009) Remote control of implanted devices through Home Monitoring™ technology improves detection and clinical management of AF. Europace. 11:54-61.

[20] Hindricks G, Pokushalov E, Urban L, Taborsky M, Kuck KH, Lebedev D, et al. (2010) Performance of a new leadless implantable cardiac monitor in detecting and quantifying AF: Results of the XPECT trial. Circulation: Arrhythmias and Electrophysiology 3:141-147.

[21] Buxton AE, Lee KL, Fisher JD, Josephson ME, Prystowsky EN, Hafley G. (1999) A randomized study of the prevention of sudden death in patients with coronary artery disease. New England Journal of Medicine. 341:1882-1890.

[22] Bardy GH, Lee KL, Mark DB, Poole JE, Packer DL, Boineau R, et al. (2005) Amiodarone or an implantable cardioverter-defibrillator for congestive heart failure. New England Journal of Medicine. 352:225-237.

[23] Daubert JP, Zareba W, Cannom DS, McNitt S, Rosero SZ, Wang P, et al. (2008) Inappropriate ICD Shocks in MADIT II. Journal of the American College of Cardiology. 51:1357-1365.

[24] Swerdlow CD, Ahern T, Chen PS, Hwang C, Gang E, Mandel W, et al. (1994) Underdetection of ventricular tachycardia by algorithms to enhance specificity in a tiered therapy cardioverter-defi brillator. Journal of the American College of Cardiology. 24:416–424.

[25] Duru F, Bauersfeld U, Rahn-Schonbeck M, Candinas R. (2000) Morphology discriminator feature for enhanced ventricular tachycardia discrimination in implantable cardioverter defibrillators. Pacing and Clinical Electrophysiology. 23:1365-1374.

[26] Brugada P (2006) What evidence do we have to replace in-hospital implantable cardioverter defibrillator follow-up? Clinical Research in Cardiology. 95(Supplement 3):iii3-iii9.

[27] Ip J, Waldo AL, Lip GY, Rothwell PM, Martin DT, Bersohn MM, et al. (2009) Multicenter randomized study of anticoagulation guided by remote rhythm monitoring in patients with implantable cardioverter-defibrillator and CRT-D devices: Rationale, design, and clinical characteristics of the initially enrolled cohort. The IMPACT study. American Heart Journal. 158:364-370.

[28] Carlsson J, Miketic S, Windeler J, Cuneo A, Haun S, Micus S, et al. (2003) Randomized trial of rate-control versus rhythm-control in persistent atrial fibrillation: the Strategies of Treatment of Atrial Fibrillation (STAF) study. Journal of American College of Cardiology. 41(10):1690-6.

[29] Lévy S. (2005) Internal defibrillation: where we have been and where we should be going? Journal of Interventional Cardiac Electrophysiology. 13:61-66.

[30] Santini L, Forleo GB, Romeo F. (2011) Esophageal electrical cardioversion of atrial fibrillation: when esophagus gives a help to cardiologists. Cardiology Research and Practice. 2011:983937.

[31] Manegold JC, Israel CW, Ehrlich JR, Duray G, Pajitnev D, Wegener FT, Hohnloser SH. (2007) External cardioversion of atrial fibrillation in patients with implanted pacemaker or cardioverter-defibrillator systems: a randomized comparison of monophasic and biphasic shock energy application. European Heart Journal. 28:1731–1738.

[32] Gammage MD. (2007) External cardioversion in patients with implanted cardiac devices: is there a problem? European Heart Journal 28 :1668–1669

[33] Fuster V, Rydén LE, Cannom DS, Crijns HJ, Curtis AB, Ellenbogen KA, et al. (2011) 2011 ACCF/AHA/HRS focused updates incorporated into the ACC/AHA/ESC 2006 Guidelines for the management of patients with atrial fibrillation: a report of the American College of Cardiology Foundation/American Heart Association Task Force on Practice Guidelines developed in partnership with the European Society of Cardiology and in collaboration with the European Heart Rhythm Association and the Heart Rhythm Society. Journal of American College of Cardiology. 57:101-198.

[34] Garrigue S, Barold SS, Cazequ S, Gencel L, Jaïs P, Haissaguerre M, Clémenty J. (1998) Prevention of atrial arrhythmias during DDD pacing by atrial overdrive. Pacing and Clinical Electrophysiology. 21:250–255.

[35] Gillis AM, Wyse G, Connolly SJ, Dubuc M, Philippon F, Yee R, et al. (1999) Atrial pacing periablation for prevention of paroxysmal atrial fibrillation. Circulation. 99:2553–2558.

[36] Lam CTF, Lau CP, Leung SK, Tse HF, Lee KLF, Tang MO, et al. (2000) Efficacy and tolerability of continuous overdrive atrial pacing in atrial fibrillation. Europace 2:286–291.

[37] Carlson MD, Ip J, Messenger J, Beau S, Kalbfleisch S, Gervais P, et al. (2003) A new pacemaker algorithm for the treatment of atrial fibrillation: results of the Atrial Dynamic Overdrive Pacing Trial (ADOPT). Journal of the American College of Cardiology. 20:627–633.

[38] Murgatroyd FD, Nitzsche R, Slade AK, Limousin M, Rosset N, Camm AJ, et al. (1994) A new pacing algorithm for overdrive suppression of atrial fibrillation. Pacing and Clinical Electrophysiology. 17:1966–1973.

[39] Lee MA, Weachter R, Pollak S, Kremers MS, Naik AM, Silverman R, et al. (2003) The effect of atrial pacing therapies on atrial tachyarrhythmia burden and frequency. Journal of the American College of Cardiology. 41:1926–1932.

[40] Adler S, Ziegler P, Koehler J, Holbrook R, Hettrick DA. (2001) Post mode switch overdrive pacing algorithm reduces atrial tachyarrhythmia recurrence in patients with bradycardia and atrial tachyarrhythmias. Circulation. 104:II-624.

[41] Platonov PG. (2007) Interatrial conduction in the mechanisms of atrial fibrillation: from anatomy to cardiac signals and new treatment modalities. Europace 9:vi10-vi16.

[42] Bailin SJ, Adler S, Giudici M. (2001) Prevention of chronic atrial fibrillation by pacing in the region of Bachmann's bundle: results of a multicenter randomized trial. Journal of Cardiovascular Electrophysiology 12:912–917.

[43] Padeletti L, Pieragnoli P, Ciapetti C, Colella A, Musilli N, Porciani MC, et al. (2001) Randomized crossover comparison of right atrial appendage pacing versus interatrial septum pacing for prevention of paroxysmal atrial fibrillation in patients with sinus bradycardia. American Heart Journal, 142:1047–1055.
[44] Saksena S, Prakash A, Ziegler P, Hummel JD, Friedman P, Plumb VJ, et al. (2002) Improved suppression of recurrent atrial fibrillation with dual-site right atrial pacing and antiarrhythmic drug therapy. Journal of the American College of Cardiology. 40:1140–1150.
[45] Adler SW, Wolpert C, Warman EN, Musley SK, Koehler JL, Euler DE. (2001) Efficacy of pacing therapies for treating atrial tachyarrhythmias in patients with ventricular arrhythmias receiving a dual-chamber implantable cardioverter defibrillator. Circulation. 104:887–892.
[46] O Souza, S Gursoy, F Simonis, G Steurer, E Andries, P Brugada (1992) Right-sided versus left-sided radio frequency ablation of the His bundle. Pacing and Clinical Electrophysiologhy. 15:1454–1459.
[47] Kalbfleisch SJ, Williamson B, Man KC, Vorperian V, Hummel JD, Calkins H, et al. (1993) A randomized comparison of the right- and left-sided approaches to ablation of the atrioventricular junction American Journal of Cardiology. 72:1406–1410.
[48] Brignole M. (2000) Ablate and pace: palliating the symptoms? American Journal of Cardiology. 86:4K-8K.
[49] Brignole M, Gianfranchi L, Menozzi C, Alboni P, Musso G, Bongiorni MG, et al. (1997) Assessment of atrioventricular junction ablation and DDDR mode-switching pacemaker versus pharmacological treatment in patients with severely symptomatic paroxysmal atrial fibrillation: a randomized controlled study. Circulation. 96:2617–2624.
[50] Kay GN, Ellenbogen KA, Giudici M, Redfield MM, Jenkins LS, Mianulli M, Wilkoff B. (1998) The Ablate and Pace Trial: a prospective study of catheter ablation of the AV conduction system and permanent pacemaker implantation for treatment of atrial fibrillation. Journal of Interventional Cardiac Electrophysiology. 2:121–135.
[51] Gasparini M, Auricchio A, Metra M, Regoli F, Fantoni C, Lamp B, et al. (2008) Long-term survival in patients undergoing cardiac resynchronization therapy: the importance of performing atrio-ventricular junction ablation in patients with permanent atrial fibrillation. European Heart Journal. 29:1644–1652.
[52] Leon AR, Greenberg JM, Kanuru N, Baker CM, Mera FV, Smith AL, et al. (2002) Cardiac resynchronization in patients with congestive heart failure and chronic atrial fibrillation: effect of upgrading to biventricular pacing after chronic right ventricular pacing. Journal of the American College of Cardiology. 39:1258–1263.
[53] Brignole M, Botto GL, Mont L, Oddone D, Iacopino S, De Marchi G, et al. (2012) Predictors of clinical efficacy of 'Ablate and Pace' therapy in patients with permanent atrial fibrillation. Heart. 98:297-302.
[54] Nowinski K, Gadler F, Jensen-Urstad M, Bergfeldt L. (2002) Transient proarrhythmic state following atrioventricular junction radiofrequency ablation: pathophysiologic mechanisms and recommendations for management. American Journal of Medicine. 113:596–602.
[55] Evans GT, Scheinman MM, Bardy G, Borggrefe M, Brugada P, Fisher J, et al. (1991) Predictors of in-hospital mortality after DC catheter ablation of atrioventricular junction. Results of a prospective, international, multicenter study. Circulation. 84:1924–1937.

[56] Ozcan C, Jahangir A, Friedman PA, Patel PJ, Munger TM, Rea RF, et al. (2001) Long-term survival after ablation of the atrioventricular node and implantation of a permanent pacemaker in patients with atrial fibrillation. New England Journal of Medicine. 344:1043–1051.
[57] Epstein AE, DiMarco JP, Ellenbogen KA, Estes NA, Freedman RA, Gettes LS, et al. (2008) ACC/AHA/HRS 2008 Guidelines for Device-Based Therapy of Cardiac Rhythm Abnormalities: a report of the American College of Cardiology/American Heart Association Task Force on Practice Guidelines. Journal of American College of Cardiology. 51:e1-62.
[58] Linde C, Leclercq C, Rex S, Garrigue S, Lavergne T, Cazeau Set al. (2002). Long-term benefits of biventricular pacing in congestive heart failure: results from the MUltisite STimulation in cardiomyopathy (MUSTIC) study. Journal of the American College of Cardiology. 40:111-118.
[59] Doshi RN, Daoud EG, Fellows C, Turk K, Duran A, Hamdan MH, Pires LA. (2005) Left ventricular-based cardiac stimulation post AV nodal ablation evaluation (the PAVE study). Journal of Cardiovascular Electrophysiology. 16:1160-1165.
[60] Brignole M, Gammage M, Puggioni E, Alboni P, Raviele A, Sutton R, et al. (2005) Comparative assessment of right, left, and biventricular pacing in patients with permanent atrial fibrillation. European Heart Journal. 26:712-722.
[61] Leclercq C, Mabo P. (2008) Cardiac resynchronization therapy and atrial fibrillation. Do we have a final answer? European Heart Journal. 29:1597–1599.
[62] Bardy GH, Lee KL, Mark DB, Poole JE, Packer DL, Boineau R, et al. (2005) Amiodarone or an implantable cardioverterdefibrillator for congestive heart failure. New England Journal of Medicine. 352:225–237.
[63] Padeletti L, Muto C, Maounis T, Schuchert A, Bongiorni MG, Frank R, et al. (2008) Atrial fibrillation in recipients of cardiac resynchronization therapy device: 1-year results of the randomized MASCOT trial. American Heart Journal. 156:520-526.
[64] Azpitarte J, Baún O, Moreno E, García-Orta R, Sánchez-Ramos J, Tercedor L. (2001) In patients with chronic atrial fibrillation and left ventricular systolic dysfunction, restoration of sinus rhythm confers substantial benefit. Chest. 120:132-8.
[65] Butter C, Winbeck G, Schlegl M et al.(2004) Management of atrial fibrillation in cardiac resynchronization therapy clinical practice of CRT: How to improve the success rate. European Heart Journal. 6: D106–D111.
[66] Chen MS, Marrouche NF, Khaykin Y, Gillinov AM, Wazni O, Martin DO, et al.(2004) Pulmonary vein isolation for the treatment of atrial fibrillation in patients with impaired systolic function. Journal of the American College of Cardiology. 43:1004–1009.
[67] Hsu LF, Jaïs P, Sanders P, Garrigue S, Hocini M, Sacher F, et al. (2004) Catheter ablation for atrial fibrillation in congestive heart failure. New England Journal of Medicine. 351:2373–2383.
[68] Gentlesk PJ, Sauer WH, Gerstenfeld EP, Lin D, Dixit S, Zado E, et al. (2007) Reversal of left ventricular dysfunction following ablation of atrial fibrillation. Journal of Cardiovascular Electrophysiology. 18: 9–14.

Section 3

Management of Complications

Chapter 6

Complications of Pacemaker Implantation

Jeffrey L. Williams and Robert T. Stevenson

Additional information is available at the end of the chapter

http://dx.doi.org/10.5772/48682

1. Introduction

Approximately 180000 patients undergo pacemaker implantation in the U.S each year [1]. In addition, the extreme elderly are the most rapidly growing segment of the U.S. [2,3] and pacemakers are commonly implanted in this population. There are reports of pacemaker implant complications (generally clinical trials reporting outcomes and incident complication rates) and fewer reports of complication rates in the extreme elderly (with a persistent exclusion of elderly patients from ongoing clinical trials [4]). A comprehensive review of pacemaker implant complications can help improve informed consent in preoperative patients. Major and minor complications are defined based upon prior reports of device-related complications. [5,6,7,8] Major complications have been defined as death, cardiac arrest, cardiac perforation, cardiac valve injury, coronary venous dissection, hemothorax, pneumothorax, transient ischemic attack, stroke, myocardial infarction, pericardial tamponade, and arterial-venous fistula. Minor complications have been defined as drug reaction, conduction block, hematoma or lead dislodgement requiring reoperation, peripheral embolus, phlebitis, peripheral nerve injury, and device-related infection. This chapter will include discussion of common and uncommon complications of pacemaker implantation including associated incidence as well as the associated radiographs and common clinical signs of these complications.

2. Demographics of pacemaker implantation

From 1993 to 2006, 2.4 million patients received a primary pacemaker and 69,000 pacemaker generator changes; women comprised 49% of pacemakers. [1] A review of studies involving pacemaker implantation in adults reveals an average age range of 69-86 years with approximately 30-40% of patients aged > 80years [9,10]. There is a tendency for higher percentage of female patients as age increases; a prior study from our Heart Rhythm Center [11] examined pacemaker implant outcomes of extremely elderly patients (>80years) with an average implant age of 86 and revealed 61% of implants were performed in females.

3. Preprocedural issues

3.1. Preoperative risk assessment

As with all surgical interventions requiring anesthesia, recognizing and managing comorbid conditions preoperatively helps to mitigate the risks during and immediately after pacemaker implantation. The association of heart failure and other structural heart disease with cardiac conduction system disease as well as the expanding role of biventricular pacemakers specifically indicated for patients with symptomatic congestive heart failure means that there is an inherently high risk population of patients frequently served in the EP lab. Indeed, CHF increases the risk of all surgery. A decreased LVEF has been found to be a predictor of perioperative mortality and morbidity, with the highest risk group being those with an EF < 35%; the very patients brought to the lab for resynchronization therapy. Pre-procedural management of CHF is not only integral to our practice but vitally important to the safety of the procedure. Patients certainly should not be in a state of decompensated heart failure.

3.2. Infection

Patients who present with systemic infection and positive blood cultures carry the highest risk of infection. Infection of implantable devices is one of the most feared complications due to the dismal prognosis of untreated infections and risk of device removal. Often we are asked to evaluate patients for bradyarrhythmias when they happen to be identified at the time of hospitalization for infectious etiologies such as pneumonia and urosepsis as well as post cardiac surgery. Pre-implant evaluation for potential sources of infection is critical. The estimated rate of infection of permanent endocardial pacing leads is between 1 and 2%, however the range is from under 1 percent to greater than 10%. In the PEOPLE study [12], device infection requiring removal was correlated to fever within 24 hours of device implant, temporary pacing prior to implant, and early reintervention for lead revision or hematoma evacuation. The likelihood of infection was nearly doubled by the presence of a temporary system. The association with temporary intravenous pacing wires certainly implies an association with any indwelling lines including central lines and PICC lines. The duration of hospitalization prior to implant was not correlated to higher risk of infection. Infections were negatively correlated with de-novo implantation and perioperative antibiotic prophylaxis. The latter intervention is considered controversial. Of 28,860 Danish patients [13], 3.6% had a lead related complication by 3 months. Risk factors for lead related complications included operator inexperience (<25 implants).

3.3. Procedural management of iodinated contrast agents

3.3.1. Contrast Induced Nephropathy (CIN)

Contrast-induced nephropathy is a surprisingly common complication of radio-contrast procedures occurring in 15% of cases. It is defined as an absolute increase in creatinine of 0.5mg/dl (in patients starting under 2) or an increase of 25% of baseline and typically peaks at 48-72 hours after exposure. Creatinine may remain above baseline for 7-14 days. Naturally, the best way avoid this complication is to abstain from its use. Single and dual lead pacing systems can safely be implanted without the use of contrast at all; Prior data from our Heart Rhythm Center [11] revealed that contrast was used in 55 of 92 (59.8%) of the pacemaker implantations with a mean intravenous contrast usage of 9.6cc. We often use contrast to ensure that the subclavian /axillary venous system is patent and to help guide venous access. No contrast was used for generator changes and there were no contrast reactions. CRT implantation may require contrast agents to define the coronary (CS) anatomy. The vast majority of patients undergoing CRT implants are patients with heart failure and its associated comorbidities which very frequently include diabetes and chronic kidney disease, therefore a working knowledge and respect for these agents is a necessity. We typically use 5cc of iso-osmolar contrast in a 1:1 ratio with NSS and limit CS venography to 1 cine if possible. For patients with GFR 30-60ml/min, hydration can usually be achieved with 4-6 glasses of water the evening before the procedure. ACE inhibitors, ARBs, and NSAIDS can be held the day prior and day of exposure and be resumed 24 hours after exposure. For patients with a GFR <30ml/min, the above recommendations should be followed with consideration of one or both of the following: 1.) IV hydration using 1L of NaCl 0.45% with 50mEq $NaHCO_3$ (1/2 normal saline with 1 amp of sodium bicarbonate) run at 1ml/kg/hr for 12 hours. For same day procedures, this can be administered at 3ml/kg/hr for 1 hour. 2.) N-acetylcysteine 600mg PO BID the day prior and day of the procedure, totaling 4 doses. It must be noted that besides preprocedural hydration, the evidence is not conclusive that bicarbonate and acetylcysteine offer additional benefit. Treatment of CIN after evident is largely supportive and infrequently requires short-term dialysis.

CS lead placement can be performed successfully without the use of contrast in patients at risk of CIN. [8] CS lead placement at our Heart Rhythm Center without the use of contrast begins with CS access by engagement of the CS with a 5French octapolar deflectable electrophysiology (EP) catheter or hydrophilic coated 0.035" guidewire that the CS sheath is advanced over. Next, a 0.014" guidewire is advanced out distally and the entire CS is probed for LV branch vessels in 360 degree fashion; we then work proximally and if no braches are found (including very proximal posterolateral "bailout" vessels) then we repeat the process. We have demonstrated a 97.3% success rate in LV lead placement with these techniques. [8]

3.3.2. *Contrast allergies*

Immediate anaphylactic reactions including angioedema, bronchospasm, arterial hypotension, and shock can occur within minutes of and up to 60 minutes after injection. [14] The reported incidence of severe immediate reactions to ionic contrast material (CM) is 0.1-0.4% and with newer non-ionic, low osmolar or iso-osmolar contrast is 0.02-0.04% but death rates from the two materials do not differ. [15] Although incompletely understood, direct release of histamine from circulating basophils and eosinophils is probably the primary mechanism with IgE mediated mast cell activation (i.e. true allergy) being a much less frequent secondary mechanism. A skin testing study showed that only 4% of patients with anaphylaxis symptoms had an IgE-mediated mechanism [16]. Delayed reactions from 1 hour to 7 days after injection of CM are T-cell mediated and most typically are skin reactions. [15] Patients with even mild anaphylactoid (immediate) reactions should be considered high risk in future CM administration. Indeed, a distinction between immediate anaphylactoid and non-immediate anaphylactoid reactions may be more clinically relevant than a history of mild, moderate, and severe reactions. [17] For purposes of reporting, CM reactions are graded 1-3. Grade 1 reactions include one episode of nausea/vomiting or sneezing, grade 2 reactions being fever/chills, hives, and more severe nausea/vomiting, and grade 3 reactions are potentially life-threatening and include angioedema, bronchospasm, laryngospasm, pulmonary edema, hypotension, and shock.[18] It is common practice to pre-medicate with corticosteroids with or without H1 blockers in patients with a history of moderate or severe immediate reactions, despite the fact that randomized trials comparing pretreatment strategies are severely lacking. No trials of pre-treatment have tested a steroid-antihistamine combination which is the most commonly utilized. [18] In a consensus document published by Marcos et al in 2001, 91% of survey respondents administered corticosteroids at least 11 hours prior to CM administration (though dose frequency varied from 1-3x) and 55% used an H1 blocker (diphenhydramine 25-50mg) typically administered once. [14] H2 blockers are used, but rarely. In a meta-analysis including 10,011 patients with no history of contrast allergy, routine pre-treatment with steroids alone reduced respiratory symptoms after contrast injection (frequently ionic, high osmolar) from 1.4% to 0.4% and Grade III symptoms from 0.9% to 0.2%. Only a "double dose" steroid regimen reduced Grade III symptoms. [18] In this same cohort, there were no "disastrous" consequences. Cutaneous manifestations were more often prevented by H1 antagonists and respiratory symptoms show improvement with steroid pretreatment. [18] Essential information to be sought from the patient prior to administration of contrast is history of previous CM reaction, asthma, renal insufficiency, diabetes, and metformin therapy. [19]

Routine pre-medication of all patients to receive CM is probably not warranted given the overall low incidence of a reaction; in fact some have advocated abandoning this procedure all together. [18] Patients with a history of severe CM allergy who will likely need IV CM injection should probably receive pre-exposure prophylaxis with corticosteroids as well as H1 antagonists although strong evidence of benefit is lacking. [16] The likely mechanism for the benefit of corticosteroids is a reduction in circulating basophils and eosinophils available for direct activation. If CM administration cannot be delayed for 4-6 hours after steroid injection, some would omit use and administer only H1 blockers. [19] One can also consider the addition of H2 antagonists such as ranitidine but evidence is also lacking. Low or iso-osmolar contrast such as ioxaglate, iohexol, or ioversol should be used due to the lower overall incidence of reactions in patients with a history of asthma or a CM allergy. The specific CM causing the prior reaction should be sought and avoided if possible. Cutaneous allergic testing can be performed on patients with a history of anaphylactic reactions and a "skin test negative" CM should be used but it should be noted that only a fraction of those patients will have a positive skin test.[15,18] The ESUR guidelines on prevention of CM reactions recommend Prednisone 50mg PO at 13, 7, and 1 hours prior or methylprednisolone 32mg orally 12 and 2 hours prior to exposure to CM in addition to diphenhydramine 50mg IV, IM, or PO 1 hour prior to exposure. Despite this, reactions are reported in those with prior reactions with corticosteroid pretreatment.

3.4. Thyroid

Hypothyroidism has been found in 0.5-0.8% of the population demonstrated by elevated serum levels of thyroid-stimulating hormone (TSH) or decreased serum thyroxine levels. [20] Undiagnosed (and hence untreated) hypothyroidism can lead to major perioperative complications including severe hypotension or cardiac arrest following induction of anesthesia, extreme sensitivity to narcotics and anesthetics with prolonged unconsciousness and hypothyroid coma following anesthesia and surgery. [20] Ideally, hypothyroidism is caught early and thyroxine administered until the patient is euthyroid (generally, 4-6weeks).

Hyperthyroidism affects approximately 0.2% of men and 2% of women and may cause atrial fibrillation, congestive heart failure and thrombocytopenia. [21] In addition, anesthetic drugs may be affected by the hypermetabolic state of hyperthyroidism. When total intravenous anesthesia is used (often at our center when high frequency jet ventilation is used to minimize respiratory motion), propofol infusion rates should be increased to reach anesthetic blood concentrations because the clearance of propofol is increased in hyperthyroid patients. [21] Supportive management of thyroid crisis includes hydration, cooling, inotropes and steroids. Beta-blockade and antithyroid drugs are used as the first line of treatment.

Generally, more thyroid related perioperative complications stem from hypothyroidism as opposed to hyperthyroidism however, recognition of either prior to implantation is important. Our Heart Rhythm Center generally obtains TSH prior to all device implantation and allows 4-6weeks for the patient to become euthyroid prior to proceeding with surgery. Emergent cases with thyroid abnormalities require close coordination with anesthesiology and will generally be undertaken with general anesthesia.

4. In-hospital complications

4.1. Sedation / airway:

Less than 20% of electrophysiology (EP) programs in the United States exclusively use anesthesia professionals for procedural sedation. [22] Minor complications (e.g., atelectasis, fever, vascular congestion) may simply be reflective of common postoperative pulmonary complications (PPC's) seen after general anesthesia. Atelectasis can be seen on CT scan in up to 90% of patients who are anesthetized [23] and PPC's have been found to occur in 9.6% of patients. [24]. There are data to suggest that patients undergoing invasive EP procedures may require deep conscious sedation that often is converted to general anesthesia;[25] thus, the use of general anesthesia (including HFJV) during EP procedures may enhance patient safety.[26,27] The advantage of general anesthesia was mostly studied in patients undergoing complex procedures, such as AF ablation, where precise electroanatomical mapping is required. There is not much data supporting the use of general anesthesia (which may increase costs) versus conscious sedation in routine PM implantations. In our center, we often use general anesthesia with a laryngeal mask airway to minimize patient movement during LV lead implantation.

4.2. Pneumothorax

Pneumothorax may occur in as many as 3-4% [28,29] and as few as 0-1% [8,10,11,30,31,32] but generally ranges from 1-3% (5,9,33,34,35,36,37] of patients undergoing pacemaker implantation. Routine chest radiographs are often performed immediately after pacemaker implantation though clinical signs of pneumothorax include hypoxia, shortness of breath, pleuritic pain, and hypotension. Figure 1 depicts the radiographic appearance of small, medium, and large pneumothoraces. Figure 2 depicts a pseudopneumothorax that resulted from external artifact; close review of radiographs by radiologists can limit false-positive pneumothorax interpretations. Emergent treatment of pneumothorax includes decompression of the pressure tension by thoracentesis or chest tube. Oftentimes, high concentrations of inspired oxygen can lead to a resolution of a pneumothorax that comprises less than 30% lung volume. (38) This conservative treatment of pneumothorax can reduce morbidity and duration of hospitalization and avoid invasive drainage procedures. The traditional treatment of patients with traumatic hemo- or pneumo-thoraces has been an insertion of a chest tube (CT). CT have larger caliber than pigtail catheters and can cause significant trauma during insertion, cause pain, prevent full lung expansion, and worsen pulmonary outcomes. [39] Pigtail catheters, smaller and less invasive than chest tubes, have been used successfully in patients with nontraumatic pneumothorax. Pigtail catheters have demonstrated a non-significant increase (11% vs 4% for CT) in the tube failure rate (defined by a requirement for an additional tube or by recurrence requiring intervention) [39].

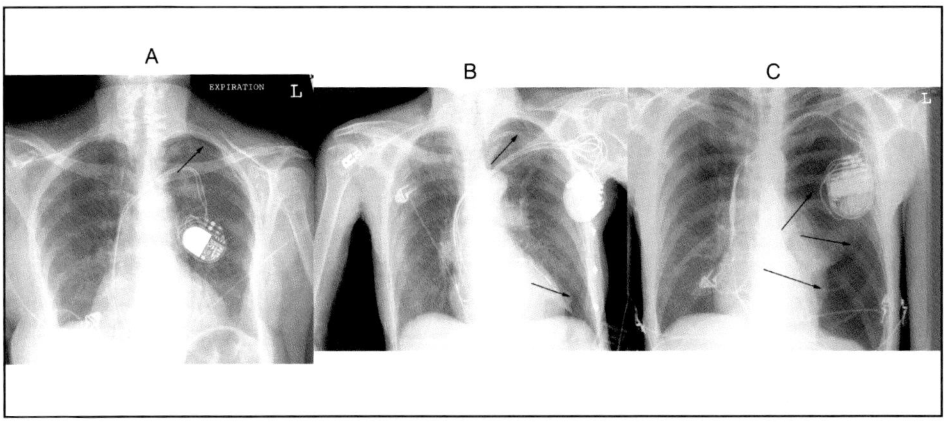

Figure 1. Examples of Pneumothoraces, Small (A), Medium (B), and Large (C). The edge of the pneumothorax is indicated by the arrows. A small left apical pneumothorax is shown in A. A moderate-sized apical and basilar pneumothorax is shown in B. An almost complete collapse of the left lung is shown in C. Please note that examples shown in B and C are from defibrillator implantations.

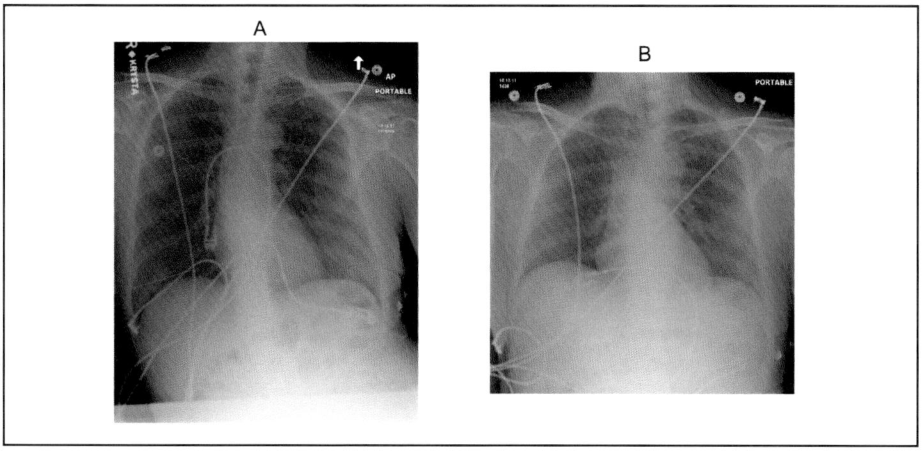

Figure 2. Pseudopneumothorax after removal of temporary internal jugular vein temporary pacemaker. Figure A shows an outline (arrows) that appears to indicate a pneumothorax in an asymptomatic patient. Repeat CXR indicates that initial findings have resolved (with no intervention) and was likely external artifact from gown or skin.

4.3. Vascular access and hemothorax

The axillary venous approach has been associated with less frequent pneumothorax and subclavian crush syndrome. [40,41] The axillary vein is the continuation of the basilica vein that terminates immediately beneath the clavicle at the outer border of the first rib, at which point it becomes the subclavian vein. [42] Direct subclavian venous punctures are associated with increased rate of pneumothorax [5] while cephalic vein cutdown has been associated with the lowest rate of pneumothorax and lead damage. [33,31] Fluoroscopic-guided, first rib approach to axillary vein access is the most effective means to access the vessel while minimizing the risk of pneumothorax. [42] A prior study did examine pacemaker implantation complication rates of 632 consecutive implants at a single non-community institution.[33] They found a 0.6% rate of hemothorax with a substantially large incidence of complications experienced by low-volume (<12 implants per year) implanters.

Hemothorax can be caused by pacemaker lead placement (more frequently atrial lead perforation) as well as vascular access damage to the subclavian and axillary veins as well as the vena cava. Figure 3 depicts a post-implant CXR of a hemothorax from damage to the superior vena cava during upgrade of dual chamber pacemaker to biventricular defibrillator. This patient experienced pain during passage of the introducer placed over a guidewire seen in inferior vena cava with subsequent development of right pleural effusion. The injury was believed to have occurred during passage of CS guiding catheter introducer over the wire. Recognition of new effusions should be treated as possible procedural related hemothorax and surgical consultation is warranted.

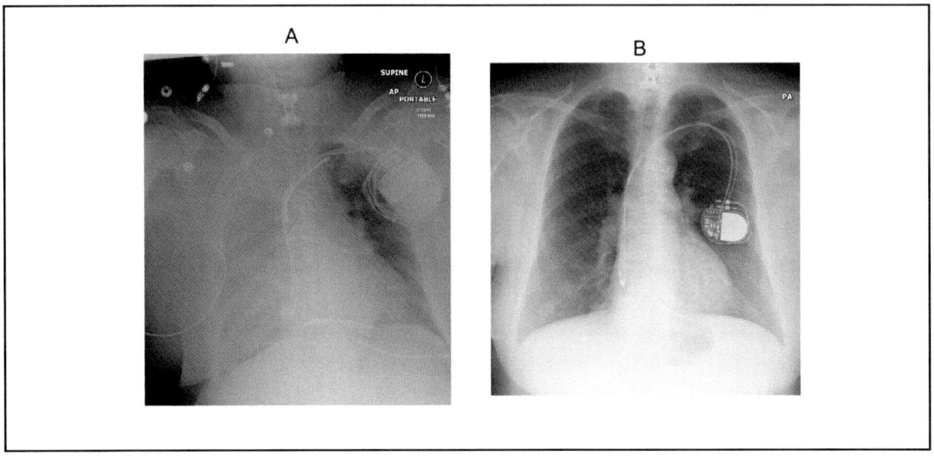

Figure 3. Hemothorax after Device Implantation (A) From Wire/Sheath Trauma to the Superior Vena Cava. The right hemithorax has a layered effusion with blunting of the right costophrenic angle. Image B depicts the preoperative radiograph prior to upgrade of pacemaker to defibrillator.

4.4. Perforation / tamponade

Perforation (both acute and subacute) has been reported to occur in up to 1% of pacemaker implantations. [5,8,10,31,32,35,36,37] In addition, asymptomatic subclinical perforation may occur in 15% of patients after device implantation. [43] Symptoms of perforation include pleuritic chest pain from pericarditis, diaphragmatic or intercostal muscle stimulation and, in the presence of pericardial effusion, patients may develop shortness of breath and hypotension as tamponade develops. [44] Others signs/symptoms of perforation include right bundle-oid paced QRS morphology (though we have seen RBBB configuration and diaphragmatic stimulation in RV apical lead position) or friction rub after implant. If perforation is suspected, urgent evaluation of the patient and device function is warranted though lead parameters are often within normal limits. [44] Figure 4 shows examples of coronary sinus damage that can occur during LV lead implantation. Figure 5 depicts right ventricular lead perforations. Cardiac surgery is typically not required for a majority of patients diagnosed with cardiac perforation from a pacemaker implantation. Rather, most cases can be managed with pericardiocentesis for symptomatic effusions and repositioning of the lead in the EP laboratory with close cardiothoracic surgical collaboration. [45,46,44] Figure 6 shows a large cardiac silhouette developing after pacemaker implantation that was due to large pericardial effusion. The effusion was treated with pericardiocentesis (with no evidence of reaccumulation) and did not require lead repositioning. Though perforation and subsequent tamponade are infrequent complication of pacemaker implantation, they can be responsible for significant patient morbidity and mortality. The risks of perforation cannot be underestimated; death from tamponade with subsequent cardiac arrest was responsible for 21.8% of the mortality in a worldwide study of perforation after ablation for atrial fibrillation. [47]

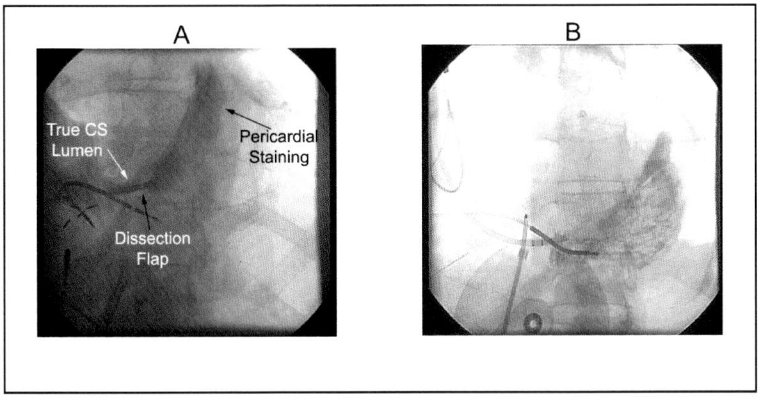

Figure 4. Damage to the coronary sinus during left ventricular lead implantation. Image A depicts a dissection/perforation flap and the resulting pericardial staining from engaging the coronary sinus with a deflectable electrophysiology recording catheter. Image B shows a similar instance of pericardial staining with no focal dissection flap or perforation. Both patients underwent successful LV lead implantation at the time.

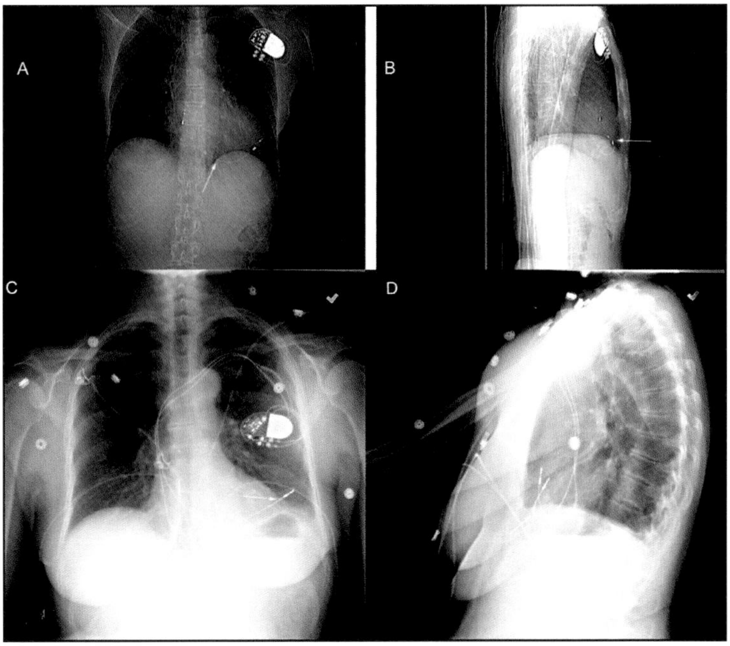

Figure 5. Examples of Right Ventricular Pacemaker Lead perforation. Images A and B depict an RV lead perforation that exits the right ventricular base in A (arrow) and reenters near the right ventricular apex in B (arrow). Images C and D depict an right ventricular apical perforation. The lead is seen exiting the cardiac silhouette in C (arrow); the lateral view (D) depicts an abrupt change in lead course (arrow) that is often seen in right ventricular apical perforations as the lead courses posteriorly in the pericardial space.

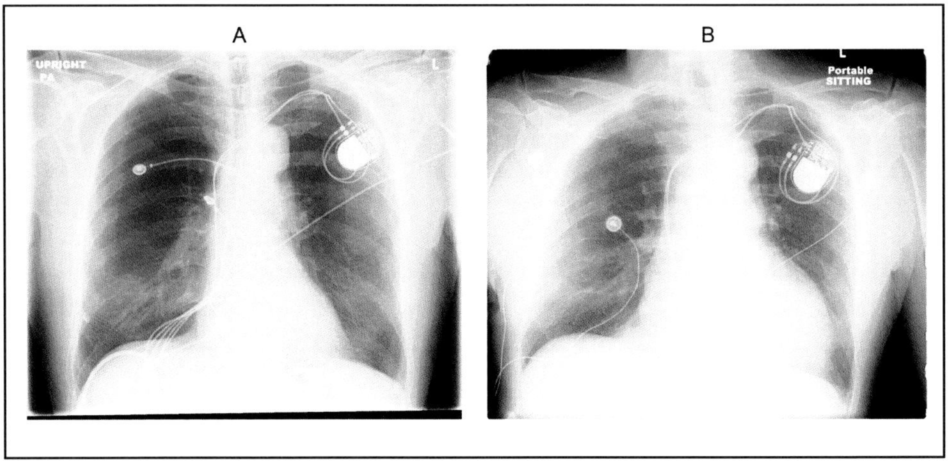

Figure 6. Chest radiograph appearance of large pericardial effusion after RV lead perforation. Immediate post-implant CXR (A) shows normal appearance of the cardiac silhouette. Two weeks post-operative CXR performed because patient reported symptoms of chest pressure (B) shows enlarged cardiac silhouette. Patient responded to pericardiocentesis with no lead repositioning.

4.5. Complications of Left Ventricular (LV) lead placement via the coronary sinus

The emergence of resynchronization therapy has led to an increase in attempts at left ventricular lead placement via the coronary sinus. The MIRACLE study program [48] reported a 91.6% success rate for LV lead placement, while COMPANION [49] revealed an 89% success rate for LV lead placement. Another report indicated a similar 92% success rate with LV lead placement. [50] Though we counsel our patients on a LV lead placement success rate at 88-92%, our center demonstrated a 97% success rate (64 of 66 patients) with LV lead placement within the range from 2:30 to 5:30 o'clock in the left anterior oblique (LAO) view. [8]

Complications of biventricular pacing, specifically LV lead placement, include cardiac perforation, coronary sinus dissection, electrical trauma (damage to the native conduction system), failure to place the lead, dislodgement of the lead, and diaphragmatic stimulation. [51] CS dissections or perforations, cardiac perforations, or cardiac vein dissection or perforation was reported in 45 of 2078 (2%) in the MIRACLE study program. [48] Figure 4 depicts damage done to the coronary sinus during LV lead implantation. Loss of LV capture and diaphragmatic stimulation leading to interruption of resynchronization therapy has been found to occur in 10% and 2% of patients, respectively. [52] The development of new LV leads with up to 4 electrodes offer the possibility of numerous pacing vectors that can minimize loss of capture and diaphragmatic stimulation.

4.6. Arrhythmias (SVT, VT, VF)

The incidence of sustained atrial, pacemaker-mediated and ventricular rhythm disturbances after pacemaker implantation is low. [53]. In patients without prior atrial arrhythmias, Jordaens et al found early atrial fibrillation (during the first week) in 2 of 112 patients and late atrial fibrillation was seen in seven patients, flutter in one, yielding a total incidence of 8.9% for 22 months. There were no significant differences with respect to age, etiology, electrocardiographic diagnosis, pacing history, or the measured intracardiac P wave between the group with and the group without atrial fibrillation. Ventricular fibrillation has been reported to occur in 0.1% of all patients undergoing pacemaker implantation and up to 0.6% of patients aged > 90 years undergoing pacemaker implantation. [10]

It has been reported that ventricular tachyarrhythmias may be present in 12-31% of patients months to years after pacemaker implantation [54] but this may reflect underlying substrate issues. However, there are several situations where pacemaker implantation may cause the ventricular tachyarrhythmias. These include pacemaker lead irritation of the right ventricular inflow [55] and outflow tracts [56], pacemaker stimulus on T wave [57], reentrant circuit around endocardial pacemaker lead [58] and bradycardia-dependent VT facilitated by long pause caused by myopotential inhibition of a VVI pacemaker. [59]

4.7. Death

In-hospital death generally occurs in less than 1% of pacemaker implantations [5,8,10,11,37] however there is a concern that death is underreported as some studies do not specifically mention perioperative death. [9, 30,31,32, 33] The most common causes of confirmed device related in-hospital deaths are perforations (subclavian artery, brachiocephalic trunk, right atrium, and right ventricle). The most common cause of non-device related in-hospital deaths is myocardial infarction as well as less commonly pulmonary embolism, stroke, heart failure, and sepsis. [60]

4.8. Pocket hematoma

The incidence of pocket hematoma has been reported at 4.9% and leading to prolonged hospitalization in 2.0% of all patients. [61] Reoperation for pocket hematoma was required in 1.0% of patients. High-dose heparinization, combined acetylsalicylic acid (ASA)/thienopyridine treatment after coronary stenting, and low operator experience were independently predictive of hematoma development. [61] In addition, development of postoperative hematoma places the patient at elevated risk of device infection. [62] There is data to suggest that warfarin causes fewer pocket complications than heparin products. Specifically, temporarily interrupting anticoagulation is associated with increased thromboembolic events, whereas cessation of warfarin with bridging anticoagulation is associated with a higher rate of pocket hematoma and a longer hospital stay. [63]

4.9. Hospital lengths of stay

There is little data available on average length of stays post pacemaker implantation. An estimate of 2-3days as an average length of stay post implant can be made from the available studies. [5,8,11,37] There is evidence that complications cause a substantial increase in the length of stay up to 16days. [64] The mean complication costs are $4345 ± $1540 for pacemaker lead revision, $24,459 ± $14,585 for pacemaker infection, and $6187 ± $2631 for hematoma evacuation. [64]

5. Subacute post-implant complications (< 30days)

5.1. Pacemaker and lead function / failures

Electrocardiographic signs of pacemaker malfunction can be grouped into four categories: failure to capture, failure to output, undersensing, and inappropriate pacemaker rate. Sensing abnormalities may occur in 3% of patients, failure to capture in 1%, and failure to capture and inappropriate pacemaker rate in another 1% of patients. [65]

5.1.1. Failure to capture

Loss of capture after pacemaker implantation has many causes: Dislodgement, Elevated Thresholds, Inappropriate Lead Placement, Fracture, Insulation Failure, Loose set screw, Exit Block (>4 weeks), Perforation, Battery/circuit Failure, Air in Pocket, and Metabolic/Drugs (Flecainide). Lead dislodgement, the most common cause of failure to capture, [65] has been reported to occur in up to 4-6% of pacemaker implantations [28,35] but is generally reported with a 1-3% incidence [5,10,11,30,32,33,34,36,37]. Figure 7A, B, and C depicts examples of right atrial, right ventricular, and left ventricular lead dislodgements that may result in loss of capture. Lead dislodgements are treated by repositioning in the EP laboratory.

5.1.2. Failure to output

Failure to pace with no obvious pacemaker output may be caused by battery or circuit failure, lead fracture, internal insulation failure, oversensing, loose set screw, or crosstalk. Random component failure is rare however, total battery depletion can occur if routine pacemaker followup is inadequate. [65] Once initial end-of-life indicators appear, there is usually a period of months before the battery reaches a critically low voltage and pacing fails. [65] The incidence of pacemaker lead fracture has been reported at 0.1% to 4.2% per patient-year and usually occurs adjacent to the generator or near the site of venous access. [66] Figure 8 shows a lead fracture discovered at reoperation when patient presented in complete heart block with no ventricular capture almost one year from pacemaker implant. Figure 9 depicts chest radiograph findings of lead fracture (failure to pace) versus a pseudofracture (normal pacing function). Finally, air in header may cause noise oversensing (as air released out of header) as shown in Figure 10. Other electrical signals that may cause

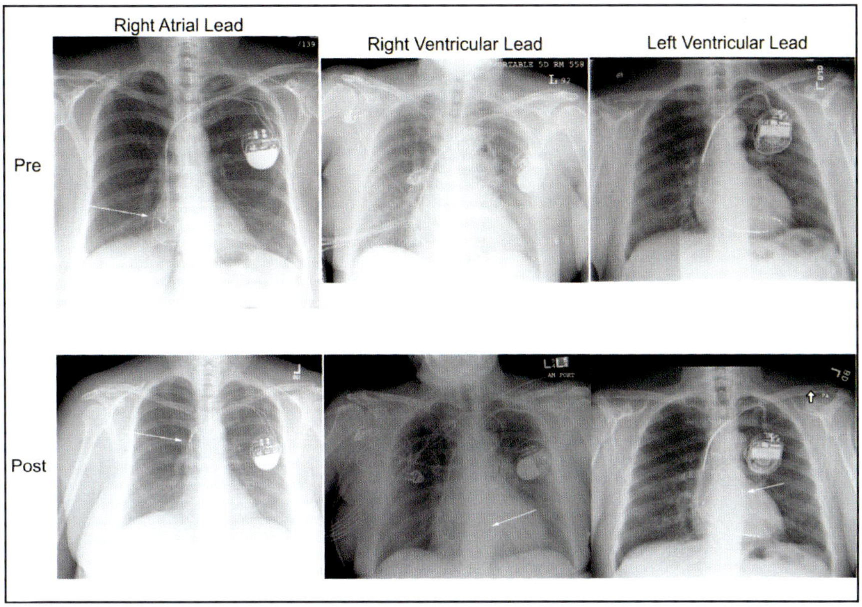

Figure 7. Right Atrial (A), Right Ventricular (B), and Left Ventricular (C) Leads Before (Pre) and After (Post) Dislodgements. Right atrial lead became dislodged after patient twiddled with device. Right ventricular lead dislodged by moving more basilar in position (arrow) one day after implant. Left ventricular lead dislodged and reseated itself in the body of coronary sinus 3 months after initial placement (arrow).

oversensing include diaphragmatic myopotentials (especially with extending bipolar sensing), T waves, P waves, and environmental noise.

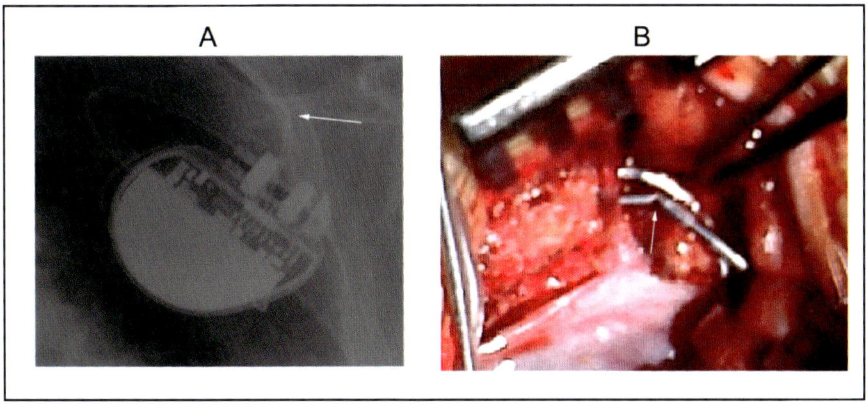

Figure 8. Right Ventricular Lead Fracture. Ventricular lead that was fractured one year after implantation resulting in failure to pace. Figure 8A shows appearance of right ventricular lead on CXR that was suspicious for fracture location (arrow). Figure 8B depicts the intraoperative appearance of lead that was likely site of fracture (arrow).

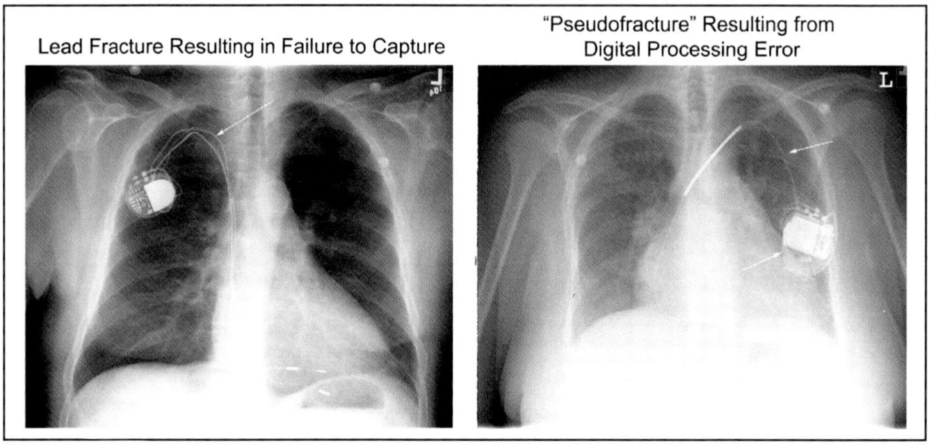

Figure 9. The radiograph in A shows a lead fracture that resulted in no capture. The radiograph in B depicts a "pseudofracture" where digital frame shift causes artifact to simulate a lead fracture in a properly functioning lead.

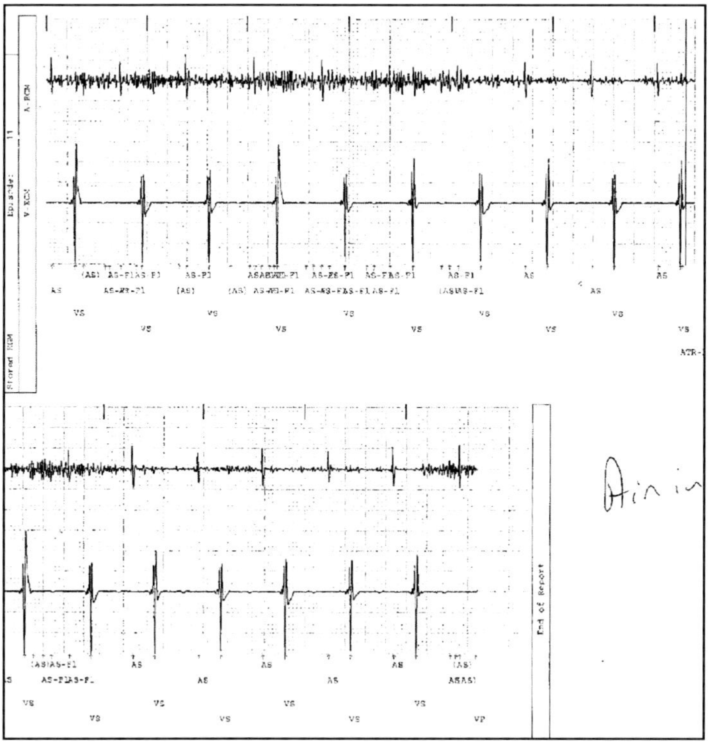

Figure 10. Noise caused by air in header. Atrial electrogram during device interrogation revealed high-frequency noise during sinus rhythm. This patient was not pacemaker dependent so there was no failure to pace.

5.1.3. *Undersensing*

Undersensing of intrinsic cardiac activity results in inappropriate pacing output that competes with intrinsic activity. Undersensing is most likely caused by lead dislodgement, poor lead position at time of implantation, or an interruption in the insulation of the pacing lead. [65]

5.2. Hospital readmission

The average rate of hospital readmission within 30 days of pacemaker implant is 4-6%. [8,11,28,35] We examined possible factors influencing readmission rates in extreme elderly undergoing pacemaker implantation. [11] Overall, increased age and Device Type (e.g., single-chamber, dual-chamber, biventricular, generator change) demonstrated a non-significant trend toward increased readmission rate. The order of decreasing significance in a multivariate analysis of readmissions was: Device Type > Age > Creatinine > Urgent/Emergent > EF > Sex > Weight.

5.3. Death

Early all-cause mortality 30-days after pacemaker implantation has been reported in 0.1-0.7% of patients. [30,5,36] Death rates may be increased (2%) in the extreme elderly aged > 80 years due to increased age-related mortality in this group. [11]

6. Late complications (> 30days)

6.1. Lead function / failures

6.1.1. *Twiddling*

Originally described in 1968 [67], twiddling refers to patient manipulation of pacemaker can or leads that may lead to malfunction. It has a reported incidence of 0.07% in a series of 17000 patients. [68] Figure 11 depicts lead orientation before and after patient twiddling resulted in lead dislodgement.

6.1.2. *Exit block*

Transient disruptions should be excluded first: metabolic and electrolyte abnormalities, drug effects, extreme hypothyroidism (myxedema), and cardiac ischemia. There is an expected rise in capture threshold in the 2-6 week period after lead placement attributed to local inflammation or foreign body reaction at the tip-tissue interface. In the era of epicardial and early endocardial leads, this was a much greater concern. Passive fixation endocardial leads have, on average, lower stimulation thresholds than active fixation leads due to lack of trauma at tissue interface. The degree that the capture threshold increases is markedly blunted with steroid eluting endocardial leads which have thus become generally preferred for their more favorable delivery characteristics having overcome the problem of

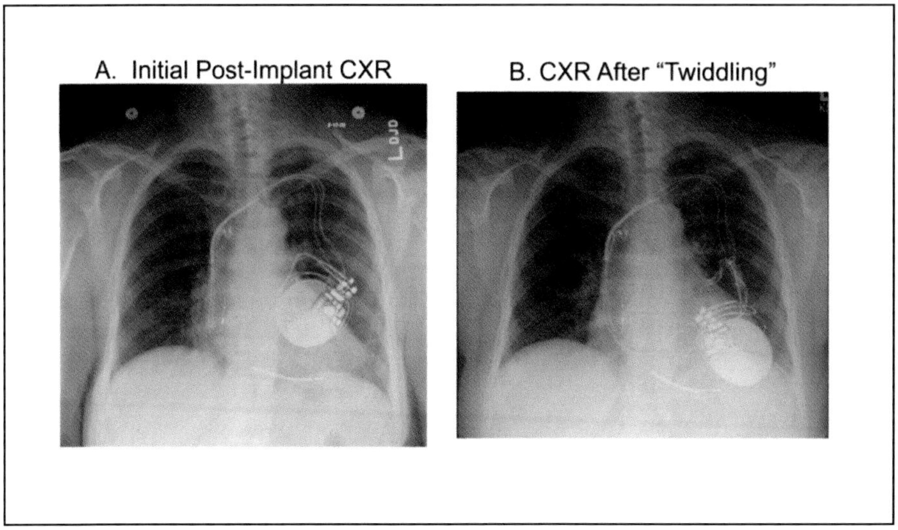

Figure 11. A and B. Lead orientation before and after patient twiddling resulted in lead dislodgement. Image A depicts the post-implant radiograph baseline lead positioning after biventricular defibrillator implant. Image B shows retracted right and left ventricular leads and leads tangled in the pocket superior to device can that is rotated.

higher stimulation thresholds. [69,70] The first randomized trial to compare a standard active fixation lead to a similar designed lead with a steroid eluting reservoir was reported in 1995. [71] Prior to that time, passive fixation leads were generally preferred because the capture threshold was relatively lower than standard active fixation leads. The disadvantage to passive fixation leads was an inability to perform atrial mapping, unreliable lateral wall stability, and requirement for placement in the atrial appendage which may be difficult in patient who have undergone bypass. The most dramatic difference in stimulation threshold between steroid eluting leads and standard endocardial leads was in the magnitude of increase in the acute phase as well as the duration of peak before returning to the chronic threshold. [71] The steroid lead returned to chronic capture threshold by week 2 whereas the non-steroid eluting lead remained above chronic threshold for 12 weeks. A non-significant increase in atrial lead dislodgements occurred with the steroid lead (0% vs 2%, p=0.58). Lower capture thresholds allow for lower programmed output to maintain 2x safety margin, ultimately improving generator longevity. A rise in capture threshold may occur beyond 6 weeks after implantation (chronic phase of lead maturation). As the threshold steadily rises, it may exceed the maximum output of the pulse generator, known as exit block. Exit block is recognized by high pacing thresholds without radiographic evidence of dislodgement. It may be related to inflammation or fibrosis at the electrode-myocardium interface and generally presents >4weeks after implantation. [65] Some patients and particularly pediatric patients are particularly prone to this phenomena and may lead to multiple lead revisions.

6.2. Device/lead advisories

A large multicenter Canadian observational study showed that the complication rate from device replacement for an advisory indication was an astounding 9.1%. [72] Of these, 5.9% required reoperation and there were 2 deaths. Naturally, the risk of an adverse outcome during replacement must be balanced by the risk of death due to device malfunction. Pacemakers and defibrillators have saved thousands of lives but as is true of all man-made devices, malfunctions have and will continue to occur. In response to a marked increase in device advisories in 2005, and to balance alarmism with protection of patients with a high risk situation, the Heart Rhythm Society (HRS), utilizing the HRS Task Force on Device Performance Policies and Guidelines published guidelines in 2006. [73] Recognizing that physicians and patients need timely and accurate information regarding device performance, arguably the most important outcome was a call for greater transparency of post market analysis and reporting of failures. Device performance is defined as the percentage of devices that are in service and functioning appropriately in living individuals over time and depends not only on the characteristics of the device but the skill of the implanting physician and caregivers following the device. [73] Data compiled from 1990-2002 from FDA annual reports showed that confirmed device malfunctions leading to device explantation were about 0.1-0.9% for pacemakers and 0.7-3.9% for ICDs. [73] Although failure rates are low, there is a negative psychological impact on patients who have a device which is under advisory, particularly if pacer dependent or if placed for a secondary indication.

To assist in communication from industry to physicians and patients it is proposed that terminology be standardized. The term "recall" was changed to "Class I Advisory" which is just short of a directive for device replacement because of a reasonable probability that malfunction could result in death or significant harm. Class II and class III recalls are subsequently referred to as advisory notices (non-life threatening malfunctions) and safety alerts (potential malfunctions). This information is disseminated from industry via standardized Physician Device Advisory Notifications and Patient Device Advisory Notifications which are also available on the manufacturer's website. Prior experience tells us the advisory information should be disseminated to physicians just before patients. Advisories should include general information about the malfunction and potential clinical implications but should acknowledge that treatment decisions should ultimately be determined by patients in consultations with physicians. The situations where device replacement is recommended are 1) When mechanism of malfunction is known and likely to be recurrent or lead to patient death, 2) The patient is pacer dependant, 3) The device was placed for a secondary prevention indication or have received appropriate therapy, 4) The device is approaching EOL. Conservative management (enhanced non-invasive and remote monitoring) should be considered when 1) The rate of malfunction is very low in non-pacer dependant patients or primary prevention without history of appropriate therapy, 2) The patient has significant comorbidities or high operative risk even when the risk of device malfunction is substantial. 3) Remote monitoring and software reprogramming can minimize risk (i.e., non physiologic noise).

6.3. Infection

Up to 60% of patients present with localized infection involving the device pocket whereas the remaining patients may present with endovascular infection but no evidence of inflammation of the device pocket. [74] Approximately 10% of patients may have intracardiac vegetations identified by transesophageal echocardiogram, though can still undergo percutaneous lead extraction safely [75]. See Figure 12 for echocardiographic image of vegetation adherent to device lead. Generally, the most common pathogen isolated is aerobic gram-positive organisms, of which 90% are Staphylococcus species, with a high rate of methicillin resistance (~50%). [74] The risk of pacemaker infection is lower than that of implantable defibrillators. The presence of epicardial leads and postoperative complications at the generator pocket are significant risk factors for early-onset ICD infection, whereas longer duration of hospitalization at the time of implantation and chronic obstructive pulmonary disease were associated with late-onset ICD infections. [62] In one of the largest studies of pacemaker infections [76], repeated operative procedures after the first pacemaker implantation were associated with a substantial incremental risk of infection. Female sex, older age, and preoperative antibiotics given at the initial implant were associated with a lower risk of later infection. The pacing mode, indication for pacing, and complexity of the procedure were not independently associated with the risk of later infection. Sixty percent of infections have been found to occur within 90days of implant [77] though a large number of infections occur during the late follow-up (>1 year post-implant) (76). Generator changes and cardiac resynchronization therapy/dual-chamber devices have also been implicated as independent predictors of infection. [77]

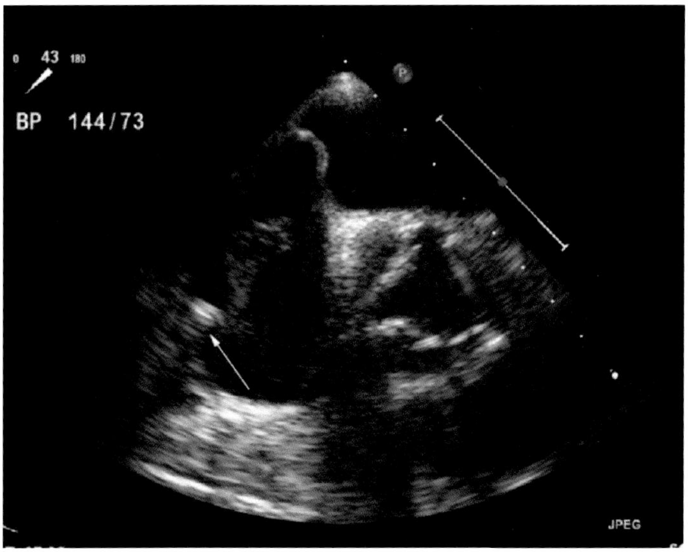

Figure 12. Transesophageal echocardiographic image of vegetation adherent to pacemaker lead. This is a short axis view showing a large, mobile vegetation (encircled) on a right ventricular lead (arrow) in a patient with persistent bacteremia.

The generally accepted means of device infection treatment is removal of the generator and all implanted leads. [78] In a large series of device extractions including 1838 leads [75], post-operative 30-day mortality was 10% though no deaths were related directly to the extraction procedure. Another series of device extractions reported a 0.5% rate of intraprocedural mortality, 4.6% rate of in-hospital mortality, and 2.6% rate of relapsing infections within 1 year of reimplantation. [74]

6.4. Pacemaker syndrome

Occurs most commonly with single chamber ventricular pacemakers (e.g., VVI or VVIR modes) and symptoms are due to loss of atrioventricular synchrony. It must be noted that pacemaker syndrome can occur with any pacing mode if AV synchrony is lost. Symptoms include malaise, weakness, cannon A waves, CP, cough, confusion, or syncope.

6.5. Venous thrombosis

Upper extremity deep venous thrombosis (or stenosis) is uncommon in the general population but venous stenosis has been seen in up to 33-64% of patients after implantation of pacing leads. [79,80] Statistically significant factors that have been associated with an increased risk include previous transvenous temporary leads [80], left ventricular ejection fraction <40% [80], systemic infection [81], absence of anticoagulation, use of hormone treatment, personal history of venous thrombosis, and presence of multiple leads. [82] Symptoms may include shoulder or neck discomfort, ipsilateral arm edema with cyanosis, dilated collateral cutaneous veins around the shoulder, or jugular vein distension. [83] Venography is considered the gold standard for diagnosis but compressive ultrasonography is an effective and economical means of confirming the clinical diagnosis. [83] Treatment may include anticoagulation (warfarin and/or heparin), extraction of old nonfunctioning lead to create a new venous channel, or venoplasty to reduce venous stenosis or allow the implantation of subsequent leads. [83,84]

7. Predicting risks for procedural complications

There is some evidence that elderly patients are at increased risk of complications following pacemaker implantation. [85] Armaganijan et al [85] found that any early complication occurred in 5.1% of patients ≥ 75 years of age compared to 3.4% of patients aged < 75 years. The concomitant use of temporary transvenous pacemakers or steroid use within 7days of implant have been shown to increase rates of post implant pericardial effusion. [45] Weaker predictors of post implant effusions were the use of helical screw ventricular leads, body mass index <20, older age, and longer fluoroscopy times. [45] Pneumothorax has been found to more common in older, lighter females. [5] A prior study examining predictors of complications in extremely elderly patients undergoing pacemaker implantation [11] found overall rates of implant complications comparable to data from younger patient populations while experiencing a higher 30day all-cause mortality (that may have been attributable to elevated all-cause mortality rates in this age-group). Multivariate analysis revealed that female sex, device type, and urgent/emergent placement demonstrated a non-significant trend toward increased rates of complication; increased age and device type demonstrated a non-significant trend toward increased readmission rate.

Higher (>12 implants/year) versus lower volume operators (<12 implants/year) have also demonstrated diverging rates of complication. [33] Finally, more complex devices (dual-chamber vs single ventricular chamber pacemakers) have been associated with higher rates of complications. [10,30,31,32,35,37] however, there is data that does not demonstrate increased rates of complications in dual-chamber devices. [9,11,34] Finally, it has been suggested that physician training (specifically, board-certification or board-eligibility in clinical cardiac electrophysiology) may result in lower rates of lead dislodgement. [7,86]

8. Conclusion

Major and minor complications occur in approximately 4-7% of patients within 30d of pacemaker implantation. [5,10,11,32,36,35] Permanent pacemakers are commonly implanted in patients over the age of 65 and this is the most rapidly growing segment of the U.S. population. That being said, pacemaker therapy is also associated with an 11-40% risk of complications in the pediatric population; the most common complications in this segment are pneumothorax, hematoma, and infection. [87] Figure 13 depicts the incidence of the most common complications after pacemaker implantation. Prompt recognition and treatment of complications after pacemaker implantation is essential for all implanting physicians regardless of background.

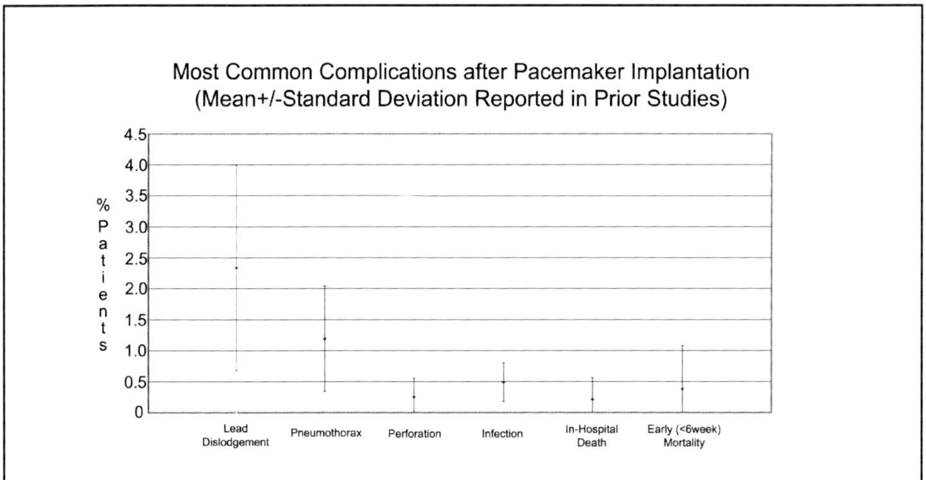

Figure 13. Most Common Complications Seen After Pacemaker Implantation. This figure depicts the most common complications seen after pacemaker implantation from available prior. The data are for complications seen within 30-42days depending upon the study parameters as referenced.

Author details

Jeffrey L. Williams and Robert T. Stevenson
The Good Samaritan Hospital, Heart Rhythm Center, Lebanon Cardiology Associates, Lebanon Pennsylvania, U.S

9. References

[1] Kurtz SM, Ochoa JA, Lau E, Shkolnikov Y, Pavri BB, Frisch D, Greenspon AJ, "Implantation trends and patient profiles for pacemakers and implantable cardioverter defibrillators in the United States: 1993-2006," Pacing Clin Electrophysiol, V. 33, No. 6 (June 1, 2010), pp. 705-11.
[2] Perls T, "Health and disease in people over 85," BMJ, V. 339 (22 December 2009), b4715.
[3] Hobbs FB, "Current Population Reports, Series P23-190, Sixty-Five Plus in the U.S.," http://www.census.gov/population/www/pop-profile/elderpop.html. Accessed 10 March 2011.
[4] Cherubini A, Oristrell J, Pla X, Ruggiero C, Ferretti R, Diestre G, Clarfield M, Crome P, Hertogh C, Lesauskaite V, Prada G-I, Szczerbinska K, Topinkova E, Sinclair-Cohen J, Edbrooke D, Mills G, "The Persistent Exclusion of Older Patients From Ongoing Clinical Trials Regarding Heart Failure," Arch Intern Med, V. 171, No. 6 (March 28, 2011), pp. 550-556.
[5] Link MS, Estes NAM, Griffin JJ, Wang PJ, Maloney JD, Kirchhoffer JB, Mitchell GF, Orav J, Goldman L, Lamas GA, "Complications of Dual Chamber Pacemaker Implantation in the Elderly," J Intervent Cardiac Electrophys, V. 2 (1998), pp. 175-179.
[6] Alter P, Waldhans S, Plachta E, Moosdorf R, Grimm W, "Complications of Implantable Cardioverter Defibrillator Therapy in 440 Consecutive Patients," PACE, V. 28 (September 2005), pp. 926-932.
[7] Curtis JP, Luebbert JJ, Wang Y, Rathore SS, Chen J, Heidenreich PA, Hammill SC, Lampert RI, Krumholz HM, "Association of Physician Certification and Outcomes Among Patients Receiving an Implantable Cardioverter-Defibrillator," JAMA, V. 301, No. 16 (April 22/29, 2009), pp. 1661-1670.
[8] Williams JL, Lugg D, Gray R, Hollis D, Stoner M, Stevenson R, "Patient Demographics, Complications, and Hospital Utilization in 250 Consecutive Device Implants of a New Community Hospital Electrophysiology Program," American Heart Hospital Journal, V. 8, No. 1 (Summer, 2010), pp. 33-39.
[9] Rosenheck S, Geist M, Weiss A, Hasin Y, Weiss TA, Gotsman MS, "Permanent Cardiac Pacing in Octogenarians," Amer J Ger Card, V. 4, No. 6 (1995), pp. 42-47.
[10] Nowak B and Misselwitz B, "Effects of increasing age onto procedural parameters in pacemaker implantation: results of an obligatory external quality control program," Europace, V. 11 (November 2008), pp. 75-79.

[11] Stevenson R, Lugg D, Gray R, Hollis D, Stoner M, Williams JL, "Pacemaker Implantation in the Extreme Elderly," Journal of Interventional Cardiac Electrophysiology, V. 33, No. 1 (January 2012), pp. 51-58.

[12] Klug D, Balde M, Pavin D, Hidden-Lucet F, Clementy J, Sadoul N, Luc Rey J, Lande G, Lazarus A, Victor J, Barnay C, Grandbastien B, Kacet S, "Risk Factors Related to Infections of Implanted Pacemakers and Cardioverter-Defibrillators," Circulation, Vol. 116, (August 2007), pp.1349-1355.

[13] Kirkfeldt RE, Johansen JB, Nohr EA, Moller M, Nielsen JC, "Risk Factors for Lead Complications in Cardiac Pacing: A Population-based Cohort of 28,860 Danish Patients," Heart Rhythm, Vol.8, No.10, (October 2011), pp.1622-1628.

[14] Marcos, SK, Thomsen, HS. "Prevention of general reactions to contrast media: A consensus report and guidelines," Eur Radiol, Vol.11, N.9 (2001), pp.1720-8.

[15] Brockow K, Christiansen C, Kanny G, Clément O, Barbaud A, Bircher A, DeWachter P, Guéant JL, Rodriguez Guéant RM, Mouton-Faivre C, Ring J, Romano A, Sainte-Laudy J, Demoly P, Pichler WJ, ENDA and the EAACI interest group on drug hypersensitivity (2005), "Management of hypersensitivity reactions to iodinated contrast media," Allergy, Vol.60, pp.150–158.

[16] Trcka J, Schmidt C, Seitz CS, Brocker EB, Gross GE, Trautman A, "Anaphylaxis to iodinated contrast materials: nonallergic hypersensitivity or IgE-mediated allergy? AJR, V. 190, No. 3 (2008), pp. 666-670

[17] Guillaume B, Kellner F, Barnig C, "Management of Patients with History of Adverse Effects to Contrast Media When Pulmonary Artery CT Angiography is Required," Radiology, V. 245 (December 2007), pp. 919-921.

[18] Tramer MR, vonElm E, Loubeyre P, Hauser C, "Pharmacologic prevention of Serious Anaphylactic Reactions Due to Iodinated Contrast Material: Systematic Review," BMJ, V.333, (September 2006), pp. 675-678.

[19] The Royal College of Radiologists, "Standards for Intravascular Contrast Administration To Adult Patients: Second Edition," London, The Royal College of Radiologists, February 2010.

[20] Murkin JM, "Anesthesia and hypothyroidism: a review of thyroxine physiology, pharmacology, and anesthetic implications," Anesth Analg, V. 61, No. 4 (April 1982), pp. 371-83.

[21] Farling PA, "Thyroid Disease," Br J Anaesth, V. 85, No. 1 (2000), pp. 15-28.

[22] Gaitan BD, Trentman TL, Fassett SL, Mueller JT, Altemose GT, "Sedation and analgesia in the cardiac electrophysiology laboratory: a national survey of electrophysiologists investigating the who, how, and why?" J Cardiothorac Vasc Anesth 2011; 25:647–659.

[23] Magnusson L and Spahn DR, "New concepts of atelectasis during general anesthesia," British J Anaesthesia, V. 91, No. 1 (2003), pp. 61-72.

[24] Lawrence VA, Hilsenbeck SG, Mulrow CD, Dhanda R, Sapp J, Page CP, "Incidence and hospital stay for cardiac and pulmonary complications after abdominal surgery," J Gen Intern Med, V. 10 (1995), pp. 671-678.

[25] Trentman TL, Fassett SL, Mueller JT, Altemose GT, "Airway interventions in the cardiac electrophysiology laboratory: a retrospective review," J Cardiothorac Vasc Anesth 2009; 23:841–5.

[26] DiBiase L, Conti S, Mohanty P, et al. General anesthesia reduces the prevalence of pulmonary vein reconnection during repeat ablation when compared with conscious sedation: Results from a randomized study. Heart Rhythm 2011; 8:368–372.

[27] Williams JL, Valencia V, Lugg D, Gray R, Hollis D, Toth JW, Benson R, DeFrancesco-Loukas MA, Stevenson R, Teiken PJ, "High Frequency Jet Ventilation During Ablation of Supraventricular and Ventricular Arrhythmias: Efficacy, Patient Tolerance and Safety," The Journal of Innovations in Cardiac Rhythm Management, 2 (2011), 1–7]

[28] Hargreaves MR, Doulalas A, Ormerod OJM, "Early Complications Following Dual Chamber Pacemaker Implantation: 10-Year Experience of a Regional Pacing Centre," Eur JCPE, V. 5, No. 3 (1995), pp. 133-138.

[29] Noseworthy PA, Lashevsky I, Dorian P, Greene M, Cvitkovic S, Newman D, "Feasibility of Implantable Cardioverter Defibrillator Use in Elderly Patients: A Case Series of Octogenarians," PACE, V. 27 (March 2004), pp. 373-378.

[30] Chauhan A, Grace AA, Newell SA, Stone DL, Shapiro LM, Schofield PM, Petch MC, "Early Complications After Dual Chamber Versus Single Chamber Pacemaker Implantation," PACE, V. 17, Part II, (November 1994), pp. 2012-2015.

[31] Wiegand UKH, Bode F, Bonnemeier H, Eberhard F, Schlei M, Peters W, "Long-Term Complication Rates in Ventricular, Single Lead VDD, and Dual Chamber Pacing," PACE, V. 26 (October 2003), pp. 1961-1969.

[32] Eberhart F, Bode F, Bonnemeier H, Boguschewski F, Schlei M, Peters W, Wiegand UKH, "Long term complications in single and dual chamber pacing are influenced by surgical experience and patient morbidity," Heart, V. 91 (2005), pp. 500-506.

[33] Parsonnet V, Bernstein AD, Lindsay B, "Pacemaker-Implantation Complication Rates: An Analysis of Some Contributing Factors," JACC, V. 13, No. 4 (March 15, 1989), pp. 917-921.

[34] Aggarwal RK, Connelly DT, Ray SG, Ball J, Charles RG, "Early complications of permanent pacemaker implantation: no difference between dual and single chamber systems," Br Heart J, V. 73 (1995), pp.571-575.

[35] Kiviniemi MS, Pirnes MA, Eranen HJK, Kettunen RVJ, Hartikainen JEK, "Complications Related to Permanent Pacemaker Therapy," PACE, V. 22 (May 1999), pp. 711-720.

[36] Ellenbogen KA, Hellkamp AS, Wilkoff BL, Camunas JL, Love JC, Hadjis TA, Lee KL, Lamas GA, "Complications Arising After Implantation of DDD Pacemakers: The MOST Experience," Amer J Card, V. 92 (September 15, 2003), pp. 740-741.
[37] van Eck JWM, van Hemel NM, Zuithof P, van Asseldonk JPM, Voskuil TLHM, Grobbee DE, Moons KGM, "Incidence and predictors of in-hospital events after first implantation of pacemakers," Europace, V. 9 (June 2007), pp. 884-889.
[38] Chadha TS, Cohn MA, "Noninvasive treatment of pneumothorax with oxygen inhalation," Respiration, V. 44, No. 2, (1983), pp. 147-52.
[39] Kulvatunyou N, Vijayasekaran A, Hansen A, Wynne JL, O'Keeffe T, Friese RS, Joseph B, Tang A, Rhee P, "Two-year experience of using pigtail catheters to treat traumatic pneumothorax: a changing trend," J Trauma, V. 71, No. 5 (Nov 2011), pp. 1104-7.
[40] Fyke FE III, "Infraclavicular lead failure: tarnish on a golden route," Pacing Clin Electrophysiol, V. 16 (1993), pp. 373-376.
[41] Magney JE, Flynn DM, Parsons JA, Staplin DH, Chin-Purcell MV, Milstein S, Hunter DW, "Anatomical mechanisms explaining damage to pacemaker leads, defibrillator leads, and failure of central venous catheters adjacent to the sternoclavicular joint," Pacing Clinical Electrophysiol, V. 16 (1993), pp. 445-447.
[42] Belott P, "How to access the axillary vein," Heart Rhythm, V. 3, No. 3 (March 2006), pp. 366-369.
[43] Hirschl DA, Jain VR, Spindola-Franco H, Gross JN, Haramati LB, "Prevalence and Characterization of Asymptomatic Pacemaker and ICD Lead Perforation on CT," PACE, V. 30 (January 2007), pp. 28–32.
[44] Wang NC, Williams JL, Jain SK, Shalaby A, "Post-Pacemaker Pulsations," Amer J Med, V 122, No. 4 (April 2009), pp. 345-347.
[45] Mahapatra S, Bybee KA, Bunch TJ, et al, "Incidence and predictors of cardiac perforation after permanent pacemaker implantation," Heart Rhythm, V. 2 (2005), pp. 907-911.
[46] Geyfman V, Storm RH, Lico SC, Oren IV JW, "Cardiac tamponade as complication of active-fixation atrial lead perforations: proposed mechanism and management algorithm," Pacing Clin Electrophysiol, V. 30 (2007), pp. 498-501.
[47] Cappato R, Calkins H, Chen S-A, Davies W, Iesaka Y, Kalman J, Kim Y-H, Klein G, Natale A, Packer D, Skanes A, "Prevalence and Causes of Fatal Outcome in Catheter Ablation of Atrial Fibrillation," JACC, Vol. 53, No. 19 (May 12, 2009), 1798–803.
[48] Leon AR, Abraham WT, Curtis AB, et al.; for the MIRACLE Study Program, "Safety of Transvenous Cardiac Resynchronization System Implantation in Patients with Chronic Heart Failure: Combined Results of Over 2000 Patients from a Multicenter Study Program," J Am Coll Cardiol, 2005;46(12):2348–56.
[49] Bristow MR, Saxon LA, Boehmer J, et al., "Cardiac-Resynchronization Therapy with or without an Implantable Defibrillator in Advanced Chronic Heart Failure for the

Comparison of Medical Therapy, Pacing, and Defibrillation in Heart Failure (COMPANION) Investigators," N Engl J Med, 2004;350(21):2140–50.

[50] D'Ivernois C, Lesage J, Blanc P, "Where are left ventricular leads really implanted? A study of 90 consecutive patients," Pacing Clin Electrophysiol, 2008;31(5):554–9.

[51] Ellery SM and Paul VE, "Complications of biventricular pacing," European Heart Journal Supplements, V. 6, Supp. D (2004), pp. D117-D121.

[52] Knight BP, Desai A, Coman J, Faddis M, Yong P, "Long-term retention of cardiac resynchronization therapy," JACC, V. 44, No. 1 (July 7, 2004), pp. 72-77.

[53] Jordaens L, Robbens E, Van Wassenhove E, Clement DL, "Incidence of arrhythmias after atrial or dual-chamber pacemaker implantation," Eur Heart J, V. 10, No. 2 (Feb 1989), pp. 102-107.

[54] Faber TS, Gradinger R, Treusch S Morkel C, Brachmann J, Bode C, Zehender M, "Incidence of ventricular tachyarrhythmias during permanent pacemaker therapy in low-risk patients results from the German multicentre EVENTS study," European Heart Journal, V. 28, No. 18 (2007), pp. 2238–2242.

[55] Datta G, Sarkar A, Haque A, "An Uncommon Ventricular Tachycardia due to Inactive PPM Lead," ISRN Cardiology, V. 2011 (2011), Article ID 232648, 3 pages.

[56] Bohm A, Pinter A, Preda I, "Ventricular tachycardia induced by a pacemaker lead," Acta Cardiologica, V. 57, No. 1 (2002), pp. 23–24.

[57] Freedman A, Rothman MT, Mason JW, "Recurrent ventricular tachycardia induced by an atrial synchronous ventricular-inhibited pacemaker," Pacing and Clinical Electrophysiology, V. 5, No. 4 (1982), pp. 490–494.

[58] Li W, Sarubbi B, Somerville J, "Iatrogenic ventricular tachycardia from endocardial pacemaker late after repair of tetralogy of Fallot," Pacing and Clinical Electrophysiology, V. 23, No. 12 (2000), pp. 2131–2134.

[59] Iesaka Y, Pinakatt T, Gosselin AJ, Lister JW, "Bradycardia dependent ventricular tachycardia facilitated by myopotential inhibition of a VVI pacemaker," Pacing and Clinical Electrophysiology, V. 5, No. 1 (1982), pp. 23–29.

[60] Schulza N, Puschelb K, Turkc EE, "Fatal complications of pacemaker and implantable cardioverter defibrillator implantation: medical malpractice?" Interactive CardioVascular and Thoracic Surgery, V. 8 (2009), pp. 444–448.

[61] Wiegand UKH, LeJeune D, Boguschewski F, Bonnemeier H, Eberhardt F, Schunkert H, Bode F, "Pocket Hematoma After Pacemaker or Implantable Cardioverter Defibrillator Surgery: Influence of Patient Morbidity, Operation Strategy, and Perioperative Antiplatelet/Anticoagulation Therapy," CHEST, V. 126, No. 4 (October 2004), pp. 1177-1186.

[62] Sohail MR, Hussain S, Le KY, Dib C, Lohse CM, Friedman PA, Hayes DL, Uslan DZ, Wilson WR, Steckelberg JM, Baddour LM; Mayo Cardiovascular Infections Study Group, "Risk factors associated with early- versus late-onset implantable

cardioverter-defibrillator infections," J Interv Card Electrophysiol. V. 31, No. 2 (Aug 2011), pp. 171-83.

[63] Ahmed I, Gertner E, Nelson WB, House CM, Dahiya R, Anderson CP, Benditt DG, Zhu DWX, "Continuing warfarin therapy is superior to interrupting warfarin with or without bridging anticoagulation therapy in patients undergoing pacemaker and defibrillator implantation," Heart Rhythm, V. 7, No. 6 (June 2010), pp. 745-749.

[64] Ferguson TB Jr, Ferguson CL, Crites K, Crimmins-Reda P, "The additional hospital costs generated in the management of complications of pacemaker and defibrillator implantations," J Thorac Cardiovasc Surg, V. 111 (1996), pp. 742-752.

[65] Hayes DL and Vlietstra RE, "Pacemaker Malfunction," Annals of Internal Medicine, V. 119, No. 8 (October 15, 1993), pp. 828-835.

[66] Alt E, Volker R, Blomer H, "Lead fracture in pacemaker patients," Thoracic Cardiovasc Surg, V. 35 (1987), pp. 101-104.

[67] Bayliss CE, Beanlands DS, Baird RJ, "The pacemaker-twiddler's syndrome: a new complication of implantable transvenous pacemakers," Can Med Assoc J, V. 99 (1968), pp. 371–3.

[68] T. Fahraeus and C. J. Hoijer, "Early pacemaker twiddler syndrome," Europace, Vol. 5 (July 2003), pp.

[69] Ellenbogen KA, Wood MA, Gilligan DM, Zmijewski M, Mans D and The CAPSURE Z Investigators (1999), "Steroid Eluting High Impedance Pacing Leads Decrease Short and Long-Term Current Drain: Results from a Multicenter Clinical Trial," Pacing and Clinical Electrophysiology, V.22 No.1 (January 1999), pp. 39-48.

[70] Fortescue EB, Berul Cl, Cecchin F, Walsh EP, Triedman JK, Alexander ME, "Comparison of Modern Steroid-Eluting Epicardial and Thin Transvenous Pacemaker Leads in Pediatric and Congenital Heart Disease Patients," J Interv Card Electrophysio, V.14, No.1 (October 2005), pp.27-36.

[71] Crossley GH, Brinker JA, Reynolds D, Spencer W, Johnson B, Hurd H, Touder L, ZmijewskinM, "Steroid Elution Improves the Stimulation Threshold in an Active-Fixation Atrial Permanent Pacing Lead," Circ V. 92 (1995), pp.2935-2939.

[72] Gould, PA. Outcome of Advisory ICD replacement: One year follow-up. Heart Rhythm Vol5, No12, December 2008.

[73] Carlson MD, Wilkoff, BL. Recommendation from the HRS task force on device performance policies and guidelines. Heart Rhythm 2006;3:1250-1273.

[74] Tarakji KG, Chan EJ, Cantillon DJ, Doonan AL, Hu T, Schmitt S, Fraser TG, Kim A, Gordon SM, Wilkoff BL et al, "Cardiac implantable electronic device infections: Presentation, management, and patient outcomes," Heart Rhythm V. 7, No. 8 (August 2010), pp. 1043-1047.

[75] Grammes JA, Schulze CM, Al-Bataineh M, Yesenosky GA, Saari CS, Vrabel MJ, Horrow J, Chowdhury M, Fontaine JM, Kutalek SP, "Percutaneous pacemaker and implantable cardioverter-defibrillator lead extraction in 100 patients with intracardiac

vegetations defined by transesophageal echocardiogram," J Am Coll Cardiol, V. 55, No. 9 (March 2010), pp. 886-94.

[76] Johansen JB, Jørgensen OD, Møller M, Arnsbo P, Mortensen PT, Nielsen JC, "Infection after pacemaker implantation: infection rates and risk factors associated with infection in a population-based cohort study of 46299 consecutive patients ," Eur Heart J, V. 32, No. 8 (April 2011) pp. 991–998.

[77] Nery PB, Fernandes R, Nair GM, Sumner GL, Ribas CS, Menon SM, Wang X, Krahn AD, Morillo CA, Connolly SJ, Healey JS, "Device-related infection among patients with pacemakers and implantable defibrillators: incidence, risk factors, and consequences," J Cardiovasc Electrophysiol, V. 21, No. 7 (July 2010), pp. 786-90.

[78] Wilkoff BL, "How to treat and identify device infections," Heart Rhythm, V. 4 (2007), pp. 1467–1470.

[79] Oginosawa Y, Abe H, Nakashima Y, "The incidence and risk factors for venous obstruction after implantation of transvenous pacing leads," Pacing Clin Electrophysiol, V. 25 (2002), pp. 1605-1611.

[80] DaCosta SS, Scalabrini NA, Costa A, Caldas JG, Martinelli FM, "Incidence and risk factors of upper extremity deep vein lesions after permanent transvenous pacemaker implant: A 6-month follow-up prospective study," Pacing Clin Electrophysiol, V. 25 (2002), pp. 1301-1306.

[81] Bracke F, Meijer A, Van Gelder B, "Venous occlusion of the access vein in patients referred for lead extraction: Influence of patient and lead characteristics," Pacing Clin Electrophysiol, V. 26 (2003), pp. 1649-1652.

[82] van Rooden CJ, Molhoek SG, Rosendaal FR. Schalij MJ, Meinders AE, Huisman MV, "Incidence and risk factors of early venous thrombosis associated with permanent pacemaker leads," J Cardiovasc Electrophysiol, V. 15 (2004), pp. 1258-1262.

[83] Rozmus G, Daubert JP, Huang DT, Rosero S, Hall B, Francis C, "Venous Thrombosis and Stenosis After Implantation of Pacemakers and Defibrillators," J Interv Cardiac Electrophysiol, V. 13 (2005), pp. 9-19.

[84] Worley SJ, Gohn DC, Pulliam RW, Raifsnider MA, Ebersole B, Tuzi J, "Subclavian venoplasty by the implanting physicians in 373 patients over 11 years," Heart Rhythm, V. 8, No. 4 (April 2011), pp. 526-533.

[85] Armaganijan LV, Toff WD, Nielsen JC, Andersen HR, Connolly SJ, Ellenbogen KA, Healey JS, "Are Elderly Patients at Increased Risk of Complications Following Pacemaker Implantation? A Meta-Analysis of Randomized Trials," Pacing Clin Electrophysiol, Epub ahead of Print, (2011 Oct 31).

[86] Cheng A, Wang Y, Curtis JP, Varosy PD, "Acute Lead Dislodgements and In-Hospital Mortality in Patients Enrolled in the National Cardiovascular Data Registry Implantable Cardioverter Defibrillator Registry," J Am Coll Cardiol, V. 56 (2010), pp. 1651-1656.

[87] Czosek RJ, Meganathan K, Anderson JB, Knilans TK, Marino BS, Heaton PC, "Cardiac rhythm devices in the pediatric population: Utilization and complications," Heart Rhythm, V. 9, No. 2 (Feb 2012), pp. 199-208.

Chapter 7

Device-Related Endocarditis and Infected Leads Extraction: The Dark Side of The Moon

Michele Rossi, Giuseppe Musolino, Giuseppe Filiberto Serraino and Attilio Renzulli

Additional information is available at the end of the chapter

http://dx.doi.org/10.5772/48463

1. Introduction

Cardiac rhythm management devices are being increasingly implanted worldwide not only for symptomatic bradycardia, but also for the management of arrhythmia and heart failure (Adabag et al. 2011; COMPANION Investigators 2004; Multicenter Automatic Defibrillator Implantation Trial Investigators 1996; Sudden Cardiac Death in Heart Failure Trial Investigators 2005). The benefit of cardiac resynchronization therapy (CRT) with permanent pacemakers (PPM) as first invasive step to treat the failing heart (Adabag et al. 2011; COMPANION Investigators 2004) and the survival advantage of internal cardiac defibrillator (ICD) in patients with end stage heart failure compared with medical therapy alone (Multicenter Automatic Defibrillator Implantation Trial Investigators 1996; Sudden Cardiac Death in Heart Failure Trial Investigators 2005), have supported a more liberal implantation policy of these devices. Moreover the widespread use of the trans-catheter aortic valve implantation (TAVI) for the percutaneous treatment of severe aortic stenosis, in high risk patients that would, otherwise, deemed inoperable by conventional surgery, has carried along a high post procedural implantation rate of PPMs in this elderly subgroup of patients (Bates et al. 2011; D'Ancona et al. 2011). It seems logical to expect an increased rate of device related infections to follow the boom of PPMs and ICDs implantation in the last two decades (Voigt et al. 2006). Of the 400,000 -500,000 permanent pacemaker leads implanted worldwide each year, around 10% may eventually fail or become infected, becoming potential candidates for removal (Byrd et al. 1999). Device infections can be local, involving the insertion site of PPM or ICD box, or systemic because of the spreading along the PPM leads and, in worst case scenario, lead to septic shock and device-related endocarditis. Device-related endocarditis has been reported in 23% of infected PPMs, the remainder being pocket infections (Sohail et al. 2007). The infection can spread over the cardiac structures and typically involves the tricuspid valve. Right-sided endocarditis accounts for only 5–10 % of cases of infective endocarditis (Chan et al. 1989) and occurs predominantly in selected patient's subgroup, such as: intravenous drug users, patients with pacemakers, ICD or central venous lines and with congenital heart diseases (Robbins et al. 1986). The tricuspid valve can show massive vegetations with or without valve regurgitation (figure 1).

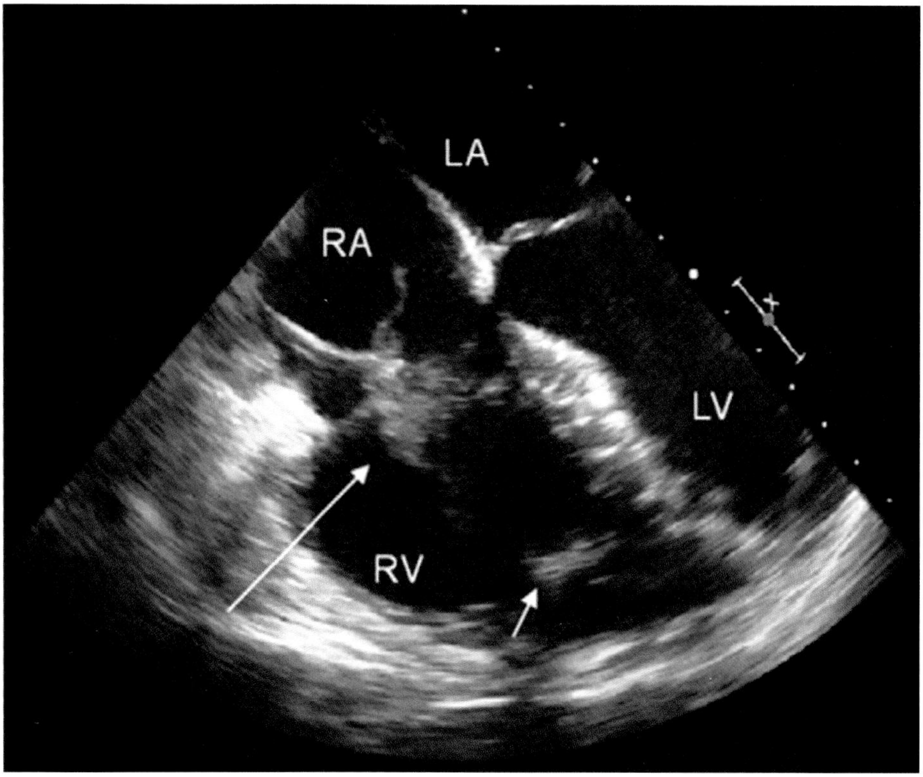

LA: left atrium; LV: left ventricle; RA: right atrium; RV: right ventricle.

Figure 1. [1]Transesophageal echocardiography –four chamber view - shows multiple vegetations on the tricuspid valve (long arrow) and pacing leads (short arrow).

This chapter will focus on the presentation, diagnosis and management of device-related endocarditis and explore different extraction techniques - both percutaneous and surgical.

2. Device-related endocarditis

Mortality rates for infected PPM devices range from 31% to 66% when the device is not explanted (Cacoub et al. 1998). Better outcomes, with mortality rates of 18% or less, have been reported when a combined management with device removal and antimicrobial therapy is adopted (Klug et al. 1997). Pacemaker related sepsis or endocarditis is a class I

[1]From Rossi et al. with permission.

indication for lead extraction, according to the recently updated device infection guidelines (Baddour et al. 2010). Standard treatment includes removal of infected PPM device combined with six weeks of antimicrobial therapy. Management of device-related endocarditis is challenging and requires collaborative efforts between cardiologists, surgeons, and infective disease specialists.

2.1. Clinical presentation

The presentation can be acute, with onset of symptoms in the first 6 weeks after the last procedure on the implant site, or chronic, with >6 weeks from the last procedure on the implant site to the onset of symptoms. In the acute form, the short time elapsed between PM implantation and the occurrence of infection facilitates the diagnosis. The vast majority of patients will have systemic symptoms from septic shock to fever, pneumonia, pulmonary embolism, associated with local signs of infection at the PM site. In the chronic form, the delay between the onset of symptoms and the implant time makes it difficult to diagnose PM-lead infection. Often delays in diagnosis of chronic device-related endocarditis are related to the fact that PM-lead infection was not considered in the differential diagnosis or because, possible clues were ignored: for example, blood cultures positive for S. epidermidis were erroneously considered contamination of the specimens (Klug et al. 1997). The most common chronic presentation would be fever or chills with asthenia, and wasting, sometimes associated with symptoms and signs of low tract respiratory infection (cough, expectoration, bronchitis, pneumonia, pulmonary abscess, pleural effusion). History of pulmonary embolism, arthralgia, spondylitis or signs of local infection at the PM site could be present. The diagnosis of systemic infection related to PM-lead infection must be systematically considered in the presence of chronic fever, recurrent bronchitis, or pulmonary infection or in case of recurrent or persistent evidence of infection at the implant site (Klug et al. 1997). More over endocarditis of the right heart should be specifically excluded, regardless the presence or absence of tricuspid regurgitation (Love et al. 2000).

2.2. Diagnosis

Patients will have elevated markers of inflammation. Erythrocyte sedimentation rate (ESR) and CRP will be elevated, often along with high withe cell count (WCC) due to an increase in polymorphonuclear cells. Positive blood cultures will confirm the diagnosis. Blood cultures should be taken on 3 consecutive days and integrated with cultures at the site of battery pocket if appropriate (wounds, local infection, or PM exteriorization). The Duke criteria are useful to define systemic infection related to PM-lead infection (tab.1), but as suggested by Klug et al (1997), the importance of some clinical criteria, should, probably, be highlighted, such as, local symptoms of infection at the PM site and pulmonary infections, to facilitate the diagnosis (tab.2).

Chest roentgenogram will often show signs of pulmonary infection or pleural effusion. Echocardiography is essential to confirm the diagnosis and to clarify whether treatment will require removal of the infected pacing system. However, a single negative transthoracic echocardiogram (TTE) is not enough to exclude the diagnosis of lead-related endocarditis. Although TTE has about 80% sensitivity in the detection of vegetations in the right heart (Love et al. 2000), often patients present with PM-lead–related endocarditis with intact tricuspid leaflets (Klug et al. 1997). This is the reason why a transoesophageal echocardiogram (TOE) should always be performed in the diagnostic algorithm when device-related endocarditis is suspected. Ventilation perfusion pulmonary scintigraphy can corroborate the diagnosis showing multiple septic lung embolisms. It is wise to perform also a wider range of investigations to exclude other sources of infection. These will normally include a dental pantomogram, sinus radiographs and abdominal ultrasound.

Definite infective endocarditis
Pathological criteria
Microorganisms: demonstrated by culture or histology in vegetation, in a vegetation that has embolized, or in intracardiac abscess, or
Microorganisms demonstrated by culture of the lead
Clinical criteria(as listed in Table 2)
Two major criteria, or
One major and three minor criteria, or
Five minor criteria
Possible infective endocarditis
Findings consistent with infective endocarditis that fall short of "definite" but not "rejected"
Rejected
Firm alternate diagnosis explaining evidence of infective endocarditis, or
Resolution of infective endocarditis syndrome, with antibiotic therapy for ≤4 days, or
No pathological evidence of infective endocarditis at surgery or autopsy, with antibiotic therapy for ≤4 days

Table 1. [2] Modified Duke Criteria for Diagnosis of Infective Endocarditis on PM Leads

[2]From Klug et al. with permission

Major criteria
Positive blood culture for infective endocarditis
Typical microorganisms for infective endocarditis from two separate blood cultures
Streptococcus viridans, Streptococcus bovis, HACEK group, or
Community-acquired *Staphylococcus aureus* or enterococci, in the absence of a primary focus, or
Persistently positive blood culture, defined as microorganism consistent with infective endocarditis from Blood cultures drawn >12 hours apart, or
All of three or a majority of four or more separate blood cultures, with first and last drawn at least 1 hour apart
Evidence of endocardial involvement:
Positive echocardiogram for infective endocarditis:
Oscillating intracardiac mass on PM leads or on the endocardial structure in contact with PM leads
Abscess in contact with PM leads
Minor criteria
Fever >38°C
Vascular phenomena: arterial embolism, septic pulmonary infarcts, mycotic aneurysm, intracranial hemorrhage, Janeway lesions
Immunologic phenomena: glomerulonephritis, Osler nodes, Roth spots
Echocardiogram: consistent with infective endocarditis but not meeting major criterion as noted previously (sleevelike appearance)
Microbiological evidence: positive blood culture but not meeting major criterion as noted previously.

Table 2. [3] Definition of Terms Used in the Proposed Modified Diagnostic Criteria

2.3. Pathophysiology

It is commonly accepted that the most common portal of entry to develop device-related endocarditis is the subcutaneous site of insertion of the pacing system. Extension along the lead into the vascular system is the usual explanation for the localization of the infection to the lead. Bacterial colonization of the lead during the course of bacteremia whose origin is not related to the pacing system might be possible but has been less well documented. Staphylococci are responsible for the vast majority of these infections, especially S. epidermidis in the chronic group and S. aureus in the acute group. A fungal infection is rare and more subtle to indentify. Fungal endocarditis is associated with high mortality and usually presents with scant growth of the microorganism in blood cultures (Figure 2). A

[3] From Klug et al. with permission

high index of suspicion for fungal endocarditis should be maintained in individuals with implantable pacemakers and fever of an uncertain source, especially in the context of negative blood cultures(Leong 2006). However, there is a 20-30% of device-related endocarditis with negative BC (Klug et al. 1997).

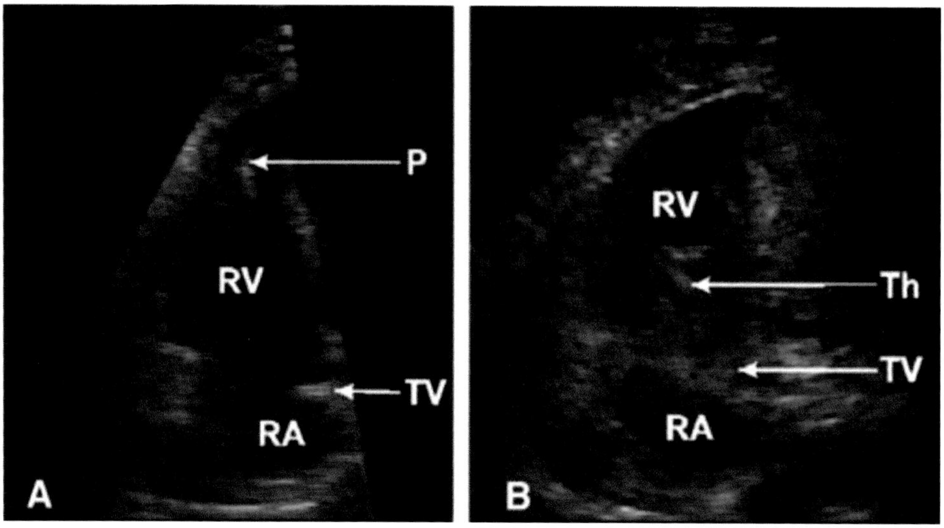

Figure 2. [4]A: Transthoracic echocardiogram of the right atrium (RA), tricuspid valve (TV) and right ventricle (RV) demonstrating a pacemaker lead (P) and no valvular vegetations. B: Second transthoracic echocardiogram of the right heart, seven weeks after the initial echocardiogram, demonstrating a right ventricular pacemaker lead thrombus (Th)

2.4. Management

The removal of the entire pacing system should be performed immediately rather than attempting prolonged antibiotic therapy alone. As in the study by Camus et al, the high rate of uncontrolled infection or relapse among patients with septicemia in relation to PM-material infection confirms the need for (Camus et al. 1993). Moreover immediate removal of the entire pacing system should be performed in all cases both for systemic infection related to PM-lead contamination and for infection of the PM pocket or the subcutaneous part of the lead (Panidis et al. 1984). Cultures of the leads and of the PM should be done after the extraction.Complete PPM or ICD removal should be performed when patients undergo valve replacement or repair for infective endocarditis, because the pacing system could serve as a nidus for relapsing infection and subsequent seeding of the surgically treated heart valve. Hardware removal is not required for superficial or incisionalinfection at the pocket site if there is no involvement of the device, 7-10 days of antibiotic therapy with an oral agent with activity against staphylococci is reasonable (Baddour 2010).

[4]From Leong et al. with permission.

3. Technique of extraction: Surgical or percutaneous?

After implantation, transvenous device leads usually undergo fibrotic encapsulation by activation of different cellular and humoral mechanisms (Esposito et al. 2002). The ensuing fibrotic lead adhesions tend to increase over time. Young patients, however, usually develop fibrotic adhesions earlier than elderly. On the contrary, systemic lead infection seems to counteract or dissolve fibrotic adherences. Current literature suggests that, the best outcome is achieved with percutaneous removal of infected devices by applying external traction on the leads (Sohail et al. 2007; Ruttmann et al. 2006). However, while simple traction is often successful in newly placed leads, it can be problematic with chronic leads and cause catastrophic complications, ranging from septic embolic phenomena to tricuspid valve injury, subclavian vein laceration, hemothorax, pocket hematoma, massive hemorrhage, and lead fracture requiring urgent surgical intervention (Sohail et al. 2007; Ruttmann et al. 2006; Panidis et al. 1984). Damage to the left sided cardiac structures is rare but may be a complication of an infected lead extraction, manifesting as iatrogenic ventricular septum disruption with consequent aortic valve leaflet prolapse and massive acute aortic regurgitation (fig.3)(Rossi et al. 2011).

Chronically implanted leads are fixed to the myocardium by fibrous tissue. Fibrous scar tissue may also encase the lead along its course. Furthermore, fragility of the lead and its tendency to break when extraction force is applied to overcome resistance imparted by the scar tissue add to the challenge of lead extraction. Thus, selecting the appropriate extraction procedure for chronically implanted leads is an important issue.

3.1. Percutaneous extraction

The removal of the entire pacing system should be performed in one session. Newpercutaneous PM and ICD lead extraction techniques have been developed to overcome the problem of a difficult extraction with the aim to reduce damage to the cardiac structures produced by the simple counter traction. Telescoping mechanical sheaths and locking stylets were introduced during the late 1980s and early 1990s. Special tools for femoral lead extraction soon followed. They can be used though a superior approach (jugular or subclavian vein) using locking stylet ; or via a femoral vein approach using double lasso catheters (Needle's eye snare) (Byrd et al. 1999; Bracke et al. 2001; Fearnot et al. 1990). In the superior vena cava approach, a locking stylet is introduced into the lead and locked close to the distal electrode in order to apply traction directly to the tip. If gentle traction is not successful, telescoping sheaths can be advanced over the lead to disrupt fibrous binding of the lead to veins or myocardium. When necessary, the tip of the lead is freed by countertraction, the sheath being positioned against the myocardium to prevent inversion during traction on the lead. In the transfemoral approach, the pacing lead is grabbed with a deflecting guide wire or retriever through a long sheath inserted from the femoral vein. The proximal end of the lead is pulled down from the subclavian vein. Then the outer sheath is advanced over the lead to disrupt the scar tissue, as with the superior approach. When the myocardium is reached countertraction is applied.

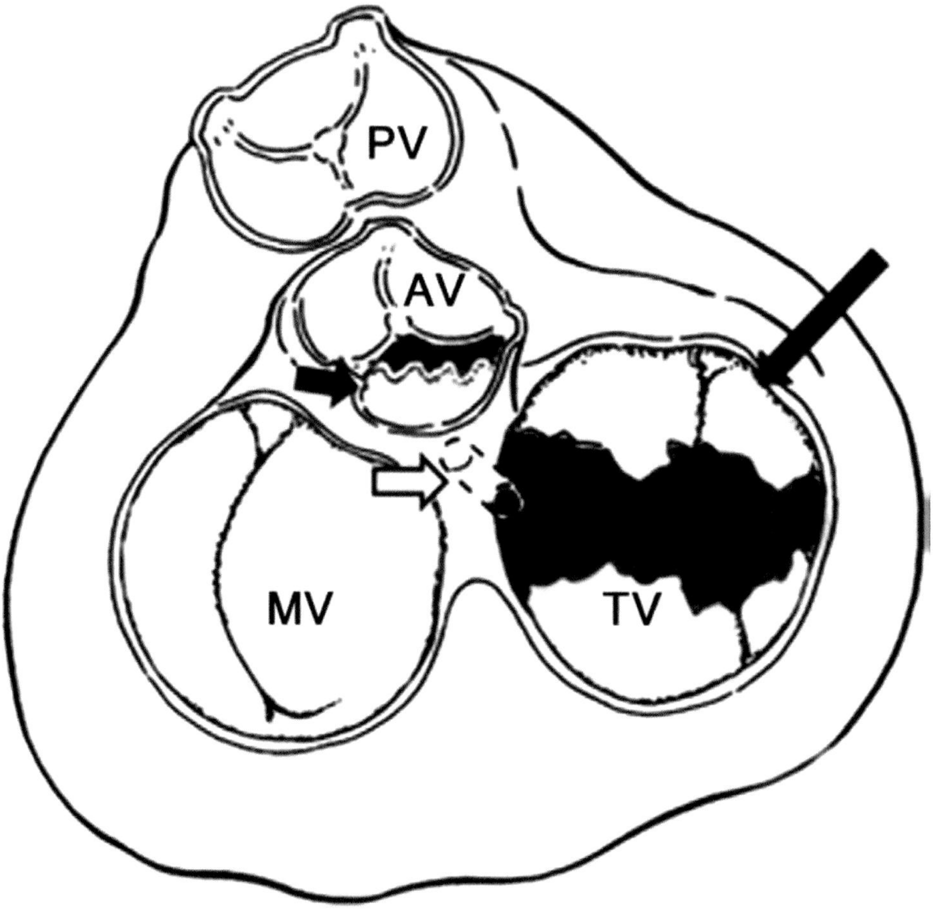

AV: aortic valve; MV: mitral valve; PV: pulmonary valve; TV: tricuspid valve.

Figure 3. [5] Four-valve view of the fibrous skeleton of the heart showing disruption of the tricuspid valve (long black arrow), ventricular septal defect (white arrow), and prolapse of the noncoronary cusp of the aortic valve (short black arrow).

3.1.1. Laser extraction

Progress has also been made in developing other systems for lead extraction powered with laser energy. The first laser-assisted lead extraction performed in 1994 was a major breakthrough. The laser extraction sheath offers a method for removal by "cutting" through scar tissue, without excessive use of force (such as with purely mechanical systems). It appears to be an efficient tool for removal of chronic implanted infected leads but its use is

[5]From Rossi et al. with permission.

Intraoperative cultures of the aortic valve and ventricular septal defect edges did not show any significant growth, supporting the hypothesis that the prolapse of the noncoronary cusp was due to lack of support on the valve structure.

associated with a high number of bleeding complications often requiring surgical revision (see section 3.3).

3.2. Surgical extraction

Surgical removal has a higher complication rate and worse outcome compared with percutaneous techniques (Klug et al. 1997). Although, in concept, the surgical approach is the cleanest way to extract an infected lead together with its vegetation without risks of pulmonary or systemic septic embolism, it is generally accepted both by surgeon and cardiologist to prefer the percutaneous extraction as first attempt. However we should not forget that the surgical population is highly selected, i.e. made of cases not suitable for percutaneous extraction or with heart damage after percutaneous attempt or with severe tricuspid valve involvement. Moreover, the presence of intracardiac vegetations alone, identifies a subset of patients at increased risk for complications and early mortality from systemic infection regardless the technique of extraction (percutaneous or surgical) and appropriate antimicrobial therapy (Grammes et al. 2010). From a review of the current literature, it appears that the indication for surgical removal is mainly limited as rescue intervention to fix complicated or failed percutaneous extraction. Surgical removal generally requires median sternotomy or thoracotomy and sometimes cardiopulmonary bypass (CBP). Nevertheless there are still patients that will benefit from a surgical removal as a first attempt rather than later, especially those with large vegetations that might obstruct the main pulmonary artery or those who need the implantation of an epicardial pacing system.

A primary surgical approach to lead removal in patients with PPM/ICD infection is recommended by the current guidelines for implantable electronic device infections and management in patients who have significant retained hardware after attempts at percutaneous removal or in patients with lead vegetations > 2 cm in diameter, because of concerns about the risk of pulmonary embolism with percutaneous lead extraction (Baddour et al. 2010). In fact, it is useful to reconsider the indication for pacing after successful extraction of the infected pacing system.Discontinuation of pacemaker treatment after lead extraction has been reported in 13–52% of patients (Bracke et al. 2001). However when permanent pacing is a must, an epicardial system is the recommended choiceespecially after valve surgery with initial hardware removal(Baddour et al. 2010). With the surgical approach, the epicardial permanent system can be easily placed at the same time of the extraction and offers the advantage of eliminating the contact between leads and systemic circulation taking the chances of infection of the new system to the ground.

3.3. Evidence-based discussion

Wilkoff et al, in a randomized control trial of 465 chronically implanted leads, achieved 94% complete removal with a laser sheath against 64% with conventional sheaths, but with an higher rate of potentially life-threatening complications (Wilkoff et al. 1999). In a multicenter study over 2338 patients, Byrd et al, reported an increased risk of failed or partial extraction with increasing implant duration, doubling every three years (Byrd et al. 1999). Kennergren et al, in a retrospective analysis of their activity on 647 lead extractions, surprisingly showed that the implantation time was not associated with extraction failure neither there was an association between implantation time and the incidence of serious complications. Actually they showed that leads can often be extracted by a superior transvenous approach with simple traction; Laser-assisted lead extraction appeared to be a useful technique to extract leads that could not be removed by manual traction but at the cost of a higher rate of bleeding complications requiring open-chest surgical revision (Kennergren et al. 2009). Alt et al, achieved total removal of 81% of 150 leads, without major complications with the use of only locking stylets (Alt et al. 1996). Tokunaga et al, performed a surgical removal without CBP after a failed extraction using the Excimer Laser Sheath Extraction System (Tokunaga et al. 2011). The authors highlight the potential risk of perforation and lethal bleeding complications using this tool and suggest a close backup by a cardiovascular surgeon. Neuzi et al, in a randomized control trial (RCT) compared the safety and efficacy of transvenous pacemaker and implantable cardioverter-defibrillator (ICD) lead extraction, with an electrosurgical dissection sheath (EDS) system using radiofrequency (RF) current or standard countertraction lead removal in 120 consecutive patients (Neuzi et al. 2007). Although the EDS extraction system appeared quicker and more effective in complete removal of leads, they could not demonstrate a significant superiority versus the standard counter-traction method. Buongiorni et al, in a retrospective analysis of 1330 leads extraction, concluded that transvenous lead extraction is an effective and safe procedure. They showed how the use of the jugular approach, in the presence of free-floating or difficult exposed leads, increases both safety and success rate (Buongiorni et al. 2005). Kratz et al, in a retrospective analysis of 365 patients who underwent PPM or ICD lead removal, showed that performing a lead extraction in a protected environment, such as an operating room, allowed rapid and effective treatment of potential procedure-related complications. Actually, the use of several extraction tools, arterial line monitoring, transesophageal echocardiography, general anesthesia, and an experienced team, yielded complete extraction in more than 90% of patients, with a low complication rate and no procedurally related deaths (Kratz et al. 2010). Grammes et al, reported their experience using percutaneous leads extraction by simple traction of 1,838 infected leads with echocardiographic evidence of intracardiac vegetations. Post-operative 30-day mortality was 10%; no deaths were related directly to the extraction procedure (Grammes et al. 2010). The common message that comes from the literature is that extraction of infected PM-leads is not just a "pull and go" procedure and should be performed by expert physicians, in tertiary centres, with a cardiac surgery back up to best manage their complications.

3.3.1. Septic embolism

There is also a concern in pacemaker related endocarditis over embolisation of vegetations adhering to the lead when endovascular extraction is attempted. Klug et al, in their series of 52 patients with device-related endocarditis, suggested to chose the technique of removal (surgical versus percutaneous) on the size of the vegetations: percutaneous when vegetation size was ≤10 mm and surgical if > 10mm at transesophageal echocardiogram (Klug et al.

1997). This policy was based on previous observations by Mugge et al and by Robbins et al, who found that embolism was more frequent with vegetation size was >10 mm in endocarditis related to valve infection (Mugge et al. 1989; Robbins et al. 1986). More recently Ruttmann et al, showed that transvenous lead removal is a safe and effective even in patients with large vegetations. Embolism to the lung happens but tends to proceed mainly without complications. However there are still cases where surgical approach is preferred, such as, in presence of large vegetations that might occlude the main pulmonary artery(Ruttmann et al. 2006) or with vegetations > 2 cm in diameter (Baddour et al. 2010).

4. Conclusion

The diagnosis of endocarditis related to PM-lead infection should be systematically considered in patients with fever, history of local complications, or pulmonary pathology after PM insertion. There are two different clinical presentations: the acute form, that presents early with sepsis, often in conjunction with local signs of infection, and a chronic form, beginning several months later. The presentation may be atypical and the symptoms may occur late after the last intervention at the PM site. CRP, ESR, scintigraphy or chest CT angiogram may be of diagnostic value. TTE and TOE must be performed in search of vegetations. Immediate removal of the entire pacing system is paramount, in addition to prolonged antimicrobial therapy. We believe that multidisciplinary approach is the key to manage device-related endocarditis and good professional relationships are essential between cardiologists, surgeons, and infective disease specialists to make the appropriate decisions to best treat these complex patients. Our recommendation, in the patients' best interest, is not to embark on extracting infected leads without doing a serious ongoing individual risk–benefit analysis. Finally a word of wisdom to the future generations: even if we are moving faster towards new innovative ways to pace the heart, we will always be dealing with their complications, therefore, is worth to create a network of professionals to address them in the best possible way.

Author details

Michele Rossi, Giuseppe Musolino, Giuseppe Filiberto Serraino and Attilio Renzulli
Department of Cardiac Surgery, Magna Graecia University, Catanzaro, Italy

5. References

Adabag S, Roukoz H, Anand IS & Moss AJ. (2011). Cardiac resynchronization therapy in patients with minimal heart failure a systematic review and meta-analysis. *J Am Coll Cardiol,* Vol. 58, No. 9 (Aug 2011), pp. 935-41. ISSN 1558-3597

Alt E, Neuzner J, Binner L, Göhl K, Res JC, Knabe UH, Zehender M & Reinhardt J. (1996). Three-year experience with a stylet for lead extraction: a multicenter study. *Pacing Clin Electrophysiol.* Vol 19, No. 1, (Jan 1996), pp. 18-25. ISSN 0147-8389

Baddour LM, Epstein AE, Erickson CC, Knight BP, Levison ME, Lockhart PB, Masoudi FA, Okum EJ, Wilson WR, Beerman LB, Bolger AF, Estes NA 3rd, Gewitz M, Newburger JW, Schron EB & Taubert KA. (2010). American Heart Association Rheumatic Fever, Endocarditis, and Kawasaki Disease Committee; Council on Cardiovascular Disease in Young; Council on Cardiovascular Surgery and Anesthesia; Council on Cardiovascular Nursing; Council on Clinical Cardiology; Interdisciplinary Council on Quality of Care; American Heart Association. Update on cardiovascular implantable electronic device infections and their management: a scientific statement from the American Heart Association. *Circulation*. Vol. 121, No. 3, (Jan 2010), pp. 458-77. ISSN 1524-4539

Bardy GH, Lee KL, Mark DB, Poole JE, Packer DL, Boineau R, Domanski M, Troutman C, Anderson J, Johnson G, McNulty SE, Clapp-Channing N, Davidson-Ray LD, Fraulo ES, Fishbein DP, Luceri RM & Ip JH; Sudden Cardiac Death in Heart Failure Trial (SCD-HeFT) Investigators. (2005) Amiodarone or an implantable cardioverter-defibrillator for congestive heart failure. *N Engl J Med*, Vol. 352, No.3 (Jan 2005), pp. 225-37. Erratum in: *N Engl J Med*. Vol. 352, No. 20 (May 2005), pp. 2146. ISSN1533-4406

Bates MG, Matthews IG, Fazal IA & Turley AJ. (2011). Postoperative permanent pacemaker implantation in patients undergoing trans-catheter aortic valve implantation: what is the incidence and are there any predicting factors? *Interact Cardiovasc Thorac Surg*. Vol 12, No.2, (Feb 2011), pp. 243-53. ISSN 1569-9285

Bongiorni MG, Giannola G, Arena G, Soldati E, Bartoli C, Lapira F, Zucchelli G & Di Cori A. (2005). Pacing and implantable cardioverter-defibrillator transvenous lead extraction. *Ital Heart J*. Vol. 6, No. 3, (Mar 2005), pp. 261-6. ISSN 1129-471X

Bracke FA, Meijer A & van Gelder LM. (2001). Pacemaker lead complications: when is extraction appropriate and what can we learn from published data? *Heart*. Vol. 85, No.3, (Mar 2001), pp. 254-9. ISSN 1468-201X

Bristow MR, Saxon LA, Boehmer J, Krueger S, Kass DA, De Marco T, Carson P, DiCarlo L, DeMets D, White BG, DeVries DW & Feldman AM; Comparison of Medical Therapy, Pacing, and Defibrillation in Heart Failure (COMPANION) Investigators. (2004). Cardiac-resynchronization therapy with or without an implantable defibrillator in advanced chronic heart failure. *N Engl J Med*, Vol. 350, No. 21 (May 2004), pp. 2140-50. ISSN 1533-4406

Byrd CL, Wilkoff BL, Love CJ, Sellers TD, Turk KT, Reeves R, Young R, Crevey B, Kutalek SP, Freedman R, Friedman R, Trantham J, Watts M, Schutzman J, Oren J, Wilson J, Gold F, Fearnot NE & Van Zandt HJ. (1999). Intravascular extraction of problematic or infected permanent pacemaker leads: 1994-1996. U.S. Extraction Database, MED Institute. *Pacing Clin Electrophysiol*. Vol. 22, No.9, (Sep 1999), pp. 1348-57. ISSN 0147-8389

Cacoub P, Leprince P, Nataf P, Hausfater P, Dorent R, Wechsler B, Bors V, Pavie A, Piette JC & Gandjbakhch I. (1998). Pacemaker infective endocarditis. *Am J Cardiol*. Vol. 82, No.4, (Aug 1998), pp. 480-4. ISSN 0002-9149

Camus C, Leport C, Raffi F, Michelet C, Cartier F & Vilde JL. (1993). Sustained bacteremia in 26 patients with a permanent endocardial pacemaker: assessment of wire removal. *Clin Infect Dis*. Vol. 17, No. 1, (Jul 1993), pp. 46-55. ISSN 1058-4838

Chan P, Ogilby JD & Segal B. (1989). Tricuspid valve endocarditis. *Am Heart J*. Vol. 117, No.5, (May 1989), pp. 1140-6. ISSN 0002-8703

D'Ancona G, Pasic M, Unbehaun A & Hetzer R. (2011). Permanent pacemaker implantation after transapical transcatheter aortic valve implantation. *Interact Cardiovasc Thorac Surg*. Vol. 13, No. 4 (Oct 2011), pp. 373-6. ISSN 1569-9285

Esposito M, Kennergren C, Holmström N, Nilsson S, Eckerdal J & Thomsen P. (2002). Morphologic and immunohistochemical observations of tissues surrounding retrieved transvenous pacemaker leads. *J Biomed Mater Res*. Vol. 63, No.5, (Sept 2002), pp. 548-58. ISSN 0021-9304

Fearnot NE, Smith HJ, Goode LB, Byrd CL, Wilkoff BL & Sellers TD. (1990). Intravascular lead extraction using locking stylets, sheaths, and other techniques. *Pacing Clin Electrophysiol*. Vol. 13, No. 12 Pt 2, (Dec 1990), pp. 1864-70. ISSN 0147-8389

Grammes JA, Schulze CM, Al-Bataineh M, Yesenosky GA, Saari CS, Vrabel MJ, Horrow J, Chowdhury M, Fontaine JM & Kutalek SP. (2010). Percutaneous pacemaker and implantable cardioverter-defibrillator lead extraction in 100 patients with intracardiac vegetations defined by transesophageal echocardiogram. *J Am Coll Cardiol*. Vol. 55, No. 9, (Mar 2010), pp. 886-94. ISSN 1558-3597

Kennergren C, Bjurman C, Wiklund R & Gäbel J.(2009) A single-centre experience of over one thousand lead extractions. *Europace*. Vol. 11, No.5, (May 2009), pp. 612-7. ISSN 1532-2092

Klug D, Lacroix D, Savoye C, Goullard L, Grandmougin D, Hennequin JL, Kacet S & Lekieffre J. (1997). Systemic infection related to endocarditis on pacemaker leads: clinical presentation and management. *Circulation*. Vol. 95, No.8, (Apr 1997), pp. 2098-107. ISSN 0009-7322

Kratz JM, Toole JM. (2010). Pacemaker and internal cardioverter defibrillator lead extraction: a safe and effective surgical approach. *Ann Thorac Surg*. Vol. 90, No. 5, (Nov 2010), pp. 1411-7. ISSN 1552-6259

Leong R, Gannon BR, Childs TJ, Isotalo PA & Abdollah H. (2006). Aspergillus fumigates pacemaker lead endocarditis: a case report and review of the literature. *Can J Cardiol*. Vol. 22, No. 4, (Mar 2006), pp. 337-40. ISSN 0828-282X

Love CJ, Wilkoff BL, Byrd CL, Belott PH, Brinker JA, Fearnot NE, Friedman RA, Furman S, Goode LB, Hayes DL, Kawanishi DT, Parsonnet V, Reiser C & Van Zandt HJ. (2000). Recommendations for extraction of chronically implanted transvenous pacing and defibrillator leads: indications, facilities, training. North American Society of Pacing and Electrophysiology Lead Extraction Conference Faculty. *Pacing Clin Electrophysiol*. Vol. 23, No. 4 Pt 1, (Apr 2000), pp. 544-51. ISSN 0147-8389

Moss AJ, Hall WJ, Cannom DS, Daubert JP, Higgins SL, Klein H, Levine JH, Saksena S, Waldo AL, Wilber D, Brown MW & Heo M. (1996). Improved survival with an implanted defibrillator in patients with coronary disease at high risk for ventricular arrhythmia. Multicenter Automatic Defibrillator Implantation Trial Investigators. *N Engl J Med*. Vol. 335, No. 26, (Dec 1996), pp. 1933-40. ISSN 0028-4793

Mügge A, Daniel WG, Frank G & Lichtlen PR. (1989). Echocardiography in infective endocarditis: reassessment of prognostic implications of vegetation size determined by the transthoracic and the transesophageal approach. *J Am Coll Cardiol*. Vol. 14, No.3, (Sep 1989), pp. 631-8. ISSN 0735-1097

Neuzil P, Taborsky M, Rezek Z, Vopalka R, Sediva L, Niederle P & Reddy V. (2007). Pacemaker and ICD lead extraction with electrosurgical dissection sheaths and standard transvenous extraction systems: results of a randomized trial. *Europace*. Vol. 9, No.2, (Feb 2007), pp. 98-104. ISSN 1099-5129

Panidis IP, Kotler MN, Mintz GS, Segal BL & Ross JJ. (1984). Right heart endocarditis: clinical and echocardiographic features. *Am Heart J*. Vol. 107, No.4, (Apr 1984), pp. 759-64. ISSN 0002-8703

Robbins MJ, Frater RW, Soeiro R, Frishman WH & Strom JA. (1986). Influence of vegetation size on clinical outcome of right-sided infective endocarditis. *Am J Med*. Vol. 80, No. 2, (Feb 1986), pp. 165-71. ISSN 0002-9343

Robbins MJ, Soeiro R, Frishman WH & Strom JA. (1986). Right-sided valvular endocarditis: etiology, diagnosis, and an approach to therapy. *Am Heart J*. Vol. 111, No. 1, (Jan 1986), pp. 128-35. ISSN 0002-8703

Rossi M, Pirone F, Nair S & Trivedi U. (2011). Massive acute aortic regurgitation after infected pacemaker lead removal: a word of caution. *Ann Thorac Surg*. Vol. 92, No.2, (Aug 2011), pp. e29-31. ISSN 1552-6259

Ruttmann E, Hangler HB, Kilo J, Höfer D, Müller LC, Hintringer F, Müller S, Laufer G & Antretter H. (2006). Transvenous pacemaker lead removal is safe and effective even in large vegetations: an analysis of 53 cases of pacemaker lead endocarditis. *Pacing Clin Electrophysiol*. Vol. 29, No.3, (Mar 2006), pp. 231-6. ISSN 0147-8389

Sohail MR, Uslan DZ, Khan AH, Friedman PA, Hayes DL, Wilson WR, Steckelberg JM, Stoner S & Baddour LM. (2007). Management and outcome of permanent pacemaker and implantable cardioverter-defibrillator infections. *J Am Coll Cardiol*. Vol. 49, No.18, (May 2007), pp. 1851-9. ISSN 1558-3597

Tokunaga C, Enomoto Y, Sato F, Kanemoto S, Matsushita S, Hiramatsu Y, Aonuma K & Sakakibara Y. (2012). Surgical removal of infected pacemaker leads without cardiopulmonary bypass after failed extraction using the Excimer Laser Sheath Extraction System. *J Artif Organs*. Vol. 15, No. 1, (Mar 2012), pp. 94-8. ISSN 1619-0904

Voigt A, Shalaby A & Saba S. (2006). Rising rates of cardiac rhythm management device infections in the United States: 1996 through 2003. *J Am Coll Cardiol*. Vol. 48, No.3, (Aug 2006), pp. 590-1. ISSN 1558-3597

Wilkoff BL, Byrd CL, Love CJ, Hayes DL, Sellers TD, Schaerf R, Parsonnet V, Epstein LM, Sorrentino RA & Reiser C. (1999). Pacemaker lead extraction with the laser sheath: results of the pacing lead extraction with the excimer sheath (PLEXES) trial. *J Am Coll Cardiol*. Vol. 33, No. 6, (May 1999), pp. 1671-6. ISSN 0735-1097

Chapter 8

Mechanism and Management of Pacing Lead Related Cardiac Perforation

Sanjay Kumar, Haidar Yassin, Opesanmi Esan,
Adam S. Budzikowski and John T. Kassotis

Additional information is available at the end of the chapter

http://dx.doi.org/10.5772/48630

1. Introduction

1.1. Incidence and time course for cardiac perforation

Cardiac perforation due to a pacemaker or defibrillator lead occurs at a rate of 0.4–2.0%. Since first described [1], the overall incidence has decreased significantly. The reported incidence of this complication has been as low as < 1 % to as high as 15% [2-4]. Of 4,280 permanent pacemaker (PPM) implants only 50 (1.2%) patients developed a significant effusion and symptoms consistent with a perforation [5]. The incidence of this complication from the time of surgery decreases over time. By convention, a perforation detected within 24 hours, is classified as acute. If detected within 30 days of implantation (usually 5 days- 4 weeks), it is referred to as early (sub-acute); and, those detected after 30 days referred to as late, delayed or chronic perforation. The majority of perforations manifest within a year but rarely cases have been reported as late as five years following implantation. [6]

1.2. RV perforation

1.2.1. Modeling of RV perforation

In order to develop perforation resistant leads, several models of myocardium - lead interaction have been developed. Lead related factors that affect propensity for perforation include lead thickness as well as stiffness. Refinement of the current lead technology produce leads with both a reduced thickness and stiffness. In experimental model [7] bipolar leads with silicone rubber insulation had lower stiffness as compared with those coated with polyurethane. While a lower stiffness is a desirable property, it results in a thinner lead with a higher penetration pressure (force per unit area). In a porcine perforation model [8] studying the effect of cylindrical punches, of variable diameter, on RV wall tissue the penetration pressure (force/cross sectional area) decreases as a function of an increasing punch diameter. The penetration pressure decreased by approximately 25 % as the punch diameter was doubled. **(Figure 1)**

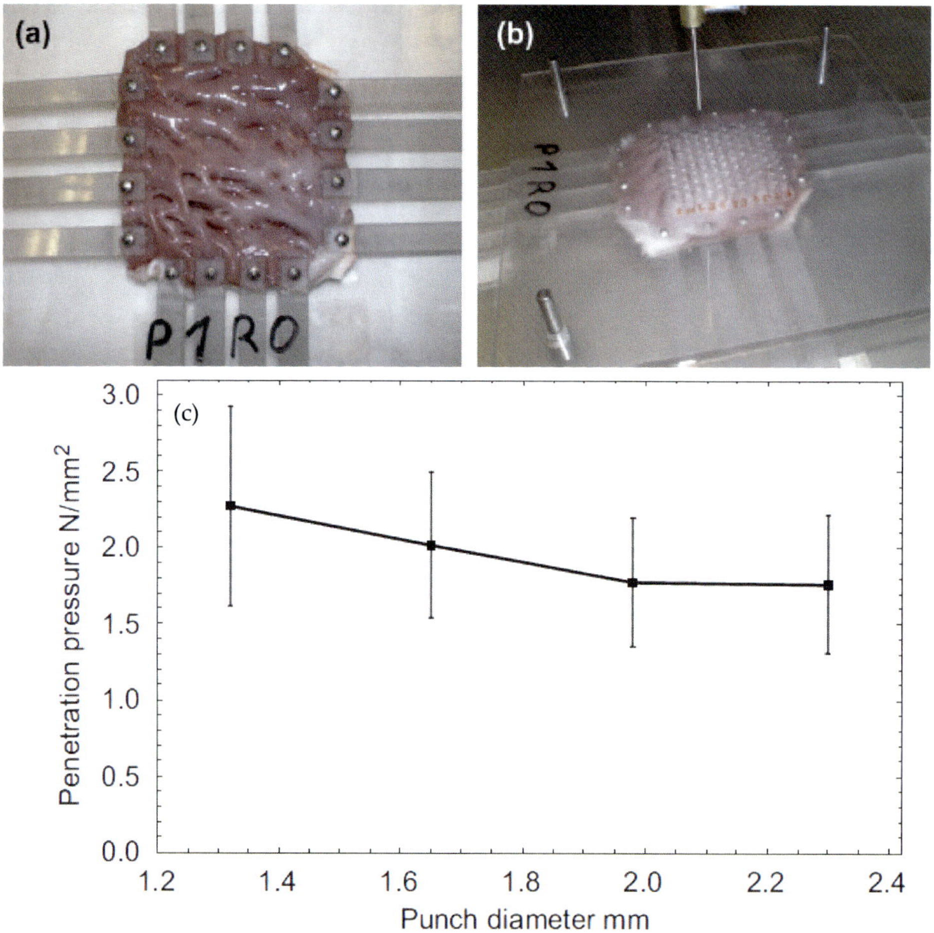

Figure 1. Figures show the porcine specimen of RV free wall fixed to the grips (a) and specimen bi-axially stretched to its testing conditions (b). Figure (c) shows penetration characteristics of the right ventricular myocardium. Penetration pressure (penetration force divided by punch cross section) with respect to the punch diameter. "(With permission from Gasser TC: Journal of Biomechanics. 42:629-633, 2009.)

Myocardium related factors which contribute to the perforation risk include the wall thickness and the viscoelastic properties of the tissue. Experimental data suggest that the myocardium is anisotropic (with the highest stiffness in the direction of the fiber's longitudinal orientation), non-linear, nearly elastic and exhibiting heterogeneity throughout a particular chamber (e.g. RV) [9].

The interaction between the lead tip and myocardium is complex, varies with the cardiac cycle, and changes over time. The lead tip penetrates the tissue, creating a fissure between local fibers. The lead wedges into this "crack", expanding the opening over time [7]. This is illustrated by the detection of a "crack" (fissure) both by light and electron microscopy, see **Figures 2, 3**. However, it should be noted that when a "crack" splits the plane of fibers, compared to a punch, there is higher likelihood of closure due to the opposing forces of the myocardium, which act to seal the fissure. This may explain why many perforations are subclinical. Despite advancements in the knowledge of the lead-tissue interaction and advances in lead technology, this complication has still not been eliminated.

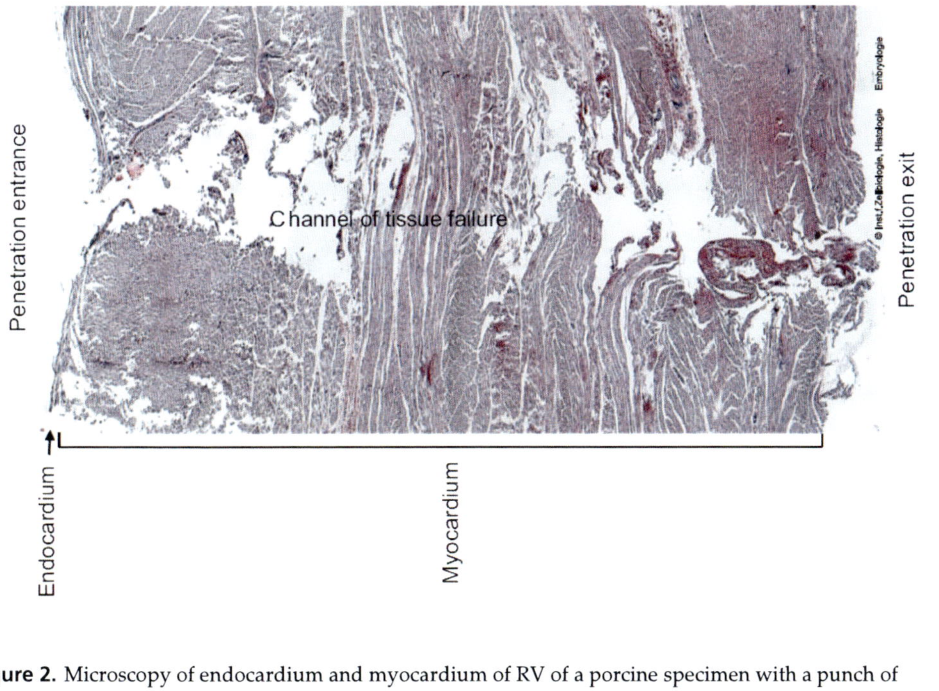

Figure 2. Microscopy of endocardium and myocardium of RV of a porcine specimen with a punch of 2.3 mm diameter. Picrosirius red stain illustrates tissue failure through the different layers of the ventricular tissue. "(With permission from Gasser TC: Journal of Biomechanics. 42:629-633, 2009.)

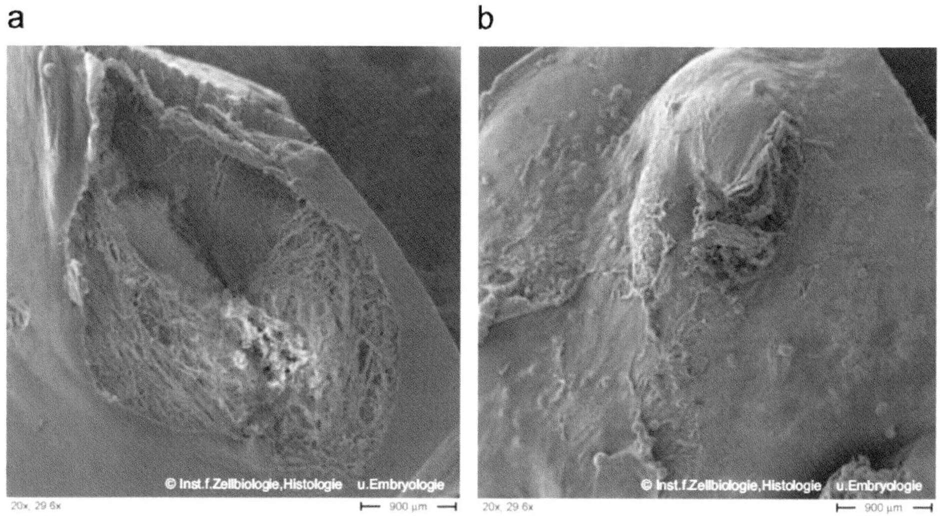

Figure 3. Electron microscopy images taken from the (a) entrance and (b) exit of the punch illustrating a splitting mode failure and the presence of remaining deformations respectively. "(With permission from Gasser TC: Journal of Biomechanics. 42:629-633, 2009.)

1.2.2. Free wall perforation

Hirschl et al studied the incidence of an asymptomatic lead perforation, by computed tomography and correlated with electrophysiologic data. Out of 100 consecutive PPM and intra-cardiac defibrillator (ICD) implantations, right ventricular (RV) perforation was less common (6% vs. 15%) than right atrial (RA) perforation, respectively [4]. However, in a recent study of 2,385 patients undergoing an electrophysiology study as well as pacemaker lead insertion, 7 (0.3%) patients experienced an RV perforation compared to only 1 (0.04%) RA perforation [10]. The predisposition to develop an RV perforation was a function of RV location; explained in part by the heterogeneous nature of the RV. The RV resembles a pyramidal structure with the interventricular septum (IVS) located posteriorly and the free wall located anteriorly. The RV free wall is thinner (<0.5 cm) than the septum (ranging from 0.6 to 0.9 cm) [11], accounting for the higher risk of perforation. Positioning leads in the RV IVS may not only reduce the risk of perforation but reduce the degree of QRS widening, possibly minimizing asynchrony. In the majority of cases the perforating lead is contained within the pericardium, however, in rare cases the lead can migrate along the pericardium traversing the diaphragm into the abdominal cavity. **Figure 4 and 5** (chest x-ray and CT scan) illustrate an example of a RV free wall perforation.

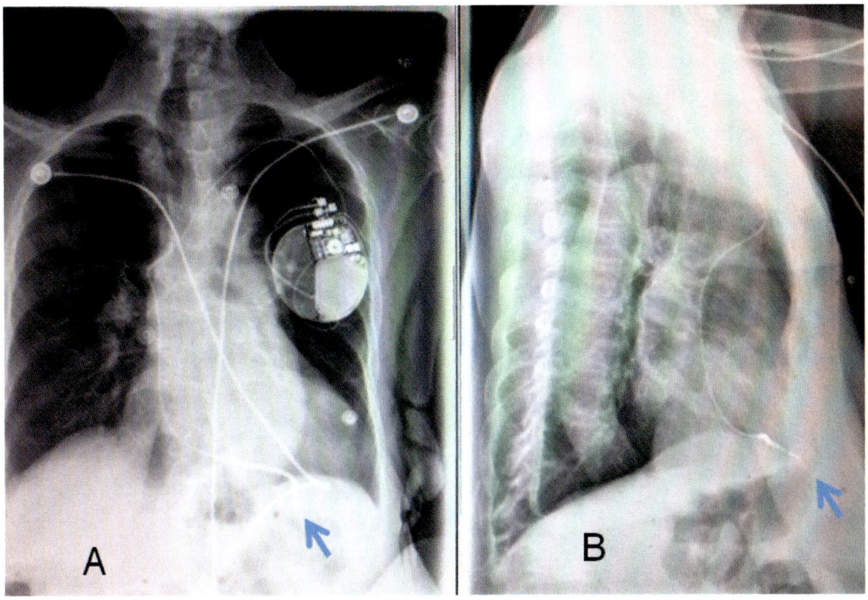

Figure 4. RV lead (arrows) perforating through the RV and sharply pointing below the diaphragm in PA view (A) and the lead is excessively close to the sternum and gastric air under the left hemidiaphragm in lateral view (B).

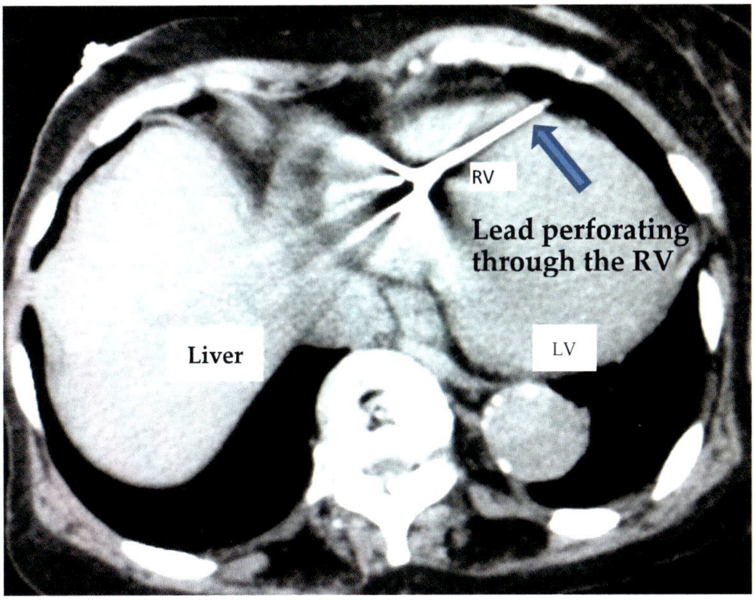

Figure 5. Axial view of CT scan of chest of the same patient in figure 4, showing the RV lead perforation through the RV apex. RV=right ventricle, LV=left ventricle

1.2.3. Migration to the LV cavity

As a consequence of the thicker IVS, direct perforation through the septum and migration of lead tip into the left ventricle (LV) is rare [12]. However, the RV PPM lead may end up in LV due to mal-positioning during implantation. A common route for the lead to access the LV is a patent foramen ovale [13] or atrial septal defect [14]. These patients may remain asymptomatic for a long time, and often lead malposition is detected incidentally. It can be detected by fluoroscopy or chest radiography, presence of right bundle branch block (RBBB) with pacing on electrocardiogram (ECG) or when the patient presents with symptoms of a peripheral embolism (e.g. cerebrovascular accident) [14]. LV epicardial pacing may result when the electrode perforates through the RV apex migrating and remaining along the LV epicardial surface [15].

1.3. RA perforation

The RA is more susceptible to perforation as compared to the RV, attributable to the thinner wall of the atrium [4]. Thicker electrodes and active fixation leads are more likely to cause this form of perforation. Most commonly, one observes RA appendageal perforation. Age, gender, device type and anticoagulation status appear to increase the risk for perforation [16]. The lead may traverse through the pericardium into the lung field. Although, surgical intervention may be needed most cases are treated with percutaneous drainage or simple lead repositioning.

1.4. Coronary Sinus (CS) dissection/perforation

CS perforation is a relatively rare complication during pacemaker implantation. The rate of CS perforation has seen an upturn with increased CS cannulation during LV lead insertion for cardiac resynchronization therapy (CRT). The incidence of CS dissection and CS perforation have been reported to vary from 2%-4%, 0.3%-2%, respectively [17]. Cardiac tamponade and pericarditis have been reported with a CS perforation [18].

In the early experience with PPM implantation the CS was selected for the purpose of RA pacing, affording a more stable catheter position. With a high perforation risk, tamponade and thrombosis, complicating lead insertion with CS manipulation, the RA became the preferred site. Enhanced stability with the RA appendage as the preferred site occurred once active fixation leads became mainstream. **Figure 6** shows a CS lead perforating through the body of coronary sinus. During CRT, LV pacing is achieved by placing an electrode via the os of the CS to one of its tributaries. This procedure may result in a CS dissection. The overwhelming majority of CS dissections are without incident, with the dissection flap sealed by blood flow within the CS. Even if contrast extravasates out of the CS, the low perfusion pressure within the CS prevents any significant bleeding. In the majority of cases the true lumen of the CS can be re-accessed. The lead serves to tamponade the dissection or perforation and the procedure can proceed with successful lead placement. Serial echocardiograms are needed to assure any significant pericardial blood accumulation. If significant blood accumulation occurs within the pericardium this can be relieved via a percutaneous approach, very rarely patients require surgical drainage.

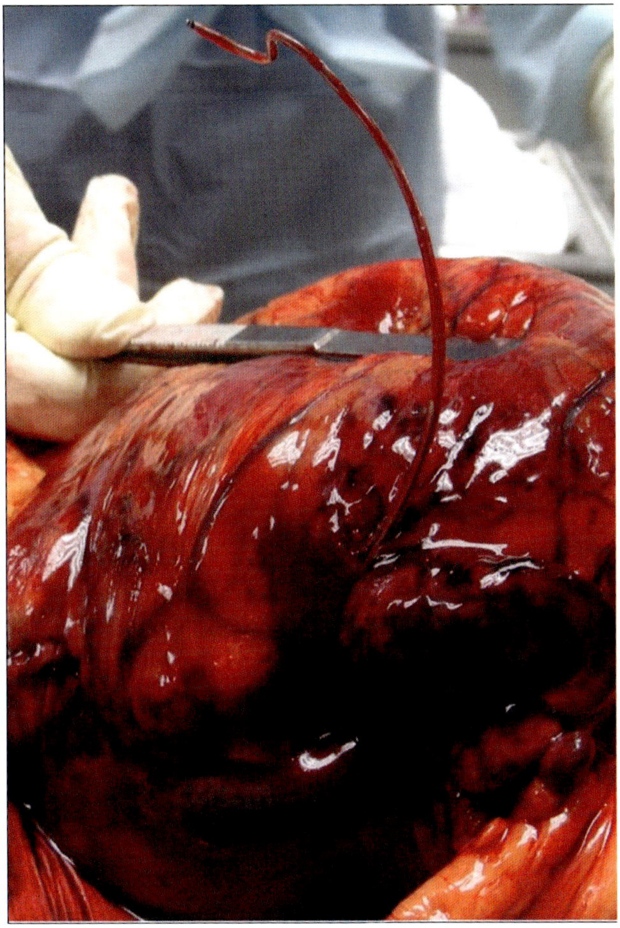

Figure 6. CS lead is perforating through coronary sinus as seen during autopsy. Patient was asymptomatic and died for unrelated reason. Courtesy of Jenny Libien, MD. Department of Pathology, SUNY Downstate. Brooklyn, NY.

1.5. Great vessel injury/dissection

Transvenous leads can be placed through various venous access sites, including, axillary, subclavian or cephalic veins. Innominate or internal jugular veins have been used as well. Lead placement via persistent left sided superior vena cava has been reported [19] and in such cases implantation could be challenging. These electrodes are designed to traverse the circulation from the point of vessel entry proximal to the generator to the targeted cardiac chamber. As one can imagine, injury can theoretical occur anywhere through this entire route.

Commonly, venous injury, hematoma or even inadvertent arterial puncture can occur during the time of implantation and usually respond to compression. Perforation of the innominate vein has been reported and is attributed to its curvaceous course. This tortuosity increases with age, with a higher predisposition in the elderly [20]. The use of the internal jugular vein was associated with complications in 3 out of 92 implantations, including one patient who suffered permanent recurrent laryngeal nerve injury and two with thrombophlebitis. [21]

2. Diagnostic approach

2.1. Presentation and symptoms

Manifestations of a cardiac perforation depend largely on the site, presence and rate of accumulation of pericardial fluid. Approximately 1%-7% of patients present acutely; 1% present early and 0.1% present as a late perforation. [2] Acute perforations often present with chest pain, dyspnea and signs of pericardial effusion or tamponade. Asymptomatic perforations are not infrequent and as a result the diagnosis is often delayed. The most common presentation of a delayed perforation is a hemopericardium (with or without cardiac tamponade), pericarditis, diaphragm or chest wall muscle stimulation, loss of capture and pneumothorax [22]. Penetration to the superior mediastinum may result in largyngeal nerve injury. Rarely patient's may present with a mediastinal bleed.

The presentation of patients with cardiac perforation can be variable; therefore, a high index of suspicion needs to be maintained for a rapid diagnosis. Patients present with chest pain, shortness of breath, presyncope or syncope. The physical examination may reveal signs of cardiac tamponade (hypotension, tachycardia, elevated jugular venous pressure, distant heart sounds, pulsus paradoxus etc.), friction rub, ascites or leg edema. In addition, signs of pneumothorax or pleural effusions may be noted. On ECG, a new RBBB may be noted, suggesting insertion or migration of the lead into the LV cavity, occasional penetration into the epicardium.

2.2. Analysis of interrogation data

Upon suspicion of a perforation the device should be interrogated immediately. Routine device checks are performed to ensure normal pacing and or sensing function. A thorough device evaluation can be helpful in increasing one's suspicion of lead migration. In many instances one will detect an alteration in pacing function. New onset diaphragmatic, pectoralis or intercostal muscle stimulation with intermittent or constant failure to sense and capture should increase ones suspicion of a lead migration and possible perforation. However, one should keep in mind that a normal interrogation does not exclude the presence of a cardiac perforation.

2.3. Use of remote monitoring for the early detection of a perforation

Most of the current defibrillators and some PPMs have the capacity for home monitoring. They routinely transmit data regarding rhythm and system integrity at set time intervals. In the correct setting, abnormalities in the transmitted data should increase one's level of supposition for a perforation. A perforation often leads to a change in impedance and/or pacing threshold with a loss of capture. Several published reports have shown that early detection of a perforation was made via home monitoring. The perforations were detected 12 days and 4 weeks, respectively, following the insertion of the device [20, 21]. With growing support for the use of home monitoring the number of cases diagnosed via this modality is expected to grow.

2.4. Imaging studies

Multi-detector computed tomography (MDCT) is the imaging modality of choice in diagnosing a lead perforation, identifying the pericardial effusion while, assisting in the therapeutic approach. However, a simple chest x-ray (preferably postero-anterior and lateral view) should be the starting point in the diagnosis of a cardiac perforation. An enlarged cardiac silhouette, pneumothorax, pleural effusion can also be supportive in making the diagnosis. Usually the lead tip should be within 3 mm of the cardiac border; if the tip extends outside the cardiac border, a perforation should be suspected. Physicians should familiarize themselves with the expected position of the RA or RV leads. In this regard, a baseline x-ray is useful. If a lead deviates significantly from its original or expected position or has developed an unusual contour, one should suspect perforation. **Figure 7** shows the normal cardiac anatomy with respect to pacing leads. On a frontal radiograph, the tip of the right ventricular lead should be seen to the left of the spine. On the lateral view, it should traverse anteriorly towards the RV [23]. However, in some centers leads are preferentially positioned in RV outflow tract (free wall or septal aspect). In these cases a left lateral view (45 degree) x-ray would display the RV lead to be pointing to the left in the case of free wall and to the right in case of septal positioning of the lead. Similarly, a left lateral x-ray would show the RV lead projecting anteriorly in case of free wall or posteriorly in case of septal positioning of the lead. [24]

Fluoroscopy plays an important role during positioning of the leads. In this regard the implanter needs to have a thorough understanding of flouroscopic anatomy, in order to confirm proper positioning and detect a mal-positioned lead. In the case of a perforation, the lead electrodes can extend outside of the cardiac silhouette and not move with the contraction of the heart [22]. Further clues to the early detection of a cardiac perforation include: an unexplained decrease in blood pressure; a decreased pulsatility of the cardiac silhouette; an increase in the size of the cardiac silhouette; and, an abnormal position of lead relative to pericardial outline [23].

Echocardiography is widely available and easily performed to detect a cardiac perforation. Echocardiography can detect pericardial fluid, cardiac tamponade, malposition as well as extension through the myocardium but rarely is able to identify the extra-cardiac presence of the lead. [25] On occasion the perforation may not cause any detectable pericardial effusion or there may be poor data acquisition, hence the absence of an effusion does not rule out a cardiac perforation.

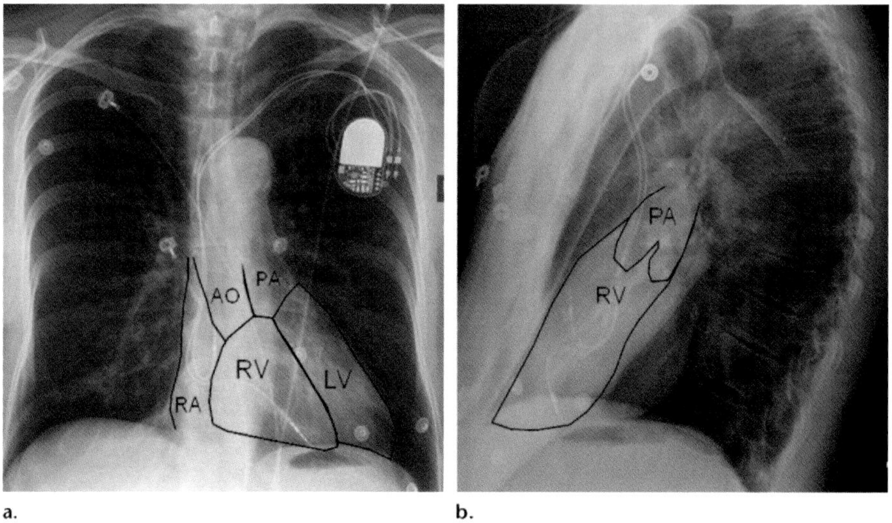

Figure 7. Normal cardiac anatomy. Frontal (a) and lateral (b) chest radiographs show the aorta (AO in a), left ventricle (LV in a), main pulmonary artery *(PA)*, right atrium (*RA* in a), and right ventricle (RV). "(With permission from Aguilera AL: Radiographics. 31:1669-1682,2011.)

3. Lead design and propensity for perforation

3.1. Active vs. passive fixation leads

The type of lead fixation mechanism contributes to the risk of perforation. Studies have shown that active fixation (screw-in) leads are associated with a higher risk of perforation, related to lead thickness and over-torquing. It has been speculated that the newer, thinner leads, exert a higher force per unit area on the endocardium, and exhibit a higher incidence of delayed perforations [25]. In addition, the tip force and the myocardial counterforce are variable, changing over time and with each cardiac cycle. When the lead tip force exceeds the counterforce a perforation can occur. On the other hand, passive fixation lead placed in vulnerable region of the RV (apex) may exhibit an even higher risk of perforation compared to the active fixation leads. It is speculated that successful insertion of a passive fixation lead uses the RV apex, whose trabeculations are used to anchor the lead; however, this represents the most vulnerable zone within the chamber. The higher incidence of perforation associated with active fixation leads may be attributed to the mere fact that we are actively "screwing" the lead into the RV wall, making sure we have adequate tissue contact by monitoring the current of injury.

3.2. Defibrillation lead size and risk of perforation

Recent studies have reported a surprisingly high incidence of cardiac perforation with small body (7F) active fixation defibrillator leads (Riata) as compared to Sprint Fidelis leads (3.8% vs. 0%) [23]. The reasons for higher perforation rate are largely unknown but may include lead design and breeches in structural integrity [26]. Another important property in assessing the propensity of a lead to perforate is "thickness". Older manufactured leads were thicker than the newer models. Thicker leads are stiffer and exert a higher pressure on the cardiac tissue thus associated with higher cardiac perforations.

3.3. Preformed J shape lead design and risk for retained wire perforation

One of the first and most serious lead recalls involved the Accufix atrial pacing lead which was recalled due to a high risk of J retention wire fracture. The J wire fracture protruded with time through the insulation resulting in a high rate of atrial perforation [27], **(Figure 8).** Many of these leads needed to be extracted and were associated with a significant morbidity and mortality, due to the friability of the lead. Temporary atrial and ventricular epicardial pacing wires are routinely placed after cardiac surgery. These wires are routinely removed from patients prior to discharge. They are pulled and cut at skin level and allowed to retract into the pericardial sac. These wires can migrate to the RV extend into the pulmonary artery [28] or migrate to the left atrium and subsequently to the carotid arteries [29].

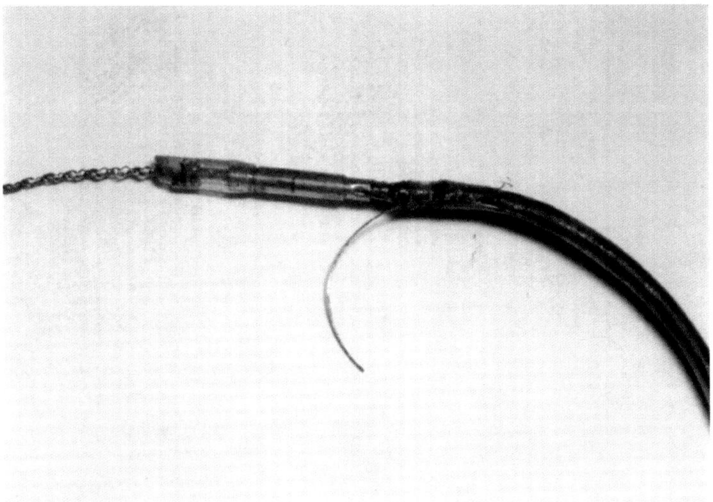

GOROG D A , LEFROY D C Heart 2000;83:563-563

Figure 8. J-retention wire protruding through the insulation. (With Permission from Gorog DA: Heart. 83:563-563, 2000.)

4. Patient risk factors and risk for perforation

Cardiac perforation may be associated with intrinsic myocardial, as well as, patient-specific factors rendering this, rather uncommon complication more predictable. Mahapatra et al [5] have investigated the risk factors for the development of symptomatic pericardial effusion consistent with cardiac perforation in more than 4,000 patients. The multivariate analysis identified variables associated with perforation included: steroid use (HR 3.2); temporary pacemaker wire insertion (HR 2.7); active-fixation leads (HR 2.5); low body-mass index (HR 2.5); advancing age (HR 1.4); and, longer fluoroscopy times (HR 1.3). Predictors with a lower perforation potential included, a pulmonary artery pressure >35 mm Hg (probable protective effect of hypertrophied RV) and BMI>30 (univariate predictor only). Interestingly, steroid use is associated with cardiac atrophy, mediated by a muscle specific protein called muscle ring finger-1 [30].

The specific lead type, site of implantation, and the occurrence of traumatizing factors may result in a higher incidence of RV perforation. Although factors, such as defibrillator leads, excessive slack during lead implantation, smaller diameter leads with higher resistance, chest wall trauma especially soon after implantation and multiple shocks delivered around the time of implantation are yet to be validated, they remain important considerations when one considers the predisposition to perforation. It has previously been suggested that RV free wall and/or apical insertions, especially in the elderly are associated with higher perforation rate attributed to the thinner wall in that region, which atrophies with age. In addition, the use of anticoagulants may increase the risk of perforation.

5. Implantation techniques to minimize the risk of perforation

Certain steps should be taken to reduce the incidence of lead related cardiac perforation. It is imperative that in obtaining an informed consent, patients should be made aware of the symptoms to watch for following a surgery for a more rapid recognition of complications. Only experienced implanters with highly trained personnel, in dedicated electrophysiology laboratories, should perform these procedures.

Careful patient selection and avoidance of temporary pacing wires would be helpful in reducing this complication. In addition, selection of more compliant (less stiff) leads, wider lead tip area and placement in the RV septum can further reduce this risk. It has also been suggested that excessive slack on the lead after placement can increase the tension on the free wall resulting in a late perforation. Post-procedure, a high index of suspicion needs to be maintained; while the clinical examination, routine chest x-ray, ECG and pacemaker interrogation including remote monitoring can help expedite the diagnosis.

6. Management of lead perforation

The management of cardiac perforation depends on the timing of this complication. Acutely, the pacing lead can be repositioned and the patient is monitored with serial echocardiography. The risk of bleeding during removal of a lead increases rapidly in non-acute perforations. Subacute or delayed perforation is dealt with on a case by case basis. In some cases, when the cardiac perforation is asymptomatic or not associated with pacing/sensing malfunction or mediastinal bleeding or if the risk of lead removal outweighs the non-removal, the lead can be left in place. Patients can be observed and watched for lead migration and at that point lead extraction could be performed. [16, 30, 31] Simple lead positioning can be utilized in some cases especially in acute or early stages when minimal fibrotic adhesions facilitate repositioning. [32] If there is bleeding within or outside of the mediastinum, accompanied by lung or other vascular damage, especially if the lead was recently implanted, the lead should be explanted surgically to insure adequate surgical correction of the problem.

6.1. Non-thoracotomy approach

Active Fixation leads can be removed transvenously under direct fluoroscopic visualization. However, an Expert Consensus Statement published by the Heart Rhythm Society [33] recently classifies following conditions as class III indication for transvenous extraction of non-functional leads. They cited the following in their decision: lead removal is not indicated in patients with a known anomalous placement of leads through structures other than normal venous and cardiac structures, (e.g. subclavian artery, aorta, pleura, atrial or ventricular wall or mediastinum) or through a systemic venous atrium or systemic ventricle. Additional techniques including surgical backup should be deployed in the appropriate clinical scenario. Simple perforations can be managed with a percutaneous approach. In one series of 11 patients with an RV perforation, in 10 patients, the leads were removed by simple traction under fluoroscopic guidance in the operating room with surgical backup support. In one patient, surgical intervention was required after a pericardiocentesis, underscoring the need for close monitoring [34]. In the analysis of 33 consecutive patients who developed cardiac perforation with associated with tamponade, within 24 hours of procedure (electrophysiology or device implant), nineteen (58%) patients were managed conservatively with intravenous fluid and pressor support. Fourteen (42%) required a pericardiocentesis. The authors suggested that in the setting of acute tamponade associated with a large pericardial effusion (> 2 cm), associated with RV diastolic collapse, pericardiocentesis would likely be needed. As a less invasive measure, video assisted thoracoscopy surgery (VATS) with adjuvant anterior minimally invasive anterior thoracotomy has also been used [35].

6.2. Thoracotomy approach

A surgical approach is recommended when cardiac tamponade is the presenting feature, complicating a lead extraction or an anomalous approach to lead implantation is present. Passive fixation leads are bulky and have tines potentially worsening damage if the leads are "pulled" transvenously.

During the procedure the lead tip is freed up from the tissue, and then the body of the lead is removed transvenously. Surgeons can also place epicardial leads as an alternative approach. It is recommended that pericardium be cleansed after extracting the contents of the hemopericardium to reduce the risk of future constrictive pericarditis [36). A surgical approach results in an increased hospital stay and its concomitant risks. In this regard the use of VATS with adjuvant anterior minimally invasive anterior thoracotomy appears promising in reducing the hospital stay and its associated morbidities.

7. Summary

The overall incidence of a cardiac perforation as a result of a transvenous lead insertion is low. Perforations can exhibit a range of manifestations, from asymptomatic to life-threatening. In order to minimize complications, temporary pacing lead placement should be avoided unless absolutely necessary. Extreme caution should be used when implanting a device in patients who are on steroids or anticoagulants. Once perforation is detected the management depends on the duration of implant (acute vs. chronic), accompanying findings (tamponade or pneumothorax) and the type of lead. In the case of an acute perforation, leads can be repositioned under fluoroscopy. Hemopericardium with tamponade can be managed via percutaneous pericardiocentesis and on occasion may require surgical drainage.

Abbreviations

BMI= body mass index
CRT= cardiac resynchronization therapy
CS= coronary sinus
CT= computerized tomography
ECG= electrocardiogram
FDA= federal drug administration
IVS= interventricular septum
HR= hazard risk
LV= left ventricle
PPM or ppms= pacemaker or pacemakers
RA= right atrium
RBBB= right bundle branch block
RV= right ventricle
VATS= video assisted thoracoscopy surgery

Author details

Sanjay Kumar, Haidar Yassin, Opesanmi Esan, Adam S. Budzikowski and John T. Kassotis*
Division of Cardiovascular Medicine, Clinical Cardiac Electrophysiology Section, SUNY Downstate, Brooklyn, NY, USA

8. References

[1] Barold SS, Center S. Electrographic diagnosis of perforation of the heart by pacing catheter electrode. Am J Cardiol. 1969 Aug;24 (2):274-8.
[2] Ellenbogen KA, Wood MA, Shepard RK. Delayed complications following pacemaker implantation. Pacing Clin Electrophysiol. 2002 Aug;25 (8):1155-8.
[3] Sivakumaran S, Irwin ME, Gulamhusein SS, Senaratne MP. Postpacemaker implant pericarditis: incidence and outcomes with active-fixation leads. Pacing Clin Electrophysiol. 2002 May;25 (5):833-7.
[4] Hirschl DA, Jain VR, Spindola-Franco H, Gross JN, Haramati LB. Prevalence and characterization of asymptomatic pacemaker and ICD lead perforation on CT. Pacing Clin Electrophysiol. 2007 Jan;30 (1):28-32.

* Corresponding Author

[5] Mahapatra S, Bybee KA, Bunch TJ, Espinosa RE, Sinak LJ, McGoon MD, et al. Incidence and predictors of cardiac perforation after permanent pacemaker placement. Heart Rhythm. 2005 Sep;2 (9):907-11.
[6] Alla VM, Reddy YM, Abide W, Hee T, Hunter C. Delayed lead perforation: can we ever let the guard down? Cardiol Res Pract. 2010;2010.
[7] Cameron J, Mond H, Ciddor G, Harper K, McKie J. Stiffness of the distal tip of bipolar pacing leads. Pacing Clin Electrophysiol. 1990 Dec;13 (12 Pt 2):1915-20.
[8] Gasser TC, Gudmundson P, Dohr G. Failure mechanisms of ventricular tissue due to deep penetration. J Biomech. 2009 Mar 26;42 (5):626-33.
[9] Forsell C, Gasser TC. Numerical simulation of the failure of ventricular tissue due to deep penetration: the impact of constitutive properties. J Biomech. 2011 Jan 4;44 (1):45-51.
[10] Aliyev F, Celiker C, Turkoglu C, Karadag B, Yildiz A. Perforations of right heart chambers associated with electrophysiology catheters and temporary transvenous pacing leads. Turk Kardiyol Dern Ars. 2011 Jan;39 (1):16-22.
[11] Lang RM, Bierig M, Devereux RB, Flachskampf FA, Foster E, Pellikka PA, et al. Recommendations for chamber quantification: a report from the American Society of Echocardiography's Guidelines and Standards Committee and the Chamber Quantification Writing Group, developed in conjunction with the European Association of Echocardiography, a branch of the European Society of Cardiology. J Am Soc Echocardiogr. 2005 Dec;18 (12):1440-63.
[12] James M, Townsend M, Aldington S. An unusual complication of transvenous temporary pacing. Heart. 2003 Apr;89 (4):448.
[13] Zaher MF, Azab BN, Bogin MB, Bekheit SG. Inadvertent malposition of a permanent pacemaker ventricular lead into the left ventricle which was initially missed and diagnosed two years later: a case report. J Med Case Reports. 2011;5 (1):54.
[14] Raghavan C, Cashion WR, Jr., Spencer WH, 3rd. Malposition of transvenous pacing lead in the left ventricle. Clin Cardiol. 1996 Apr;19 (4):335-8.
[15] Meyer JA, Millar K. Perforation of the right ventricle by electrode catheters: a review and report of nine cases. Ann Surg. 1968 Dec;168 (6):1048-60.
[16] Polin GM, Zado E, Nayak H, Cooper JM, Russo AM, Dixit S, et al. Proper management of pericardial tamponade as a late complication of implantable cardiac device placement. Am J Cardiol. 2006 Jul 15;98 (2):223-5.
[17] Azizi M, Castel MA, Behrens S, Rodiger W, Nagele H. Experience with coronary sinus lead implantations for cardiac resynchronization therapy in 244 patients. Herzschrittmacherther Elektrophysiol. 2006 Mar;17 (1):13-8.
[18] Kitamura K, Jorgensen CR, From AH. Transvenous atrial and ventricular pacing from the coronary sinus complicated by perforation and cardiac tamponade. Chest. 1971 Jul;60 (1):95-8.
[19] Innasimuthu AL, Rao GK, Wong P. Persistent left-sided superior vena cava--a pacing challenge. Acute Card Care. 2007;9 (4):252.
[20] Igawa O, Adachi M, Yano A, Miake J, Inoue Y, Ogura K, et al. Brachiocephalic vein perforation on three-dimensional computed tomography. Europace. 2007 Jan;9 (1):74-5.
[21] Brodman R, Furman S. Pacemaker implantation through the internal jugular vein. Ann Thorac Surg. 1980 Jan;29 (1):63-5.

[22] Krivan L, Kozak M, Vlasinova J, Sepsi M. Right ventricular perforation with an ICD defibrillation lead managed by surgical revision and epicardial leads--case reports. Pacing Clin Electrophysiol. 2008 Jan;31 (1):3-6.
[23] Aguilera AL, Volokhina YV, Fisher KL. Radiography of cardiac conduction devices: a comprehensive review. Radiographics. 2011 Oct;31 (6):1669-82.
[24] McGavigan AD, Roberts-Thomson KC, Hillock RJ, Stevenson IH, Mond HG. Right ventricular outflow tract pacing: radiographic and electrocardiographic correlates of lead position. Pacing Clin Electrophysiol. 2006 Oct;29 (10):1063-8.
[25] Villanueva FS, Heinsimer JA, Burkman MH, Fananapazir L, Halvorsen RA, Jr., Chen JT. Echocardiographic detection of perforation of the cardiac ventricular septum by a permanent pacemaker lead. Am J Cardiol. 1987 Feb 1;59 (4):370-1.
[26] Hauser RG, McGriff D, Retel LK. Riata implantable cardioverter-defibrillator lead failure: Analysis of explanted leads with a unique insulation defect. Heart Rhythm. 2011 Dec 28.
[27] Kay GN, Brinker JA, Kawanishi DT, Love CJ, Lloyd MA, Reeves RC, et al. Risks of spontaneous injury and extraction of an active fixation pacemaker lead: report of the Accufix Multicenter Clinical Study and Worldwide Registry. Circulation. 1999 Dec 7;100 (23):2344-52.
[28] Worth PJ, Conklin P, Prince E, Singh AK. Migration of retained right ventricular epicardial pacing wire into the pulmonary artery: a rare complication after heart surgery. J Thorac Cardiovasc Surg. 2011 Sep;142 (3):e136-8.
[29] Juchem G, Golczyk K, Kopf C, Reichart B, Lamm P. Bizarre case of migration of a retained epicardial pacing wire. Europace. 2008 Nov;10 (11):1348-9.
[30] Henrikson CA, Leng CT, Yuh DD, Brinker JA. Computed tomography to assess possible cardiac lead perforation. Pacing Clin Electrophysiol. 2006 May;29 (5):509-11.
[31] Sadamatsu K. Complication of Pacemaker Implantation: An Atrial Lead Perforation. www.intechopen.com/download/pdf/pdfs_id/13788
[32] Refaat MM, Hashash JG, Shalaby AA. Late perforation by cardiac implantable electronic device leads: clinical presentation, diagnostic clues, and management. Clin Cardiol. 2010 Aug;33 (8):466-75.
[33] Wilkoff BL, Love CJ, Byrd CL, Bongiorni MG, Carrillo RG, Crossley GH, 3rd, et al. Transvenous lead extraction: Heart Rhythm Society expert consensus on facilities, training, indications, and patient management: this document was endorsed by the American Heart Association (AHA). Heart Rhythm. 2009 Jul;6 (7):1085-104.
[34] Laborderie J, Barandon L, Ploux S, Deplagne A, Mokrani B, Reuter S, et al. Management of subacute and delayed right ventricular perforation with a pacing or an implantable cardioverter-defibrillator lead. Am J Cardiol. 2008 Nov 15;102 (10):1352-5.
[35] Welch AR, A.R., Yadav, P., Lingle, K. Subacute Right Ventricular Pacemaker Lead Perforation: Often talked about in consent forms but very rarely seen. The Journal of Innovations in Cardiac Rhythm Management. 2011;2:442-5.
[36] Saksena S. Defibrillation thresholds and perioperative mortality associated with endocardial and epicardial defibrillation lead systems. The PCD investigators and participating institutions. Pacing Clin Electrophysiol. 1993 Jan;16 (1 Pt 2):202-7.

Chapter 9

Intravascular Lead Extractions: Tips and Tricks

Spyridon Koulouris and Sofia Metaxa

Additional information is available at the end of the chapter

http://dx.doi.org/10.5772/48496

1. Introduction

The transvenous insertion of implantable pacemaker (PM) and implantable cardioverter defibrillator (ICD) leads was a major milestone in antiarrhythmic therapy with the use of cardiac devices. Indeed, based on data published over the last decade the indications for ICD therapy have further expanded [1,2] while cardiac resynchronization therapy (CRT) through bi-ventricular pacing has significantly improved mortality and quality of life in patients with heart failure and ventricular dyssynchrony [3,4,5]. Unfortunately, this exponential increase in the implantation rate of cardiac devices has been accompanied by a parallel increase in the need for explanting some of those [6]. This has been mainly attributed to the so called "increased total lead exposure time" resulting from the expanding indications for device treatments, the implantation of more leads per patient and the longer average life expectancy of device-recipients [7]. Lead removal has been performed only in limited centers from physicians with some expertise in this subject. The volume of procedures in these centers has also been increasing in a continuous manner and the techniques applied have become more and more sophisticated and effective. Indeed, the options for lead extraction were initially very limited and dedicated tools were not available. Life threatening situations such as infection with sepsis were the only reason to attempt a lead removal with these highly morbid and often ineffective techniques [8]. As a necessity to overcome these limitations a significant evolution in lead extraction technology occurred over the past 30 years. More simple, safe and efficacious techniques are nowadays widely used in clinical practice [9].

Dealing with a possible lead extraction, the main technical problems that have to be taken into consideration are: the endovascular reaction surrounding the intravenous lead, the physical characteristics of the lead affecting its removability and the lack of direct visualization along the intravascular route. Fibrotic scar tissue develops at areas of endothelial contact and engulfs the leads. This process begins with thrombus development along the lead at the time of implantation. Fibrosis of the thrombus occurs next resulting in almost complete encapsulation of the lead with a fibrin sheath within 4-5 days post implant [10,11]. Calcification of the fibrous tissue may even occur over time especially in young patients [12]. The most common adhesion sites include the venous entry site, the superior vena cava and the electrode-endocardial interface [13]. (Figure 1). In the majority of patients multiple areas of scar tissue are found. This scar resists against lead explantation and specific manipulations are needed to overcome this particular obstacle. In addition, lead to lead interaction and binding in the case of multiple leads as well as along each of the shocking coils of the ICD leads may happen, which may pose further limitations in the extraction procedure (Figure 2).

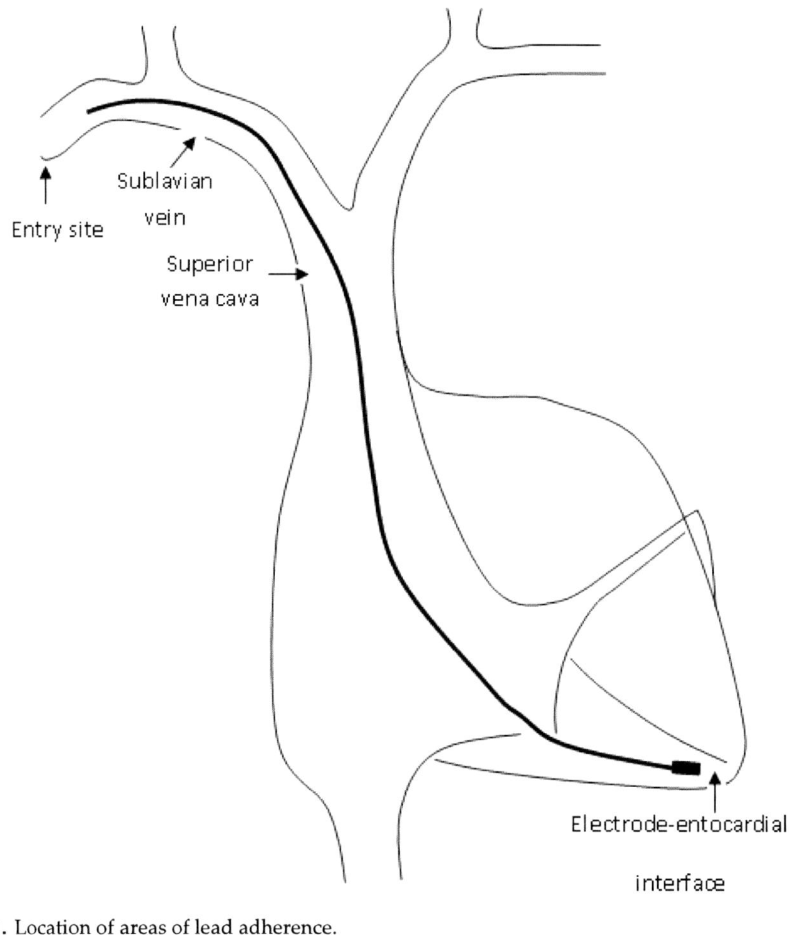

Figure 1. Location of areas of lead adherence.

On the other hand, the material and construction of the lead may promote or resist the development of scar tissue and may also largely affect the lead removability through its specific tensile strength characteristics. To combat the formation of fibrous connections, manufacturers have recently attempted to produce ICD coils coated with expanded polytetrafluoroethylene (ePTFE) or back-filled with medical adhesive (MABF). Both have been shown to be easier to extract due to decreased incidence of fibrosis on and around the filters of the coils [14]. Finally, the indirect control on the procedure from the operator due to the lack of direct visualization urges the outmost care and experience in order to avoid any major or even life-threatening consequences. Because lead extraction is not frequently performed, few high-volume centers can provide the best patient care along with opportunities for adequate physician training in this field. Both European and American Societies of Electrophysiology have set standards for training and accreditation in order to overcome these limitations. Generally, a minimum of 40 lead extractions as the primary operator is required to be considered fully trained, and 20 leads per year is needed to maintain competency [6,15].

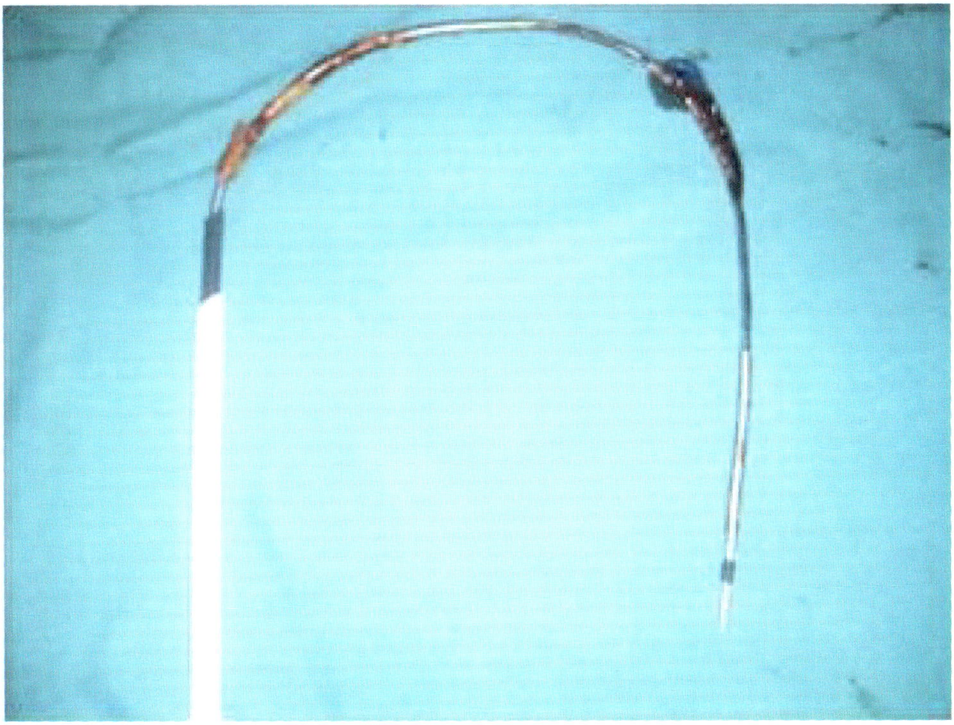

Figure 2. Extensive scarring over an extracted ICD lead.

2. Indications for lead extraction

Indications for device removal can be divided in two categories: *infectious* and *non-infectious*. Non-infectious indications include malfunctioning leads or leads which through their presence can cause harm to the patient (for example thrombosis of the superior vena), as well as leads that have to be removed in order to upgrade a device. In all published reports, infection seems to be the most common indication for lead extraction (54-60% of all extraction procedures)[16,17].

Previous reports have indicated an overall rise in the rate of device infection which might have been attributed to the wider implantation of ICDs for primary prevention of sudden cardiac death in a population whose health status is by definition relatively poor (patients post myocardial infarction with low ejection fraction and clinical signs of heart failure). Another reason could have been the subsequent generator changes whose rate has been following the increasing rate of initial implantation. Both ICD implantation and generator replacement have been clearly associated with a higher rate of device infections [18,19]. On the other hand, others have more recently reported that referrals for extraction for infection and upgrade of the device have remained relatively stable in contrast to the incidence of lead failure which seems to have decreased over the last decade (Figure 3) [20].

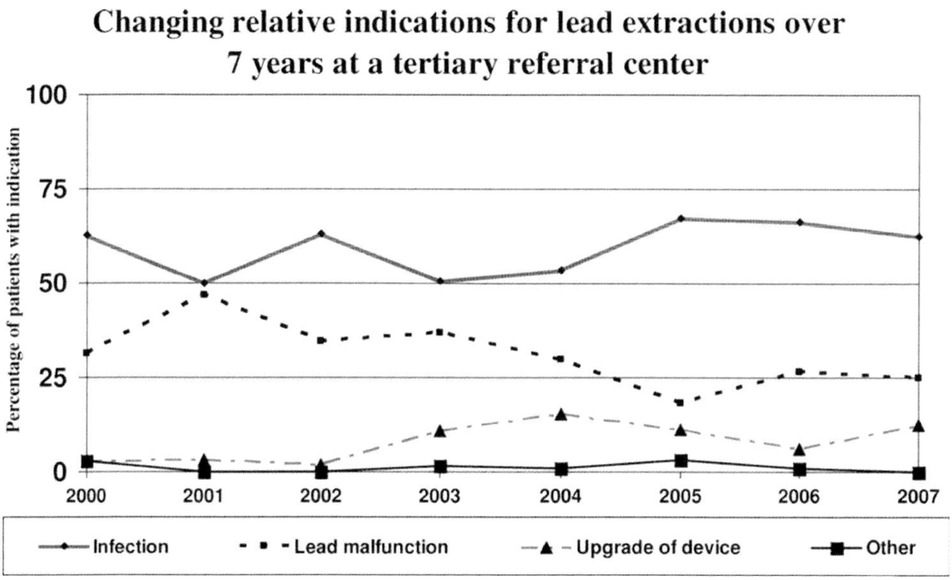

Figure 3. Indications for lead extraction in a cohort of 498 patients. There is a clear trend in the decreasing indication for lead removal due to malfunction. Referrals for extraction for infection and upgrade of the device have remained relatively stable over time (*From: Jones SO, et al. Large, single-center, single-operator experience with transvenous lead extraction: Outcomes and changing indications. Heart Rhythm 2008:5;520-525, with permission)*

The indication to remove a lead in all the above circumstances is largely dependent on patient's age, general condition, the potential of future problems, the risk to extract and the potential harmful circumstances associated with the lead presence such as subclavian or superior vena cava thrombosis. However, infection of the device regardless of its presentation makes the removal of the whole system unavoidable. This has been shown to be the only effective way to totally resolve this potentially life-threatening health problem. Staphylococcal infections dominate the responsible flora. In a recent survey Methicillin-sensitive S. aureus was found in 25% Methicillin-resistant S. aureus was found in 34% and Coagulase-negative S. species were found in 14% of the cases of pacemaker endocarditis [21]. It should be noted that even if the infection is by clinical examination found to be confined to the pocket of the device, complete removal of the system including the leads has to be performed in order to avoid future relapse of the disease in the form of endocarditis. Studies have shown that leads not thought to be infected may in fact be heavily colonized by bacteria entering the systemic circulation at the pocket site [22,23]. Indeed, the majority of extraction procedures are currently performed for infections localized to the device pocket. Nevertheless, a more widespread infection is not uncommon. In a recent review of 189 patient admitted in a single tertiary center with device infection, pocket infection was present in 52% of them while 17% had evidence of pocket infection with blood stream infection and 23% had developed device-related endocarditis [24] Finally, even in patients presenting with an erosion of the pocket, as a consequence of infection or mechanical pressure or both, the system should be considered contaminated and has to be completely removed. Of note, adherence of the generator or leads to the skin often proceeds erosion and is an indication for extraction too (Figure 4) [6,15]. Nevertheless, a few authors may still advocate a conservative approach with debridement and chronic antibiotic administration in elderly, infirmary patients with a limited life expectancy [25].

Controversy continues to exist regarding the other indications for lead removal. The risk posed by abandoned leads is relatively low. Thus many physicians would recommend simply abandoning malfunctioning leads. The opposite is however true as well. In most of the series the attempts to remove abandoned leads has been associated with a relatively low risk of complications. Accordingly, in the hands of more experienced operators non-functioning leads may become a challenge for an extraction attempt [26]. Moreover, the risk of venous obstruction seems to increase proportionally to the number of leads and this has raised some additional concerns regarding the safety of leaving "orphan" leads in place. Accordingly, the decision of explanting a non-infected lead needs to be individualized in most of the cases. The cause of malfunction is insulation defect in the majority of pacemaker lead failures [27]. In the case of ICDs, high-voltage coil failures and disruption of the polyurethane inner insulators represent the most common reason that may lead to a lead replacement. Of note, ICD lead failure rate is not at all negligible. In a recent survey failure rate reached 20% in 10-year-old leads [28].

A comprehensive list of lead removal indications has been recently published in Heart Rhythm Society expert Consensus Statement (Table 1). Nevertheless, it is important to remember that selection of the patients for lead extraction should be done on an individual case-by-case basis taking always into account the patient's clinical picture and general health status, the lead characteristics and the operator's experience along with the availability of the specific facilities and tools. Only in the case that the risk of extraction is lower in comparison to the risk of lead abandonment a procedure should be attempted.

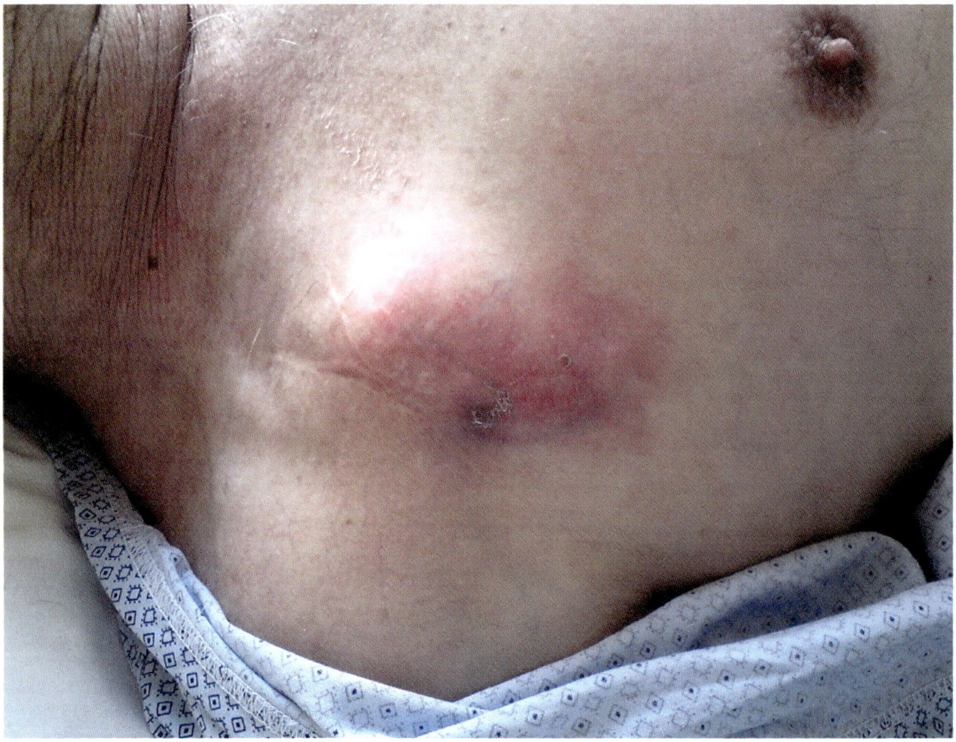

Figure 4. Device adherence to the overlying skin with initiation of erosion

3. The extraction procedure

The goal of extraction techniques of chronic pacemaker and defibrillator leads is to present an approach that is successful in extracting all leads and minimizes or eliminates complications. Separating the lead from the encapsulating inflammatory tissue is the most crucial step in this process. However, regardless of the technique that will be used, clinicians must be prepared to deal with the fact that this procedure may vary from a simple to an extremely complicated one. Thus, careful planning of the procedure along with meticulous patient preparation seems mandatory.

Indication	Class I Procedure should be performed	Class IIa Reasonable to perform procedure	Class IIb Procedure may be considered	Class III Procedure should not be performed
Infection	1. Definite infection of CIED e.g.device endocarditis or sepsis (LOE: B) 2. CIED pocket infection e.g. abscess, erosion or chronic draining sinus (LOE: B) 3. Valvular endocarditis w/o definite lead and/or device involvement (LOE: B) 4. Occult gram-positive bacteraemia (LOE: B)	Persistent occult gram-negative bacteraemia (LOE:B)		1. Superficial or incisional infection w/o involvement of device/leads (LOE: C) 2. Chronic bacteraemia due to a source other than CIED when long term suppressive antibiotics are required (LOE: C)
Thrombosis or venous stenosis	1. Clinically significant TE events associated with thrombus on lead or fragment (LOE: C) 2. Bilateral SCV or SVC occlusion precluding implant of needed TV lead (LOE: C) 3. Planned stent deployment in vein with TV lead already to avoid entrapment (LOE: C) 4. Symptomatic SVC stenosis/occlusion (LOE: C) 5. Ipsilateral venous occlusion precluding implant of additional lead when contralateral implant contraindicated (AVF, shunt or vascular access port, mastectomy) (LOE: C)	Ipsilateral venous occlusion precluding ipsilateral implant of additional lead w/o contraindication to contralateral implant (LOE: C)		

Indication	Class I Procedure should be performed	Class IIa Reasonable to perform procedure	Class IIb Procedure may be considered	Class III Procedure should not be performed
Functional leads	1. Life threatening arrhythmias due to retained leads (LOE: B) 2. Leads, due to design or failure, may pose immediate threat if left in place (LOE: B) 3. Leads that interfere with CIED function (LOE: B) 4. Leads that interfere with treatment of malignancy (radiation, surgery) (LOE: C)		1. Leads w/potential interference with CIED function (LOE: C) 2. Leads, due to design or failure, with potential threat if left in place (LOE: C) 3. Abandoned leads (LOE: C) 4. Need for MRI imaging w/o alternative (LOE: C) 5. Need for MRI conditional CIED system (LOE: C)	1. Redundant leads with <1 year life expectancy (LOE: C) 2. Known anomalous lead placement (SCA, Ao, pleura, etc) or through a systemic atrium or ventricle* (LOE: C) 3. *Can be considered w/surgical backup
Non-functional leads		1. Leads, due to design or failure, with potential threat if left in place (LOE: C) 2. CIED implant would yield >4 leads on one side or >5 leads through SVC (LOE: C) 3. Need for MRI imaging w/o alternative (LOE: C)	1. At time of indicated CIED procedure w/o contraindication to TLE (LOE: C) 2. Need for MRI conditional CIED system (LOE: C)	1. Redundant leads with <1 year life expectancy (LOE: C) 2. Known anomalous lead placement (SCA, Ao, pleura, etc) or through a systemic atrium or ventricle* (LOE: C) 3. *Can be considered w/surgical backup
Chronic pain		Severe chronic pain at device or lead insertion site with significant discomfort not manageable by medical or surgical techniques and w/o acceptable alternative (LOE: C)		

Table 1. Indications for transvenous lead extraction
Ao, aorta; CIED, cardiovascular implantable electronic device; DRE, device related endocarditis; LOE, level of evidence; SCA, subclavian artery; SCV, subclavian vein; SVC, superior vena cava; TE, thromboembolic; TLE, transvenous lead extraction; TV, transvenous; w/, with; w/o, without.

3.1. Pre-procedural and patient preparation

Extractions can be performed either in the electrophysiology / catheterization laboratory on in the operating room. The site varies according to the preference and the availability of each center [29]. In any case, a cardiothoracic surgical back up should be always immediately available to intervene in case of life threatening complications. In the presence of such a team, safety is comparable in both settings [30]. In addition to the stand-by surgeon, the required personnel include the physician performing the procedure, a "scrubbed" and a "non-scrubbed" assistant, a third "outside the door" assistant to provide equipment and assist in an emergency, anesthesia support and an x-ray technician or other personnel to operate the fluoroscopy. Regarding the instrumentation, a full range of extraction tools should be available. Additional emergency equipment that should be present in the room or immediately available includes sets for pericardiocentesis, chest drainage, vascular repair, thoracotomy, sternotomy and cardio-pulmonary bypass. In addition, equipments for transthoracic and transesophageal echocardiography, temporary pacing and general anesthesia as well as vasopressors and other emergency medications should also be available [15].

A detailed patient history should be obtained and a complete physical examination should be performed before the patient arrives to the interventional suite. Co-morbidites (anticoagulation therapy, renal impairment, allergies and antibiotic resistance) should be carefully taken into account when planning the procedure. Details about prior implantations and about the hardware in place are also mandatory. Technical characteristics of the lead should be known in advance. The vascular route has to be also explored in advance. Chest fluoroscopy can define the number, type and location of leads. Extravascular coursing can be detected through chest computed tomography [31]. Venography may be useful in case that a vascular access problem is anticipated. A transesophageal echocardiogram should be performed in all infected patients to check for vegetations. The size, shape and friability of vegetations may preclude transvenous extraction and support the decision to take the patient to the operating room. Although a clear cut-off point for the vegetation size has not been defined, many physicians would advocate surgical removal of leads of infected leads with large vegetations (>1-1,5 cm) [32],[33]. More recent evidence, however, suggests that even larger vegetations can be safely removed percutaneously [21]. Laboratory examinations should include: blood typing and crossmatch, a full blood count, coagulation profile, electrolytes, renal and liver function tests, virology screen (Hep B, C and HIV), C-reactive protein and erythrocyte sedimentation rate. A pregnancy test for young females should not be omitted [15] Finally, the patient preparation concludes with the obtaining of written informed consent.

The day of the procedure 4 packs of red blood cells should be immediately available. The patient is prepared with chlorexidine or povidone iodine and wrapped in a way to allow access ipsilaterally and contralaterally to the site of implantation, as well as to permit emergent pericardiocentesis, thoracentesis, thoracotomy, sternotomy or cardiopulmonary bypass. Large bore iv. cannulae in peripheral veins are placed bilaterally to allow for rapid fluid infusion. A percutaneous arterial line is placed for direct blood pressure monitoring. Non-invasive automated blood pressure measurements, electrocardiographic monitoring and pulse oximetry are also available throughout the procedure. Femoral venous access is obtained for possible rapid fluid administration, for potential upgrade to a transfemoral approach or to facilitate the placement of a temporary pacing electrode. For patients who are pacemaker dependent, a temporary pacemaker lead inserted via the internal jugular or the femoral vein is adequate if the system is not infected and will be immediately replaced. In the case of infected leads several strategies of inserting a longer lasting temporary lead have been described (for example placing an active fixation permanent lead through the internal jugular vein) in order to permit for an adequate lead-free interval of antibiotic administration before the permanent system will be re-implanted. The externalized pulse generator after it has been cleaned and sterilized has been successfully used for temporary pacing in some centers [34]. In patients with ICDs tachycardia therapies should be switched off in order to prevent inappropriate shocks.

3.2. Techniques and tools

Generally speaking, leads can be removed with one of the following techniques:

a. Manual traction without tools
b. Traction mediated by some sort of weight or by application of a clamp to the stretched lead
c. Mechanical sheaths, with or without the use of a locking stylet
d. Laser-assisted lead extraction, with or without the use of a locking stylet
e. Open chest extraction, with or without transvenous extraction tools
f. Thransthoracic extraction using a paraternal, subxyphoid or intercostals approach [7].

If a decision has been made to proceed via the transvenous route after the device has been opened, the pulse generator is removed and the leads to the vascular entrance are freed through careful dissection usually with the aid of electroacautery. The incision is usually performed at the site of the initial one, although some physicians make a second incision over the venous entry site of the leads. Infected pockets should undergo thorough revision and microbial cultures of the tissue should be obtained. Irrigation with hydrogen peroxide or chlorexidine and meticulous removal of all infected tissue must follow. It is not clear if a complete capsulectomy needs to be done, although this is dictated by common sense in the case an ipsilateral implantation is planned. After the leads have been dissected all the way down to the venous entry site, the anchor sleeves are removed along with any suture remnants. It is essential that the leads be completely freed and remain intact. Damaged leads can be hard to extract. When using cautery it should be kept instead that polyurethane insulation is more heat sensitive than silicone [7]. Back bleeding issues may arise when dissecting at the venous entry site. A 2-0 suture placed as a snare in the surrounding tissues may help to solve this problem.

At this stage trasvenous extraction can be successfully performed in one of the following ways applied commonly in a steward fashion:

Simple traction after the insertion of a regular stylet can be sufficient for recently implanted leads. Some experts advocate the gain of ipsilateral venous access through the introduction of a thin (i.e. 5 French) dilator and a guide wire prior to the traction attempt [3]. We do not routinely follow this practice. We simply place moderate traction on the free part of the lead trying to avoid stretching of the insulation or the induction of ectopy in the electrocardiogram. Unfortunately, there is not a priori certainty which lead will be successfully removed through this simple procedure. With traction, fibrous encapsulation often provides sufficient friction to prevent the force applied from being transmitted to the tip of the lead. When more force is needed, the tensile strength of the insulation or the conductor can be exceeded resulting in stretching or rupture. The lead may become irreversibly damaged complicating the extraction process and even leaving part of it indwelling in the venous circulation. Thus, it is of paramount importance for the lead to be removed in on piece. This can happen only if the operator has control of the body lead throughout the procedure binding the elements of the lead together. In that case, the exposed part of the lead can be used as a handle to remove its endovascular segments which will not be the case if the lead becomes distorted or elongated. Although it may be possible to snare fragments of the lead that have remained intravascularly after the main body of the lead has been removed, this may become increasingly hard at times.

Regarding the type of the lead which can be extracted by simple traction, there is always a better chance for recently implanted and active fixation than passive fixation leads, especially if they are isodiametric and can be unscrewed before extraction. Sometimes this is not feasible because the mechanism is damaged or tissue is plugging the helix. In that case manual counterclockwise rotation of the lead body may unscrew the lead. However, to achieve this, the lead body must be free of adhesions in its entire course. In the case of atrial leads, where the helix has often extended through the thin atrial wall, failure to retract the helix makes traction particularly dangerous in removing a plug of atrial tissue with subsequent tamponade. As a rule, traction should not be placed on a lead not fully unscrewed unless a cardiac surgeon is present and the operating room is ready to accept the patient.

In general, invagination of the myocardium may complicate any case of unopposed traction. Arrhythmias and hypotension can be the result of myocardial rupture, avulsion of a tricuspid valve leaflet or rupture of the superior vena cava or the subclavian veins. To avoid these complications, prolonged graded traction has been introduced. Historically speaking Bilgutay et al [35] created a graded weight and pulley system to deliver gentle traction on the externalized portion of the lead. This system required prolonged hospitalization with bed rest, increased the risk of infection and was proven frequently unsuccessful. This technique has been totally replaced nowadays from the use of locking stylets.

Traction via a locking stylet is directly applied at the tip, bypassing the conductor and the insulation. If manual traction is unsuccessful, the inner lumen is reamed with a conventional stylet to remove debris and the lead is cut approximately 5 cm from the vascular entry with a sharp scissor to maintain the shape of the spiral conductors. Care must be taken not to damage the distal lead, which should be firmly held by the assistant with his fingers or with a soft clamp if available. The central lumen of the lead is then identified and a locking stylet is inserted through it. To avoid pulling out the core and leaving the outer insulation in place, a ligature is used to tie down the insulation with the rest of the lead components and with the locking stylet. To choose the locking stylet of the appropriate size, the inner lumen diameter hat to initially be measured with the insertion of a series of gauze pins. A locking stylet of a size corresponding to the largest pin was chosen. This is not longer necessary since most of the contemporary stylets are designed to accommodate a wide range of conductor coil diameters. Locking stylets consist of a straight non-expandable wire that can be locked into the coil close to the tip of the lead. This specific design permits to focus the force of traction as close to the lead tip as possible. As a consequence, the risk of lead disruption is reduced and the likelihood of complete removal of the lead is increased [36],[37]. Several types of stylets with different locking exist. The most commonly used are: the Liberator (Cook Medical, Bloomington, Indiana, USA), the Lead Locking Device (LLD) EZ (Spectranetics, Colorado Springs, Colorado, USA) and the Extor Set (VascoMed, Binzen, Germany) (Figure 5).

The locking mechanisms of the Liberator and the Extor Set are at the distal tip of the stylet providing focal traction at the tip of the lead, whereas the LLD EZ stylet grabs the lead in multiple areas and delivers stable traction along the entire lead length. An additional advantage of both the Extor and the LLD is that they provide the ability to unlock and reposition after initial deployment. This can facilitate the advancement of the locking stylet to the lead tip in cases the later is very tortuous or has sharp bends. In that case, the clinician can advance the stylet to the obstruction, lock the stylet, free the lead at that point, unlock the stylet and advance it to the next obstruction point, repeat the maneuver and manage to reach the lead tip at the end. The Bulldog Lead Extender (Cook Medical) is a tool that can be useful if a lead cannot receive a locking stylet due to extensive damage or a solid core design. It consists of a wire with a threadable handle through which the lead is passed and secured, thereby locking the insulation and conductor to the extender. This way the exposed part of the lead is securely grasped and extended to a workable length allowing a potentially more effective direct traction.

There are still limitations to the use of a locking stylet. If the conductor is broken or distorted, e.g. with subclavian crush syndrome, it is not possible to introduce the stylet. It can also lack grip and dislocate during traction or too much force can damage the delicate locking mechanism. Further, as traction is still exerted via the distal conductor coil, this can unwind or disconnect from the electrode. As with direct traction, there is risk of invagination of the myocardium.

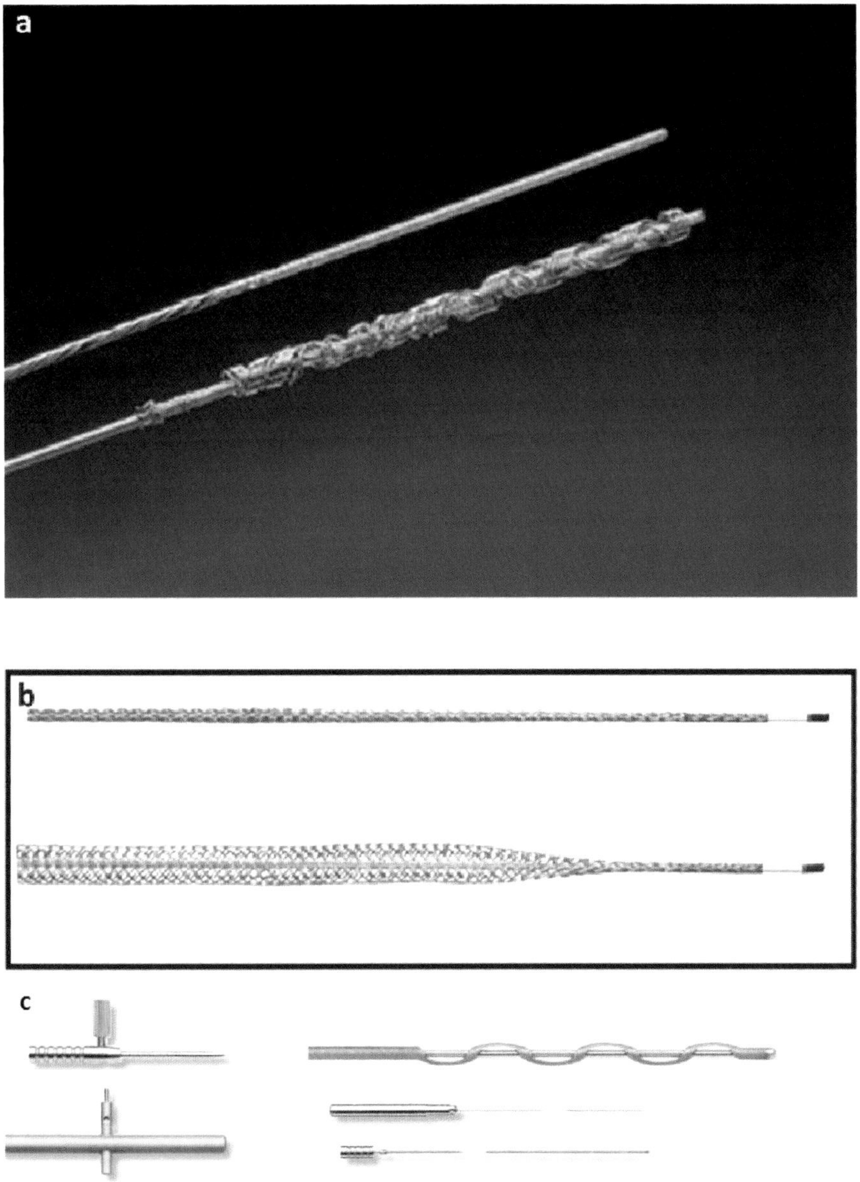

Figure 5. Various types of locking stylets. (A) The Liberator Locking Stylet (Cook Medical, Bloomington, Indiana, USA). (B) The Lead Locking Device (LLD) EZ (Spectranetics, Colorado Springs, Colorado, USA). In contrast to the Liberator locking stylet, the LLD locking stylet has a braided mesh over the entire length of a solid lead that expands when deployed. (C) The Extor Set (VascoMed, Binzen, Germany) *(from Maytine et al. The challenges of transvenous lead extraction. Heart 2011;97:425-434, modified with permission)*

Counter-pressure and Counter-traction: to overcome the limitations of a locking stylet, telescoping sheaths can be advanced over the lead with alternating counterclockwise and clockwise motions with moderate pressure. Fibrous bindings can be mechanically disrupted *(counter-pressure)*. The outer sheath also functions as a guiding catheter facilitating the movement of inner sheath and alignment of the inner sheath and the lead. It is of paramount importance to use a locking stylet at the same time, as the leads are often too fragile to withstand the traction necessary to counter the forces applied to advance the sheath. Once the distal electrode is reached, the outer sheath can be positioned against the myocardium to prevent inversion *(counter-traction)*. By pulling on the locking stylet, for several minutes if necessary, the tip of the lead is pulled inside the outer sheath. The force is thus concentrated at a small area of the scar tissue and the myocardium without gross displacement of the myocardium (Figure 6).

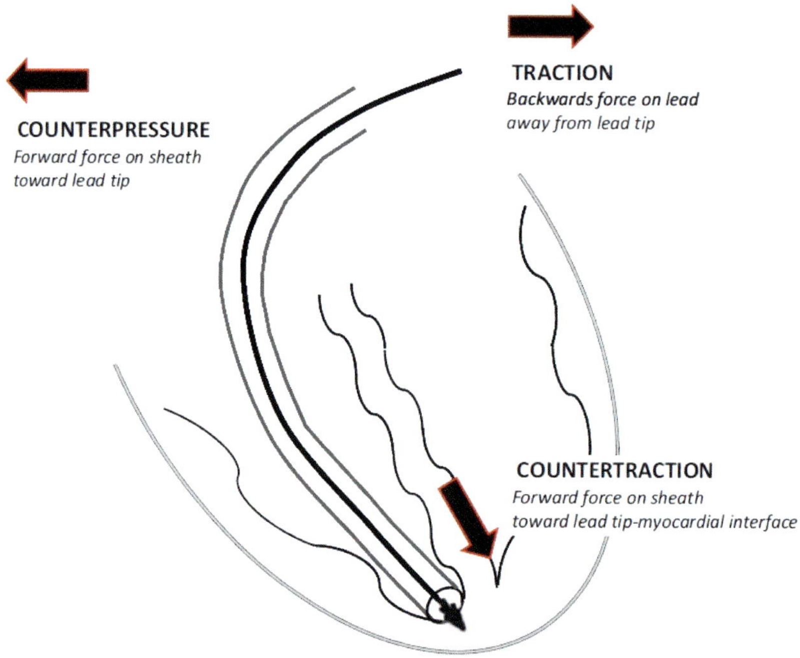

Figure 6. Schematic representation of the forces of counterpressure, traction, and countertraction. (from Maytine et al. The challenges of transvenous lead extraction. Heart 2011;97:425-434, with permission)

Telescopic sheaths are made of different materials (stainless steel, Teflon, and polypropylene) and are available in various sizes (7-16 French) (Figure 7). Sheath selection is determined by the clinical situation and the operator's preference and experience. Teflon is soft and flexible but is unable to cut through dense scar tissue, while polypropylene is stiffer and better at disrupting encapsulating scar but must be used with caution so as to avoid vascular injury. Stainless steel sheaths are employed only to deal with dense and calcified fibrosis. If despite the use of a stainless steel sheath, tight adhesions prevent further advancement to reach the tip, changing to a power sheath and/or upsizing to a larger sheath may solve the problem.

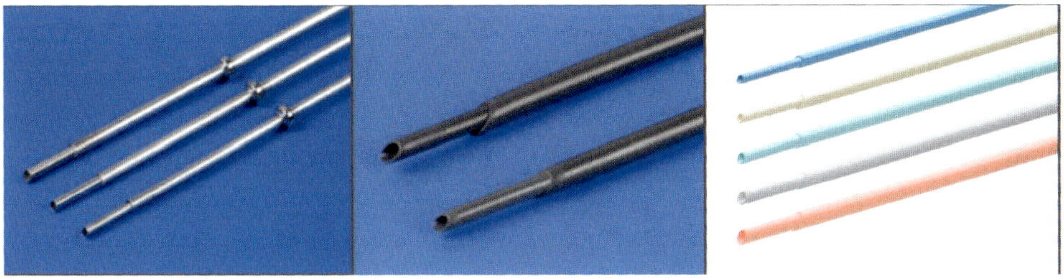

Figure 7. Various types of telescopic sheaths (from Maytine et al. The challenges of transvenous lead extraction. Heart 2011;97:425-434, with permission)

Even the removal of large vegetations (up to 4 cm) has been successfully attempted by very experienced operators with the use of 16 French sheaths [7]. Although counter-traction prevents invagination of the myocardium and diminishes the chance of rupture, perforation of the myocardium is still possible, especially in the thin-walled atrium.

Powered sheath assisted extraction: If lead removal still proves unsuccessful, a powered sheath can be used as an alternative. Powered sheaths use a source of energy to make the dissection of encapsulating fibrous tissue easier and more efficient, thus enabling the advancement of the sheath along the lead with reduced countertraction and counterpressure forces. One such powered sheath is the Excimer Laser System (Spectranetics). It consists of optic fibers spirally warped between the inner and outer tubing of the sheath. At the tip of the device the fibers are arranged in a ring. Pulsed laser light is emitted from the fibers to ablate the tissue. The device is connected to a 308 nm XeCl excimer laser (Spectranetics CVX-300), which delivers pulsed light. As the penetration depth of 308 nm light in vascular tissue is ~100 μ, it is completely absorbed in the tissue immediately in front of the tip. This results in an ablation depth, depending on the applied force, between 2 and 15 μ per pulse in the experimental setting. The influence of force is explained by increasing the mechanical effect of the micro-bubbles entrapped beneath the tip of the device in creating microscopic tears [38]. The sheath is advanced under fluoroscopic guidance over the lead body utilising the standard techniques of counterpressure and countertraction, and laser energy is delivered when encapsulating fibrous tissue halts sheath advancement. Tissue in direct contact with the sheath tip is ablated to a depth of 50 mm until the distal electrode is reached. It should be kept in mind that countertraction is still necessary to dislocate the lead tip. Great care must be paid to proper traction/countertraction techniques to prevent complications. Loss of coaxial orientation of the sheath and the lead can result in vascular injury. The leading edge of the bevel of the laser sheath should be oriented away from the vessel wall and the laser energy should be stopped before the lead tip is reached. Care must also be taken to avoid damage of the tricuspid valve. The ablation results in a shearing of the fibrous bindings, often leaving a rim of scar tissue around the lead. Compared with mechanical telescoping sheaths, laser assisted extraction results in more frequent complete lead removal and shortened extraction times without an increase in procedural risk [39]. [40].

The Perfecta Electrosurgical Dissection Sheath (Cook Medical) represents another type of powered sheath. The electrosurgical dissection sheath consists of an inner polytetrafluoroethylene (PTFE) sheath with bipolar tungsten electrodes exposed at the distal tip and an outer sheath for counterpressure and countertraction. Radiofrequency energy is delivered between the bipoles to dissect through fibrous binding sites, much like a surgical cautery tool, although the lead tip must be liberated with countertraction. In contrast to the Excimer Laser Sheath, the Electrosurgical Dissection Sheath permits a localised application of radiofrequency energy with linear rather than circumferential dissection of the encapsulating fibrous tissue. The focused and steerable dissection plane offers the potential advantages of improved precision.

However, the sheath may have to be repositioned repeatedly as a result. The Electrosurgical Dissection Sheath offers a cost effective alternative to the Excimer Laser System without compromising safety or efficacy [41].

Finally, the Evolution and Evolution Shortie Mechanical Dilator Sheaths (Cook Medical) are 'hand powered' mechanical sheaths that consist of a flexible, braided stainless steel sheath with a stainless steel spiral cut dissection tip. The sheath is attached to a trigger activation handle that rotates the sheath and allows the threaded metal end to bore through calcified and dense adhesions [42].

An inferior vena cava or transfemoral approach also named as "the inferior approach" has been developed as the alternative mode to be used often only after the approach via the implant vein ("superior approach") has failed. It is also the procedure of choice for removal of broken or cut lead with free-floating ends. This technique is an old one [43] and over the years the following tools have been developed to assist in the extraction of leads by the femoral vein:

1. The Byrd Femoral Work Station (Cook Vascular Inc, Leechburg, PA)
2. The Dotter retriever Snare
3. The Curry Loop Snare
4. The Amplatz Snares 25 mm, 25 mm (Microvena Corp)
5. The Needls Eye Snares (Cook Vascular Corp) [44] (Figure 8)

Virtually all the femoral extraction techniques use some form of snaring. Two fundamental techniques have evolved. The first uses the combination of a wire loop and catheter to snare free ends or free-floating leads. The other creates a loop around the lead to be removed when there is no free end available for simple snaring. In any case, a long sheath is introduced via the femoral vein and positioned close to the lead. Then, a retriever is inserted through the sheath to grab and secure the lead close to the tip. The isodiametric proximal part of the lead (with the connector cut off) is pulled down through the fibrous scar tissue. The outer sheath is then advanced over the doubled up lead to disrupt the scar tissue, while the lead is kept under tension by the retriever. When the sheath reaches the tip, counter-traction is applied. In comparison with the superior approach, only a short distance of scar tissue needs to be disrupted as the proximal isodiametric part of the lead can be simply pulled down. Therefore, even if no locking stylet has been used to reinforce the lead, the shorter distance to cover decreases the chance of elongating the lead. "Reversibility" is one of the most important principles to be followed with snaring techniques since the process of grasping a lead must be totally reversed and the lead freed again if necessary. If this situation cannot be reversed thoracotomy remains the only solution.

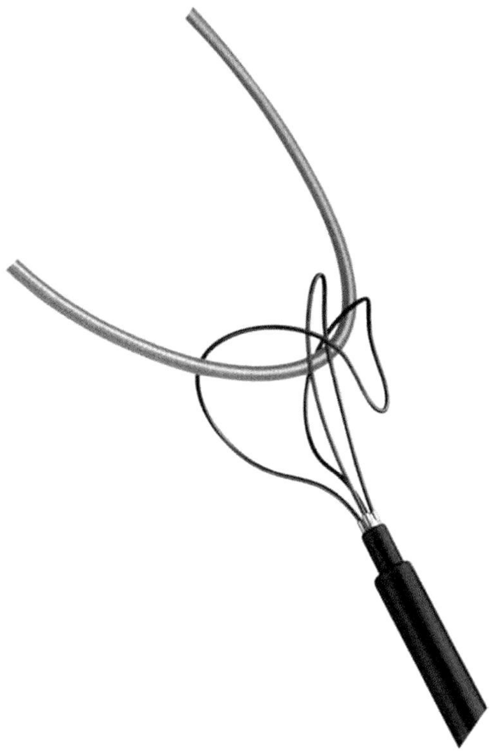

Figure 8. The Needle's Eye snaring tool

Beyond that, the main challenge of femoral retrieval remains manipulating the tools and snaring the lead in three dimensions under the guidance of two dimensional fluoroscopic imaging. The recent description of a novel technology to facilitate extraction and the maintenance of vascular access proposed a hybrid superior and inferior approach, with femoral snaring of the lead to stabilise the lead while countertraction and counterpressure are used through the right jugular vein to free the lead, reiterating the clinical importance of femoral retrieval [45],[46].

4. Complications

The major risks of transvenous lead extraction include: cardiac perforation (1-4%), emergency cardiac surgery (1-2%) and death (0.4-0.8%).[34] (Table 2). However, the risk of an individual varies according to the presence or absence of the following factors:

- Age of the patient (risk increase with advanced age)
- Gender of the patient (risk higher in female patients)
- Comorbidities
- Presence of calcifications on the leads
- Presence and size of vegetations
- Duration of implant
- Physical characteristics of the lead (fragility, condition)
- Presence of multiple leads
- Presence of ICD leads, especially with a superior vena cava coil

Major complications	Minor complications
Death	Pericardial effusion not requiring intervention
Cardiac avulsion requiring intervention (percutaneous or surgical)	Haemothorax not requiring intervention
Vascular injury requiring intervention (percutaneous or surgical)	Pocket haematoma requiring reoperation
Pulmonary embolism requiring surgical intervention	Upper extremity thrombosis resulting in medical treatment
Respiratory arrest/anesthesia related complication prolonging hospitalization	Vascular repair near implant site or venous entry site
Stroke	Hemodynamically significant air embolism
Cardiovascular implantable electronic device infection at previously non-infected site	Migrated lead fragment without sequelae
	Blood transfusion as a result of intraoperative blood loss
	Pneumothorax requiring a chest tube
	Pulmonary embolism not requiring surgical intervention

Table 2. Potential complications of transvenous lead extraction.

Complications result primarily from forces applied to separate leads from fibrous connections within the large vessels and the heart. Disruption of the superior vena cava or brachiocephalic vein is the most devastating complication of lead extraction, as it results in swift exsanguination in the thoracic cavity and is very difficult for the surgeon to control or repair. The superior vena cava has a wall thickness of sometimes <1 mm and is vulnerable for damage by the sheaths. Of note, the pathway of least resistance is the vessel wall rather than the scar. Of course, damage to the superior vena cava and its branches veins may be minimized with a femoral approach. Some have suggested the use of a large balloon to tamponade bleed from the superior vena cava until the surgeon arrives. Death can occur or emergency surgery may be needed due the above complication but also due to cardiac tamponade from cardiac rupture or due pulmonary embolism from the dislodgment of large lead vegetations. Infection with re-implantation is another potential problem to consider. Proper care of the infected pocket is essential to prevent recurrent infection. Some operators elect to leave the wound open to heal by secondary intention while others prefer tight suturing of tissues to eliminate any residual cavity. As a rule, a new device should never be placed in a previous infected pocket. However, the most important principle in preventing lead extraction complications is to avoid lead extraction by meticulous operative technique at the time of the initial implantation and by early recognition of potential problems in the immediate post-operative period [47].

5. Lead extraction success rate

The Expert Consensus of the Hearth Rhythm Society has defined the success of the lead extraction procedure in two different ways [6]: **Complete Procedural Success** has been considered the removal of all targeted leads and all lead material from the vascular space, with the absence of any permanently disabling complication or procedure related death. On the other hand as **Clinical Success** has been defined the removal of all targeted leads and lead material from the vascular space, or retention of a small portion of the lead that does not negatively impact the outcome goals of the procedure. This may be the tip of the lead or a small part of the lead (conductor coil, insulation, or the latter two combined) when the residual part does not increase the risk of perforation, embolic events, perpetuation of infection or cause any undesired outcome. Finally, the Committee defined as **Failure** the inability to achieve either complete procedural or clinical success, or the development of any permanently disabling complication or procedure related death.

Results of transvenous extraction have been repeatedly reported as associated with a high success rate of complete (>90%) or partial (>95%) removal with a concomitant low rate of complications in experienced centers [48],[49],[50]. The use of extraction sheaths ranged from 60-80% in these studies. Nevertheless, the success rate of manual only traction alone or with the use of locking stylets is not negligible ranging form 15-30% in recent studies. More recently, de Bie et al [51] reported a substantially higher clinical success rate of ~85% in >250 removal procedures with the use of manual traction without the assistance of extraction sheaths. This finding was particularly true for leads implanted > 2.6 years. Since it is not clearly defined when an attempt should be considered unsuccessful, the efficacy of these simpler techniques seem to be largely dependent of the availability of the more complex ones (i.e. telescopic or laser sheaths). That means that if an operator has a wide range of tools available, he will give up more easily on a resistant to traction lead, moving to more sophisticated techniques and strategies [51].

6. Removal of left ventricular pacing leads

Nowadays CRT is considered a standard therapy used to improve symptoms and prognosis in heart failure. Increasing evidence confirming the benefits of CRT has led to widespread implantation of CRT devices with technically challenging procedures, followed by frequent dislodgement of the coronary sinus (CS) lead or infections and requirement for extraction and re-implantation of the device. During the last decade, evolutionary changes have emerged in CS lead technology and techniques to optimize CRT function during implantation and permit the removal of left ventricular (LV) pacing leads with minor complications.

Coronary sinus lead implantation is a complex procedure with several limitations and hazards. According to several studies, the procedure is usually time consuming with long fluoroscopy times and the implantation success rate is reduced compared to conventional procedures (estimated between 90% to 97%) [52-56]. With the introduction of special delivery sheaths and the so-called 'over the wire technology' the breakthrough of LV pacing became reality in the early 2000s, yet lead stability remains problematic mainly due to different coronary sinus anatomies [57-58]. Because no muscular trabeculae is found in the CS for anchoring of the lead, the tip has to be pushed as distal as possible in a wedge position in a lateral or a postero-lateral CS branch and is typically non-actively fixated. Such an ideal position of the LV lead cannot be reached in several cases owing to small and tortuous venous anatomy, phrenic nerve stimulation or sub-optimal hemodynamics due to close proximity to the right ventricular lead. As a result, detectable CS lead dislodgement has been observed in about 4-8.6% of patients during follow-up, accompanied by loss of capture and need for repositioning [52,59,60]. To overcome these limitations, pre-shaped leads (curved in one or more dimensions) have been developed to offer stability even in proximal positions and in larger veins. Coronary sinus side branch stenting has also been performed in several occasions [61-62]. Finally, the development of an active fixation CS lead (Attain StarFix 4195, Medtronic) has also been achieved [63]. This lead body has a 55D polyurethane coating that expands into pleated loops near the electrode tip to increase its diameter and promote fixation (practically reaching stability of 100%), along with a small amount of steroid at the electrode tip to reduce inflammation in the surrounding tissue [64] (Figure 9).

In parallel to the rapid growing experience with the implantation of CS leads, a new and interesting field relating to LV pacing lead extraction and subsequent re-implantation has been developed. It should be noted, however, that in comparison to the extensive data available on conventional pacing and ICD lead extraction, the experience with LV leads is still limited. Similarly to conventional devices, infection seems to be the primary indication for removal in the case of CRT devices too. On the other hand, it might be expected that removing leads from fragile and tortuous CS vein tributaries, especially with the use of larger-bore sheaths (mechanical or laser) which may not fit into the distal branches, would lend itself to a higher risk of complications. Indeed, the high rate of hemopericardium and dense scar tissue in-growth or vein occlusion in animal models [65,66] were early findings suggesting the need for extreme care in the removal of CS leads and for detailed preoperative knowledge of the CS anatomy. Nevertheless, published data so far suggest that CS leads can be safely and successfully removed percutaneously and that CS lead extraction is not more hazardous than conventional PM/ICD lead extraction (Table 3), although post-extraction complete occlusion of the branch vein previously implanted with an LV lead followed by re-implantation complications may become a particular problem occasionally [67]. It appears that CS leads implanted for <2 years are amenable to manual traction [68] and even extraction of active fixation CS leads has been reported due to prolonged manual traction alone or careful use of a laser sheath within the CS. [69],[70],[71].

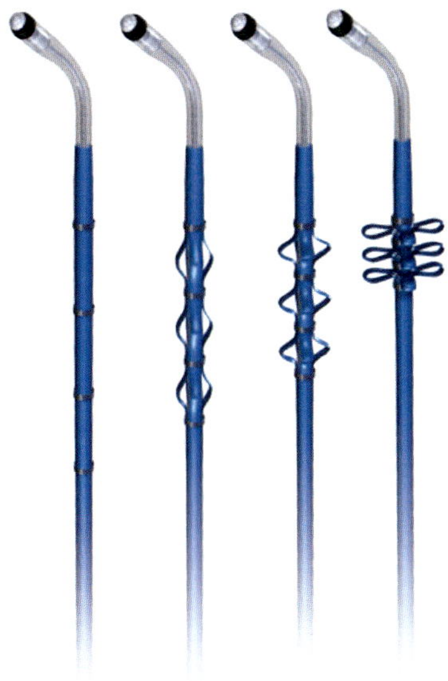

Figure 9. Medtronic Attain StarFix 4195 Coronary Sinus Lead at four stages of deployement.

All the previously mentioned techniques have been successfully used for the removal of CS infected or malfunctioning leads. Tyers et al [72] reported a series of 14 left ventricular lead extractions, all successfully removed with the use of locking stylets and powered sheaths. Bongiorni et al [73] have reported one of the earlier and larger single centre experiences on extraction of LV pacing leads: manual traction using a standard stylet only was effective in the majority of cases (73%) and mechanical dilation with polypropylene sheaths was necessary (27%) when tight adherence was found along the catheter course.

In particular, adherence in CS lead extraction was located more commonly in the systemic veins (subclavian vein 60%, innominate vein 30%, superior vena cava 20%, right atrium 20%) rather than inside the CS (10%). When areas of adherence were found inside the CS (never in its branches), dissection through a transfemoral approach was chosen and no major complications were seen. Safety and efficacy of transvenous CS lead removal was also confirmed by Di Cori et al [74] in a large, single-center experience involving extraction of 147 CS pacing leads. Nearly one-third of procedures were resistant to manual traction and thus required mechanical dilation or transfemoral approach. Complications were rare, there was no predictable pattern among manual traction or mechanical dilation removal techniques and fibrous adherence sites were also found mainly in non-CS locations (subclavian vein 66%, innominate vein 48%, superior vena cava 32%, right atrium 20% and CS 14%). Most recently, Williams et al [75] confirmed their high procedural success of 10-year experience regarding percutaneous removal of CS leads. Among 71 patients they explanted 60 CS leads and 143 non-CS leads: CS extraction had 0% operative mortality - 2.8% postprocedural mortality (in hospital <30 days) - minor complication rates 5.6% and major complication rates 1.4%. The majority of CS leads were extracted using manual traction and laser sheath dissection was required in 10% (laser was used within the CS only in two cases).

In conclusion, extensive data are available on conventional pacing and ICD lead extraction but only limited experience with LV leads exists. The LV pacing leads may be removed easily by manual traction in a large number of cases, but coronary sinus (CS) adherences may complicate extraction requiring mechanical dilation or ablative extraction techniques. In addition to CS remnant adherences, post-extraction venous occlusion might complicate the eventual re-implantation. Nevertheless, CS lead extraction seems to be not more hazardous than conventional pacemaker and defibrillator lead extraction. The evolving use of CRT in current clinical practice, is expected to improve the techniques and provide us with more data regarding the feasibility and safety of LV lead removal.

Author	CS leads extracted	infection	sepsis	malfunction	time from implant (months)	manual traction	mechanical dilation	major compli-cations	success rate
Bongiorni et al[73]	37	43.3%	29.7%	27%	19.5 ± 16.5	73%	27%	0%	100%
Williams et al[75]	60	31%	31%	38%	35.8	90%	10% (laser)	1.4%	98%
Di Cori et al[74]	147	56%	24%	20%	29±25	70%	30%	0.7%	99%
De Martino et al[77]	12	58%		42%	13.9±11.7	100%		0%	100%
Hamid et al[68]	32	56.2		43.8%	26.5±28.7	87.5%	12.5% (laser)	0%	100%
Tyers et al[72]	14				not available			7%	100%
Kasravi et al[76]	14				17.4±12.2			0%	100%

Table 3. Coronary sinus lead extraction: differences and similarities between reports

Author details

Spyridon Koulouris and Sofia Metaxa
1st Cardiology Department, Evangelismos Hospital, Athens, Greece

7. References

[1] Bardy GH, Lee KL, Mark DB, et al. Amiodarone or implantable crdioverter-defirbrillator for congestive heart failure. N Engl J Med 2005;352:225-237
[2] Moss AJ. Zareba W, Hall WJ, et al. Prophylactic implantation of a defibrillator in patients with myocardial infarction and reduced ejection fraction. N Engl J Med 2002;346:877-883
[3] Abraham WT, Fischer WG, Smith AL, et al. Cardiac reynchronization therapy in chronic heart failure. N Engl J Med 2002;346:1845-1853
[4] Bristow MR, Saxon LA, Boehmer J, et al. Cardiac-resynchronization therapy with or without an implantable defibrillator in advanced chronic heart fialure. N Engl J Med 2004;350:2140-2150
[5] Tang AS, Wells GA, Talajic M, et al, the Resynchronization–Defibrillation for Ambulatory Heart Failure Trial (RAFT) Investigators. Cardiac-resynchronization therapy for mild-to-moderate heart failure. *N Engl J Med* 2010;363:2385-2399
[6] Wilkoff BL, Love CI, Byrd BL, et al. Transvenous lead extraction: Heart Rhythm Society expert consensus on facilites, training, indications and patient management: this document was endorsed by the American Heart Association (AHA). Heart Rhythm 2009;6:1085-1104
[7] Kennergren C. A European prespective on lead extraction: Part I. Heart Rhythm 2008;5:160-162
[8] Madigan NP, Curtis JJ, Sanfelippo JF, et al. Difficulty of extraction of chronically implanted tined ventricular endocardial leads. J Am Coll Cardiol 1984;3:724-731
[9] Farooqi FM, Talsania S, Hamid S, et al. Extraction of cardiac rhythm devices: indications, techniques and outcomes for the removal of pacemaker and defibrillator leads. Int J Clin Pract 2010;64:1140-1147
[10] Robboy SJ, Harthorne JW, Leinbach RC, et al. Autopsy findings with permanent pervenous pacemakers. Circulation 1969;39:495-501
[11] Huang TY, Baba N. Cardiac pathology of transvenous pacemakers. Am Heart J 1971;83:469-474
[12] Cooper JM, Stephenson EA, Berul CI, et al. Implantable cardioverter defibrillator lead complications and laser extraction in children and youg adults with congenital heart disease: implications for implantation and management. J Cardiovasc Electrophysiol 2003;14:344-349
[13] Smith HJ, Fearnot NE, Byrd CL, et al. Five-years experience with intravascular lead extraction. Pacing Clin Electrophysiol 1994;17:2016-2020

[14] Hackler JW, Sun Z, Lindsay BD, et al. Effectiveness of implantable cardioverter-defibrillator lead coil treatments in facilitating ease of extraction. Heart Rhythm 2010;7:890-897

[15] Deharo JC, Bongiorni MG, Rozkovec A, et al. Pathways for training and accreditation for transvenous lead extraction: a European Heart Rhythm Association position paper. Europace 2012;14:124-134

[16] Smith HJ, Fearnot NE, Byrd CL, et al. Five-years experience with intravascular lead extraction. U.S. Lead Extraction Database. Pacing Clin Electrophysiol 1994:17:2016-2020

[17] Roux JF, Page P, Dubuc M, et al. Laser lead extraction: predictors of success and complications. Pacing Clin Electrophysiol 2007;30:214-20

[18] Cabell CH, Heidehreich PA, Chu VH, et al. Increasing rates of cardiac device infections among Medicare beneficiaries: 1990-1999. Am Heart J 2004;147:582-586

[19] Voigt A, Shalaby A, Saha S. Rising rates of cardiac rhythm management device infection in the United States:1996 through 2003. J Am Coll Cardiol 2006;48:590-591

[20] Jones SO, Eckart RE, Albert CM, Epstein L. Large, single-center, single-operator experience with transvenous lead extraction: Outcomes and changing indications. Heart Rhythm 2008:5;520-525

[21] Grammes JA, Schulze CM, Al-Bataineh M, et al. Paercutaneous pacemaker and implantable cardioverter-defibrillator lead extraction in 100 patients with intracardiac vegetations defined by transesophageal echocardiography. J Am Coll Cardiol 2010; 55:886-894

[22] Klug D, Wallet F, Lacroix D, et al. Local symptoms at the site of pacemaker implantation indicate latent systemic infection. Heart 2004;90:882-886

[23] Baddour LM, Epstein AE, Erickson CC, et al. Update on cardiovascular electronic device infections and their management: a scientific statement from the American Heart Association. Circulation 2010;121:458-477

[24] Sohail MR, Uslan DZ, Khan AH, et al. Management and outcome of permanent pacemaker and implantable cardioverter-defibrillator infections. J Am Coll Cardiol 2007;49:1851-1859

[25] Field M, Jones S, Epstein L. How to select patients for lead extraction. Heart Rhythm 2007;4:978-985

[26] Bracke FA, Meijer A, Van Gelder B. Pacemaker lead complications: when is extraction appropriate and what can we learn from published data? Heart 2001:85:254-259

[27] Hauser RG, Hayes DL, Kallinen LM, et al. Clinical experience with pacemaker pulse generators and transvenous leads: an 8-year prospective multicenter study. Hear Rhythm 2007;4:154-160

[28] Kleemann T, Becker T, Doenges K, et al. Annual rate of transvenous defibrillation lead defects in implantable cardioverter- defibrillators over a period of >10 years. Circulation 2007;115:2474-2490

[29] Henrickson CA, Zhang K, Brinker JA. A survey of the practice of lead extraction in the United States. Pacing Clin Electrophysiol 2010;33:721-726

[30] Franceschi F, Dubuc M, Deharo JC, et al. Extraction of transvenous leads in the operating room versus electrophysiology laboratory: a comparative study. Heart Rhythm 2011;8:1001-1005
[31] Hirschl DA, Jain VR, Spindola-Franco H, et al. Prevalence and characterization of asymptomatic pacemaker and ICD lead perforation on CT. Pacing Clin Electrophysiol 2007;30:28-32
[32] Chiu WS, Nguyen D. Pacemaker lead extraction in pacemaker endocarditis with lead vegetation: usefulness of transesophageal echocardiography. Can J Cardiol 1998;14:87-9
[33] Sohail MR, Uslan DZ, Khan AH, et al. Infective endocarditis complicating permanent pacemaker and implantable cardioverterdefibrillator infection. Mayo Clin Proc 2008;83:46-53
[34] Henrikson CA, Brikner JA. How to prevent, recognize and manage complications of lead extraction. Part III: Procedural factors. Heart Rhythm 2008;5:1352-1354
[35] Bilgutay AM, Jensen NK, Schmidt WR, et al., Incarceration of transvenous pacemaker electrode. Removal by traction, Am Heart J1969;77:377–9
[36] Fearnot NE, Smith HJ, Goode LB, et al. Intravascular lead extraction using locking stylets, sheaths, and other techniques. Pacing Clin Electrophysiol 1990;13:1864-1870
[37] Goode LB, Byrd CL, Wilkoff BL, et al. Development of a new technique for explantation of chronic transvenous pacemaker leads: five initial case studies. Biomed Instrum Technol 1991;25:50-53
[38] Gijsbers GH, van den Broecke DG, Sprangers RL, et al. Effect of force on ablation depth for a XeCl excimer laser beam delivered by an optical fiber in contact with arterial tissue under saline. Lasers Surg Med 1992;12:576-584
[39] Wilkoff BL, Byrd CL, Love CJ, et al. Pacemaker lead extraction with the laser sheath: results of the pacing lead extraction with the excimer sheath (PLEXES) trial. J Am Coll Cardiol 1999;33:1671-1676
[40] Byrd CL, Wilkoff BL, Love CJ, et al. Clinical study of the laser sheath for lead extraction: the total experience in the United States. Pacing Clin Electrophysiol 2002;25:804-808
[41] Neuzil P, Taborsky M, Rezek Z, et al. Pacemaker and ICD lead extraction with electrosurgical dissection sheaths and standard transvenous extraction systems: results of a randomized trial. Europace 2007;9:98-104
[42] Dello Russo A, Biddau R, Pelargonio G, et al. Lead extraction: a new effective tool to overcome fibrous binding sites. J Interv Card Electrophysiol 2009;24:147-150
[43] Massumi RA, Ross AN. Atraumatic nonsurgical technique for removal of broken catheters from the cardiac acvities. New Engl J Med 1967;227:195
[44] Belott PH. Lead extraction using the femoral vein. Heart Rhythm 2007;4:1102-1107
[45] Fischer A, Love B, Hansalia R, et al. Transfemoral snaring and stabilization of pacemaker and defibrillator leads to maintain vascular access during lead extraction. Pacing Clin Electrophysiol 2009;32:336-339

[46] Bongiorni MG, Soldati E, Arena G, et al. Transvenous removal of diffcult pacing and ICD leads: a new technique through the internal jugular vein. Pacing Clinc Electrophysiol 2000:23:696

[47] Henrikson CA, Brikner JA. How to prevent, recognize and manage complications of lead extraction. Part I: Avoiding lead extraction – Infectious issues. Heart Rhythm 2008;5:1083-1087

[48] Kennergren C, Bjurman C, Wiklund R, Gabel J. A single-centre experience of over one thousand lead extractions. Europace 2009;11:612–617

[49] Bongiorni MG, Soldati E, Zucchelli G, et al. Transvenous removal of pacing and implantable cardiac defibrillating leads using single sheath mechanical dilatation and multiple venous approaches: high success rate and safety in more than 2000 leads. Eur Heart J 2008;29:2886–2893

[50] Wazni O, Epstein LM, Carrillo RG, et al. Lead extraction in the contemporary setting: the LexICon Study. An observational retrospective study of consecutive laser lead extractions. J Am Coll Cardiol 2010;55:579–586

[51] de Bie M, Fouad D, Borleffs JW, et al. Trans-venous lead removal without the use of extraction sheaths, results of >250 removal procedures. Europace 2012; 14: 112–116

[52] Abraham WT, Fisher WG, Smith AL et al for the MIRACLE Study Group. Cardiac resynchronization in chronic heart failure. N Engl J Med 2002; 346: 1845-1853.

[53] Bristow MR, Saxon LA, Boehmer J et al. Comparison of Medical Therapy, Pacing and Defibrillation in Heart Failure (COMPANION) Investigators. Cardiac resynchronization therapy with or without an implantable defibrillator in advanced chronic heart failure. N Engl J Med 2004; 350: 2140-2150.

[54] Cazeau S, Leclercq C, Lavergne T et al. Multisite Stimulation In Cardiomyopathies (MUSTIC) Study Investigators. Effects of multisite biventricular pacing in patients with heart failure and intraventricular conduction delay. N Engl J Med 2001; 344: 873-880.

[55] Clelang JG, Daubert JC, Erdmann E et al. Cardiac Resynchronization – Heart Failure (CARE-HF) Study Investigators. The effect of cardiac resynchronization on morbidity and mortality in heart failure. N Engl J Med 2005; 352: 1539-1549.

[56] Azizi M, Castel MA, Behrens S, et al. Experience with coronary sinus lead implantations for cardiac resynchronization therapy in 244 patients. Herzschr Elektrophys 2006; 17: 13-18.

[57] Purerfellner H, Nesser HJ, Winter S, et al. EASYTRAK Clinical Investigation Study Group; European EASYTRAK Registry. Transvenous left ventricular lead implantation with the EASYTRAK lead system: the European experience. Am J Cardiol 2000; 86: 157K-164K.

[58] Sack S, Heinzel F, Dagres N et al. Stimulation of the left ventricle through the coronary sinus with a newly developed 'over the wire' lead system – early experiences with lead handling and positioning. Europace 2001; 3: 317-323.

[59] Leon AR, Abraham WT, Curtis AB et al. MIRACLE Study Program. Safety of transvenous cardiac resynchronization system implantation in patients with chronic

heart failure: combined results over 2000 patients from a multicenter study program. J Am Coll Cardiol 2005; 46: 2348-2356.
[60] Bulava A, Lukl J. Single-centre experience with coronary sinus lead stability and long-term pacing parameters. Europace 2007; 9: 523-527.
[61] Szilagyi S, Merkely B, Zima E et al. Minimal invasive coronary sinus lead reposition technique for the treatment of phrenic nerve stimulation. Europace 2008: 10: 1157-1160.
[62] Szilagyi S, Merkely B, Roka A et al. Stabilization of the coronary sinus electrode position with coronary stent implantation to prevent and treat dislocation. J Cardiovasc Electrophysiol 2007; 18: 303-307.
[63] Nagele H, Azizi M, Hashagen S, et al. First experience with a new active fixation coronary sinus lead. Europace 2007; 9: 437-441.
[64] Baranowski B, Yerkey M, Dresing T, et al. Fibrotic tissue growth into the extendable lobes of an active fixation coronary sinus lead can complicate extraction. PACE 2011; 34: e64-e65.
[65] Tacker WA, Vanvleet JF, Shoenlein WE, et al. Post mortem changes after lead extraction from the ovine coronary sinus and great cardiac vein. PACE 1998; 21: 296-298.
[66] Wilkoff BL, Belott P, Scheiner A, et al. Extractibility of coronary sinus defibrillation leads improves with ePTFE and medical adhesive coatings. PACE 2001; 24: 560
[67] Burke MC, Morton J, Lin AC, et al. Implications and outcome of permanent coronary sinus lead extraction and reimplantation. J Cardiovasc Electrophysiol 2005; 16: 830-837.
[68] Hamid S, Arujna A, Khan S et al. Extraction of chronic pacemaker and defibrillator leads from the coronary sinus: laser infrequently used but required. Europace 2009; 11: 213-215.
[69] Baranowski B, Yerkey M, Dresing T, et al. Fibrotic tissue growth into the extendable lobes of an active fixation coronary sinus lead can complicate extraction. Pacing Clin Electrophysiol 2011; 34: e64-e65.
[70] Hamid S, Arujuna A, Rinaldi CA. A shocking lead in the coronary sinus. Europace 2009; 11: 833-834.
[71] Curnis A, Bontempi L, Coppola G et al. Active-fixation coronary sinus pacing lead extraction: a hybrid approach. Int J Cardiol 2011; Sep 8 {Epub ahead of print}
[72] Tyers GF, Clark J, Wang Y, Mills P, Bashir J. Coronary sinus lead extraction. Pacing Clin Electrophysiol 2003; 26: 524-526.
[73] Bongiorni MG, Zucchelli G, Soldati E et al. Usefulness of mechanical transvenous dilation and location of areas of adherence in patients undergoing coronary sinus lead extraction. Europace 2007; 9: 69-73.
[74] Di Cori A, Bongiorni MG, Zucchelli G et al. Large, single-center experience in transvenous coronary sinus lead extraction: procedural outcomes and predictors for mechanical dilatation. Pacing Clin Electrophysiol 2012; 35: 215-222.
[75] Williams SE, Arujuna A, Whitaker J et al. Percutaneous lead and system extraction in patients with cardiac resynchronization therapy (CRT) devices and coronary sinus leads. Pacing Clin Electrophysiol 2011; 34: 1209-1216.

[76] Kasravi B, Tobias S, Barnes MJ, et al. Coronary sinus lead extraction in the era of cardiac resynchronization therapy: single center experience. Pacing Clin Electrophysiol 2005; 28: 51-53.

[77] De Martino G, Orazi S, Bisignani G et al. Safety and feasibility of coronary sinus left ventricular leads extraction: a preliminary report. J Interv Card Electrophysiol 2005; 13: 35-38.

Chapter 10

Emergencies of Implantable Cardioverter Defibrillator

Baris Bugan

Additional information is available at the end of the chapter

http://dx.doi.org/10.5772/47440

1. Introduction

Since the first implant in 1980, the implantable cardioverter defibrillator (ICD) has become the first line therapy for sudden cardiac death and it's technology has developed from a non-programmable device into a sophisticated multi-programmable, multi-functional device with extensive diagnostic and therapeutic options [1,2]. Programmable options of the new generation ICDs include arrhythmia detection, tachyarrhythmia therapy, pacing function, and stored intracardiac data.

An ICD consists of pulse generator, endocardial electrode, and defibrillation coils. ICD senses the rhythm and detects ventricular tachycardia (VT) and/or ventricular fibrillation (VF) and may deliver the following antitachycardia therapies [2,3]:

1. Anti-tachycardia pacing (ATP),
2. Low energy cardioversion,
3. High energy defibrillation.

All ICDs are programmed several heart rate zones to detect tachyarrhythmia. The VF zone is programmed to a rapid heart rate, often with a heart rate of ≥180 bpm. Monomorphic and stable VT may allow to program other therapy zones such as ATP. ATP may allow termination of a tachyarrhythmia via pacing impulses that are faster than the underlying VT rate and prevent defibrillator shocks (Figure 1-2) [2,4].

Randomized clinical secondary prevention trials have demonstrated the effectiveness of ICD therapy for arrhythmic death and total mortality in survivors of cardiac arrest [5]. Syncope of undetermined origin with inducible ventricular tachyarrhythmias is also indication for ICD implantation. Low incidence of sudden cardiac death and high incidence of appropriate ICD therapy has been shown in patients with syncope of undetermined origin and inducible ventricular tachyarrhythmias at follow-up [6]. Prophylactic therapy in patients at risk for sudden cardiac death (primary prevention) was first based on the results of MADIT, MUSTT, and MADIT II, then later expanded upon results from SCD-HeFT [7-9]. Multiple randomized ICD trials reported that ICD benefit increases dramatically with time [10]. Indications for ICDs have expanded considerably since approval of the first ICD in 1985 [11]. Table 1 and 2 summarizes the Class I and Class II indications for ICD implantation in adults [11,12]. In this section we discuss ICD-releated problems including implantation of device detection and therapy of VT/VF.

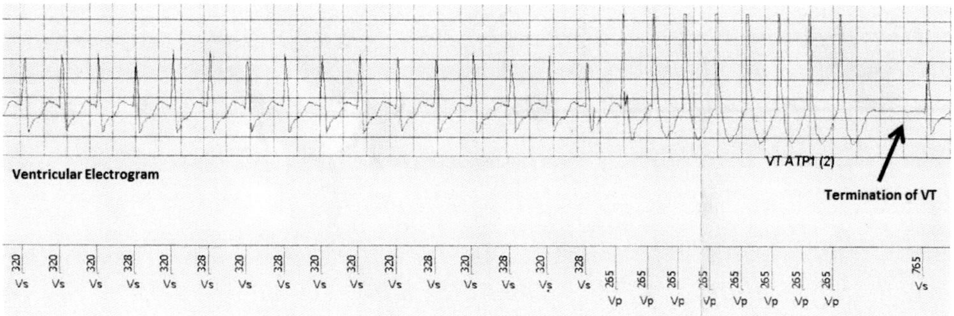

Figure 1. Stored ventricular electrogram showing a successful anti-tachycardia pacing (ATP) therapy, converting a rapid ventricular tachycardia to sinus rhythm.

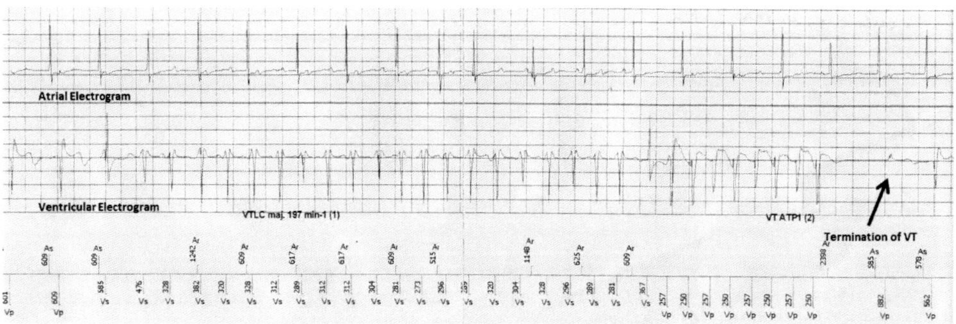

Figure 2. Stored atrial and ventricular electrogram showing a successful anti-tachycardia pacing (ATP) therapy, converting a rapid ventricular tachycardia to sinus rhythm.

Class I
1. Survivors of cardiac arrest due to VT or VF not due to a reversible cause.
2. Spontaneous sustained VT in association with structural heart disease.
3. Syncope of undetermined origin with clinically relevant, hemodynamically significant sustained VT or VF induced at EPS.

Class I
4. Patients with LVEF less than or equal to 35% due to prior MI who are at least 40 days post-MI and are in NYHA functional Class II or III.
5. Patients with nonischemic DCM who have an LVEF less than or equal to 35% and who are in NYHA functional Class II or III.
6. Patients with LV dysfunction due to prior MI who are at least 40 days post-MI, have an LVEF less than or equal to 30%, and are in NYHA functional Class I.
7. Nonsustained VT due to prior MI, LVEF less than or equal to 40%, and inducible VF or sustained VT at EPS.

Abbreviations: DCM, Dilated Cardiomyopathy; EPS, Electrophysiologic Study; LVEF, Left Ventricular Ejection Fraction; MI, Myocardial Infarction; NYHA, New York Heart Association; VF, Ventricular Fibrillation; VT, Ventricular Tachycardia.

Reproduced from Epstein AE, Dimarco JP, Ellenbogen KA et al: ACC/AHA/HRS 2008 Guidelines for device-based therapy of cardiac rhythm abnormalities. a report of the American College of Cardiology/American Heart Association task force on practice guidelines (Writing Committee to Revise the ACC/AHA/NASPE 2002 Guideline Update for Implantation of Cardiac Pacemakers and Antiarrhythmia Devices) JACC 2008;51: e1-e62.

Table 1. Indications of ICD Implantation in Adults

Class IIa
1. Unexplained syncope, significant LV dysfunction, and nonischemic DCM.
2. Sustained VT and normal or near-normal ventricular function.
3. ARVD/C who have 1 or more risk factors* for SCD.
4. HCM who have 1 or more major risk factors† for SCD.
5. Brugada syndrome who have had syncope.
6. Brugada syndrome who have documented VT that has not resulted in cardiac arrest.
7. Catecholaminergic polymorphic VT who have syncope and/or documented sustained VT while receiving beta blockers.
8. Long-QT syndrome who are experiencing syncope and/or VT while receiving beta blockers.
9. Non hospitalized patients awaiting transplantation.
10. Cardiac sarcoidosis, giant cell myocarditis, or chagas disease.
Class IIb
1. Nonischemic heart disease who have an LVEF of less than or equal to 35% and who are in NYHA functional Class I.
2. Familial cardiomyopathy associated with sudden death.
3. Long-QT syndrome and risk factors for SCD.

Class IIb
4. LV noncompaction.
5. Syncope and advanced structural heart disease in whom thorough invasive and noninvasive investigations have failed to define a cause.

Abbreviations: ARVD/C, Arrhythmogenic Right Ventricular Dysplasia/Cardiomyopathy; CABG, Coronary Artery Bypass Grafting; DCM, Dilated Cardiomyopathy; EPS, Electrophysiologic Study; HCM, Hypertrophic Cardiomyopathy; LVEF, Left Ventricular Ejection Fraction; NYHA, New York Heart Association; SCD, Sudden Cardiac Death; VF, Ventricular Fibrillation; VT, Ventricular Tachycardia.
* The risk factors include induction of VT during electrophysiological testing, detection of nonsustained VT on noninvasive monitoring, male gender, severe RV dilation, and extensive RV involvement.
† The major risk factors include prior cardiac arrest, spontaneous sustained VT, spontaneous nonsustained VT, family history of SCD, syncope, LV thickness greater than or equal to 30 mm, and an abnormal blood pressure response to exercise.
Reproduced from Epstein AE, Dimarco JP, Ellenbogen KA et al: ACC/AHA/HRS 2008 Guidelines for device-based therapy of cardiac rhythm abnormalities. a report of the American College of Cardiology/American Heart Association task force on practice guidelines (Writing Committee to Revise the ACC/AHA/NASPE 2002 Guideline Update for Implantation of Cardiac Pacemakers and Antiarrhythmia Devices) JACC 2008;51: e1-e62.

Table 2. Indications of ICD Implantation in Adults

1.1. Implantable cardioverter defibrillator related problems

In the early years, ICD's generator was implanted in the abdomen and epicardial leads and patches were placed via thoracotomy associated with significant morbidity and mortality [2]. With the new generation of endocardial leads and significant reduction in size of the devices, the procedure can be performed under local anaesthesia. Moreover, ICD generator is implanted in the pectoral region and endocardial lead is positioned at the right ventricular apex [2,3].

The ICD related problems can be classified as mechanical complications and pacing system malfunction including detection and therapy of VT/VF (Table 3). Mechanical complications are related to implantation procedure such as pneumothorax, hemothorax, subclavian artery puncture, thrombosis, pocket hematoma, infection, lead dislodgement, and myocardial perforation [3,13,14].

Venous access can be administered via the cephalic, subclavian, or axillary vein for ICD implantation and pneumothorax is mostly associated with the blind puncture approach of the subclavian vein. Review of randomized clinical trials showed that the incidence of pneumothorax was low and observed approximately 0,9% [13].

Mechanical Complications	Pacing system malfunction
Pneumothorax	Shocks delivered by the device • Inappropriate ICD Shock • Electrical Storm
Hemothorax	
Subclavian artery puncture	
Thrombosis	
Pocket hematoma	Ineffective Therapy

Mechanical Complications	Pacing system malfunction
Infection	Drug Effects on ICD
Lead dislodgement, and myocardial perforation	ICD-Pacemaker Interactions

Table 3. Implantable cardioverter defibrillator related problems

Pocket hematoma is not directly life threatening, but it may increase the risk of infection. Pocket hematoma was observed approximately 2,2% in clinical trials [13,15]. Infection is a rare complication of pacemaker and ICD implantation, with the incidence ranging from 0,8% to 5,7%. Clinical manifestations include skin infection, pocket infection, and endocarditis. Staphylococcus aureus and S. epidermidis are the most common organisms [3]. Endocarditis has a fearful mortality rate as high as 27% [16]. Randomized clinical trials demonstrated that infection rates decreased with routine use of antibiotic prophylaxis at the time of implantation or generator change and hence routine prophylaxis with antistaphylococcal antibiotics is recommended [3,17].

Venous thrombosis in the subclavian vein and superior vena cava was observed in 14% of pacemaker and ICD implantations in a prospective trial. Clinical manifestations vary from subclinical to superior vena cava obstruction syndrome [18]. Intracardiac thrombosis generally occurs in the right atrium around the lead. The size and location of the thrombus determine the clinical manifestation. Intravascular and intracardiac thrombosis may cause acute or recurrent pulmonary embolism. Treatment is usually initiated with intravenous heparinization and followed by oral anticoagulation [3].

Lead dislodgement with myocardial perforation is a rare complication with an incidence of <1% and it is defined as perforation of a device lead through the myocardium. Clinical manifestations vary from asymptomatic to sudden cardiac death [14].

Pacing system malfunction can be grouped into following categories [2,3,19].

1. Shocks delivered by the device
   a. Inappropriate ICD Shock
   b. Electrical Storm
2. Ineffective Therapy
3. Drug Effects on ICD
4. ICD-Pacemaker Interactions

2. Shocks delivered by the device

Although randomized clinical trials have demonstrated the effectiveness of ICD therapy, both appropriate and inappropriate ICD shocks are painful, physically and mentally disturbing, and potentially arrhythmogenic. In addition, inappropriate shocks are associated with a higher risk of all-cause mortality [20,21]. Even appropriate ICD shocks increase mortality, mostly due to progressive heart failure [22]. Most single shocks are appropriately delivered to therapy of VT/VF, but multiple shocks are more often classified as inappropriate [2]. When a patient presents with an ICD shock, history, physical examination, and device interrogation should be performed. Stepwise approach for patients with ICD shock is essential and the first step is to differentiate a real tachycardia from a device recorded tachycardia originating from another source (Figure 3) [2,19].

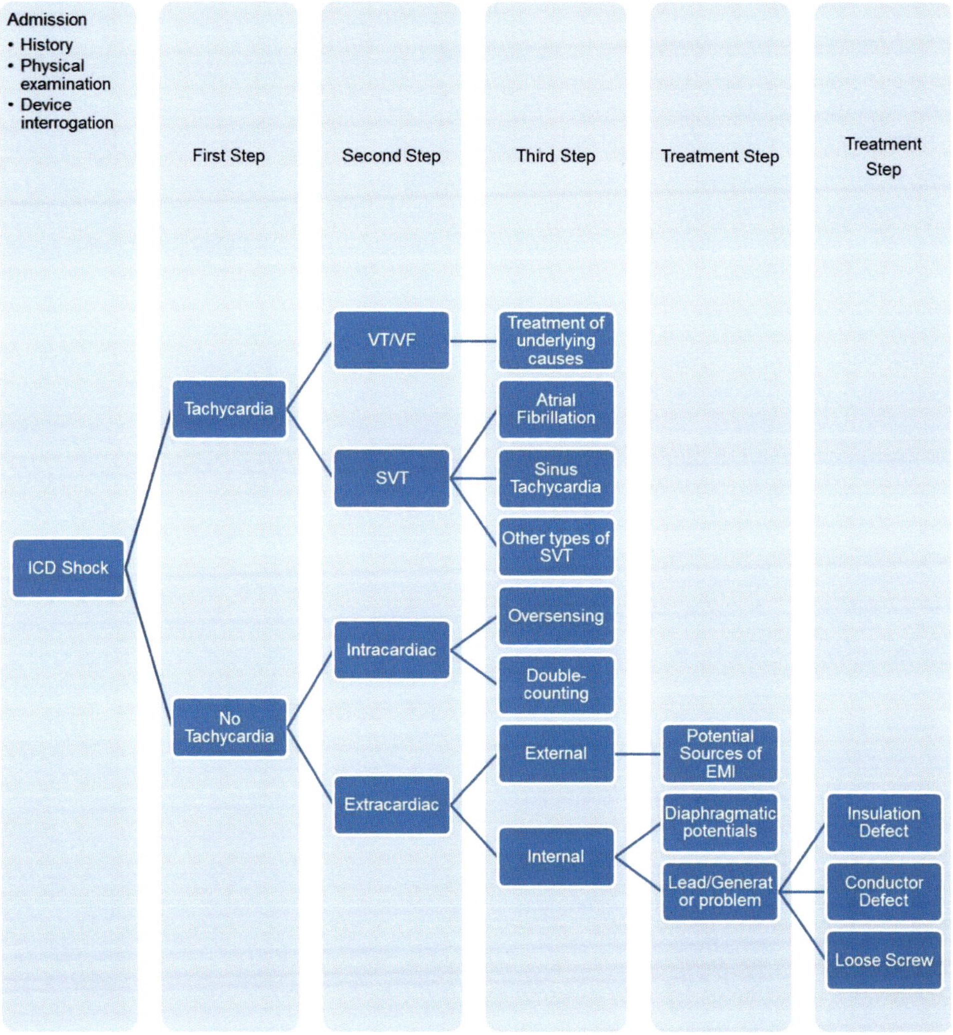

Figure 3. Stepwise Algoritm for Patients with ICD Shock. Adapted from van Erven L, Schalij MJ. Arrhythmias: Troubleshooting implantable cardioverter-defibrillator related problems. Heart 2008;94(5):649-60. Abbreviations: EMI, Electromagnetic interference; ICD, implantable cardioverter defibrillator; SVT, supraventricular tachycardia; VF, ventricular fibrillation; VT, ventricular tachycardia.

2.1. Inappropriate ICD shock

Inappropriate shock is the most common adverse effect observed among ICD patients and the incidence varies from 13% to 22% [21-24]. Inappropriate shock may be caused by misdiagnosis of supraventricular tachycardia (SVT) as VT/VF or inappropriate sensing originating from internal and external sources (Table 4) [2,21]. These sensed events must occur at a rate higher than the programmed cut-off rate [2]. Atrial fibrillation (AF) is the most common cause of inappropriate shock, followed by sinus tachycardia, atrial flutter, atrial tachycardia and less commonly other types of SVT, like atrioventricular nodal reentry tachycardia [19,25,26]. History of AF, younger age, no statin use, interim appropriate shocks, a maximal heart rate during exercise close to the detection interval, and a low cut-off rate for VT-detection have been found to be independent risk factors for inappropriate shock [21,26].

Various algorithms, including tachyarrhythmia stability, sudden onset, and morphology of rhythm have been developed to discriminate between SVT and ventricular arrhythmias. Sinus tachycardia is differentiated from VT based on sudden onset criterion. While sinus tachycardia increases gradually, VT has a sudden increase in ventricular rate. But this criterion might not differentiate slow VT from the sinus tachycardia due to minimal cycle length difference [27,28]. Stability algorithm based on regularity of VT is an effective discriminator to differantiate AF from VT; however, AF with faster ventricular rate can be regular and VT can show some irregularity. Ventricular arrhythmias have different origin and wave form, resulting in a morphology district from supraventricular rhythm. These criteria help to discriminate between SVT and ventricular arrhythmias [2]. It is important to remember that these discriminators don't work in the VF zone and hence adjusting detection intervals and therapy zones more carefully may reduce recurrent shocks. In addition, the use of medications and/or appropriate ablation procedure may prevent recurrences of SVT [19,29].

Tachycardia Related Causes	Non-Tachycardia Related Causes
Supraventricular Tachycardia • Atrial Fibrillation (most common) • Sinus Tachycardia • Atrial Flutter • Atrial Tachycardia • Other Types of Arrhythmia (like AVNRT)	Oversensing of Intracardiac Signals • Oversensingof P or T Wave • Double Counting of R Wave • Sensing of Pacemaker Artifact Oversensing of Extracardiac Signals • Conductor or Connector Defect • Myopotentials • Electromagnetic Interference

Abbreviations: AVNRT, Atrioventricular Nodal Reentry Tachycardia; ICD, implantable cardioverter defibrillator.

Table 4. Causes of Inappropriate ICD Shocks

When the device interrogation doesn't reveal a real tachycardia, the device recorded signals originate from intracardiac or extracardiac sources (Table 4) [2,30]. Oversensing of P or T wave and double counting of R wave are easily diagnosed from intracardiac electrocardiograms. T-wave oversensing occurs more frequently during exercise. A high T wave amplitude, a low R wave amplitude and younger age may contribute to T wave oversensing as a cause of inappropriate shocks. T wave oversensing and double counting of R wave can be managed by reprogramming the sensitivity level of ICD [2,30]. Device-related causes of inappropriate shocks include inappropriate sensing due to lead/device malfunction or dislodgement. Conductor defect or connector problems are associated with postural changes. Impedance may be within normal limits. On the other hand, if lead impedance is high, conductor fracture should be suspected, while low lead impedance is associated with insulation defect. Insulation defect may lead to oversensing of signals and inappropriate shocks. Upper extremity isometric exercises, deep breathing may lead to diaphragmatic oversensing and cause inappropriate shocks [2,19]. Electromagnetic interference (EMI) is recognised as high frequency, low amplitude signals that refers to noise on the ventricular channel from environmental sources. Potential sources of EMI are listed in Table 5. It is believed that using household appliances, such as televisions, radios, microwaves, toasters, and electric blankets do not effect functions of ICDs. A detailed history is useful in the diagnosis of this problem [2,19,31].

Non-Medical Sources	Medical Sources
• Electronic Article Surveillance Devices • Cellular Phones • Metal Detector Gates • Arc Welding	• Transthoracic Cardioversion • Magnetic Resonance Imaging • Radiation Therapy • Electrocautery • Lithotripsy

Table 5. Sources of Electromagnetic Interference

2.2. Electrical storm

Electrical storm refers to the occurrence of three or more episodes of VT or VF in a 24-hour period and it is associated with episodes of ATP (Figure 4) and/or multiple shocks (Figure 5) [3,32]. A patient with electrical storm should be immediately hospitalized and monitorized to determine the appropriateness of the shocks. Intravenous amiodarone is the first line therapy and the first step is to evaluate reversible causes of VT/VF such as electrolyte abnormality and ischemia. All clinicians should keep in mind that proarrhythmic effects of antiarrhythmic drugs may also lead to electrical storm. Intravenous β-blockers to suppress adrenergic stimulation, intubation and sedation, anti-ischemic therapy, intra-aortic balloon pump and ventricular assist devices for hemodynamic support have been used to suppress the ventricular arrhythmias. The ICD can be interrogated to ascertain programmed parameters to attempt pace termination of VT. Catheter ablation of VT/VF may be used as a last treatment way in selected patients [3,32,33].

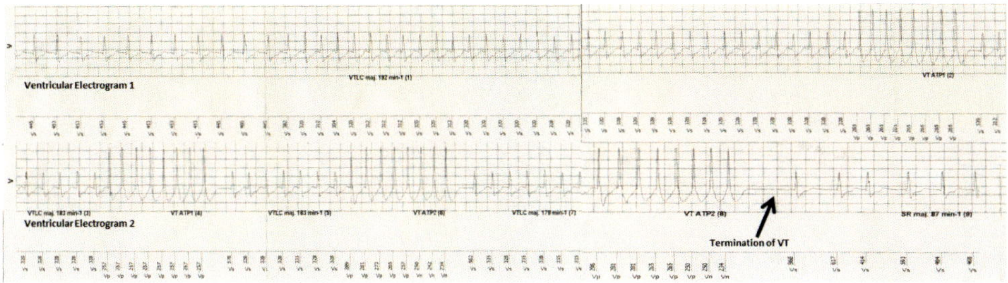

Figure 4. Continuous intracardiac electrogram recordings from interrogation of an ICD in a 56-year-old man with sustained VT. Electrical storm terminates with four episodes of ATP therapy.

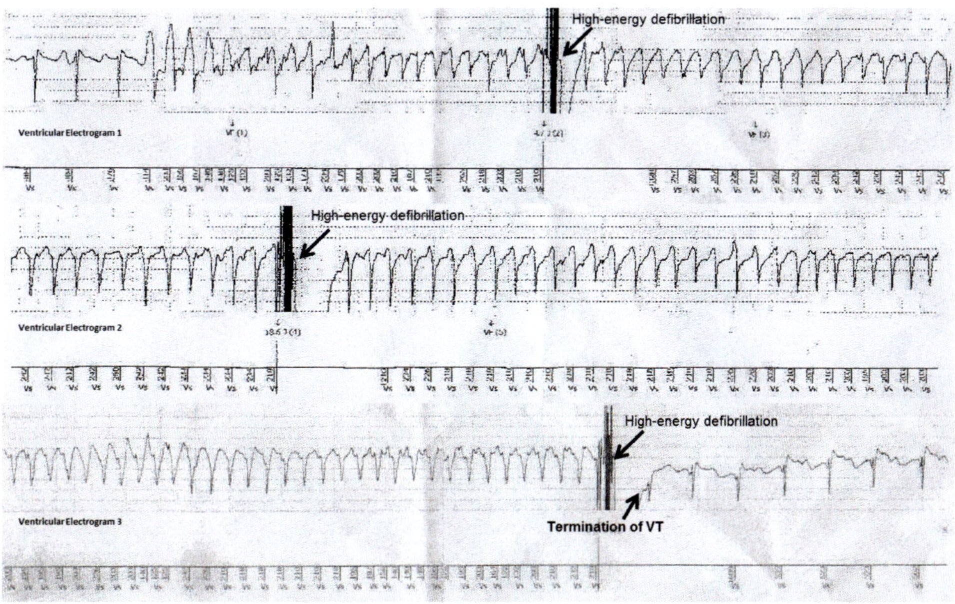

Figure 5. Continuous intracardiac electrogram recordings from interrogation of an ICD in a 62-year-old man with sustained VT. Electrical storm terminates with three episodes of high-energy defibrillation.

3. Ineffective therapy

Ineffective therapy refers to delayed or absent ICD therapy delivery during VT/VF and it can be lethal [2,3]. Undersensing and lack of detection of VT/VF, and device related problems are the main causes of ineffective ICD therapy. Lead malfunction or displacement, generator malfunction, exposure to EMI, use of antiarrhythmic drug, and pacemaker-ICD interaction may cause undersensing of VT/VF. High cut-off rate for detection, battery depletion with prolonged charge time, exposure to EMI, and slower VT may obstruct the detection of VT/VF [3]. Consequently, device failure have resulted in unnecessary deaths. Although these deaths may be infrequent, patients with an ICD should be evaluated to assess the battery status, charge time, lead integrity and function, and underlying rhythm every three months and after each exposure to EMI [3,34]. Alternatively, if remote monitoring is used, the office follow-up may be spaced out according to the recent HRS/EHRA guideline [35].

4. Drug effects on ICD

The primary indications to initiate antiarrhythmic agents in patients with ICD are suppression of the burden of the arrhythmias. Antiarrhythmic drug use has been reported to range from 49% to 69% in various trials [36]. Adding concomitant therapy with antiarrhythmic drugs to ICD patients results in following beneficial effects [3,36,37]:

1. Reduction in frequency of ICD therapy by decreasing the episodes of VT/VF or making them nonsustained,
2. Reduction of VT rate to allow ATP therapy,
3. Reduction in the frequency of recurrence of SVT to prevent inappropriate shocks,
4. Reduction in the defibrillation threshold (DFT),
5. Improvement in quality of life.

Although evidence supports above beneficial effects, the potential deleterious effects of antiarrhythmic drugs on ICD function include [3,36,37]:

1. Increased ICD discharge due to proarrhythmias or making them sustained
2. Slowing of the VT rate below cut-off detection rate for VT
3. Changing the QRS morphology that causes sensing alteration
4. Elevation of the DFT.
5. Elevation of the pacing threshold
6. Heart failure exacerbation

Drug effects on the pacing threshold vary with the class of drug and there is little or no effect on pacing threshold except class IC agents, especially flecainide [38]. The most potentially dangerous effect of drugs on ICD function is an increase in DFT that can lead to ineffective ICD therapy [3,36]. Generally, the drugs that block fast inward sodium channel and shorten the action potential duration can cause an increase in DFT, while potassium channel blocking drugs that prolong the action potential duration (e.g., sotalol) tend to decrease DFTs and these drugs are favorable choices in patients with high DFTs [3]. Class IA drugs do not seem to have significant effects on the DFT whereas class IB drugs that block fast inward sodium channel (lidocaine and mexiletine) have consistently shown elevation in DFT [3,36,39]. The effect of class IC agents on the DFT is less clear. As opposed to the class I agents, class III agents tend no effect or to lower the DFT except amiodarone. Intravenous amiodarone had no effect on DFT, while oral amiodarone was associated with an increase in DFT in animal and human studies and hence DFT should be re-evaluated whenever antiarrhythmic agents especially amiodarone is administered [3,36].

5. ICD-pacemaker ınteractions

ICD-Pacemaker interactions involve only patients with separate PM and ICD systems implanted, which is a very rare scenario nowadays. The potential adverse interaction between ICD and pacemaker include [3,40]:

1. ICD effect on pacemaker function,
2. Pacemaker effect on ICD function.

Defibrillation shocks can lead to transient failure of pacemaker sensing and pacing because of exposure of the myocardium to high current density [40]. After an ICD shock, pacemaker function needs to be evaluated as reprogramming or damage to the PM system can ocur. Bipolar pacing systems may be less sensitive to this issue. Another potential adverse effect is pacemaker reprogramming during ICD interrogation; this can be prevented by keeping adequate spatial separation between the pacemaker and ICD generators. In patients with ICDs and separate pacemakers, the pacing stimulation can cause ICD oversensing or undersensing and hence result in inappropriate therapy or failure to deliver therapy during VT/VF [3,40]. In addition, the electrical artifact between the pacemaker and the ICD lead can be oversensed by the ICD and cause inappropriate shocks [3].

6. Conclusion

Evolution of ICD technology allows accurate detection and therapy of arrhythmias, while also reducing unnecessary shocks and ineffective therapy. However, patients with ICD-related problems are increasingly encountered worldwide due the growing number of implantations. Regular outpatient follow-up is crucial to find out these problems before occurence of clinical manifestations.

Consequently, clinicians, who may not be electrophysiologists, should use stepwise approach (Figure 3), gathered from the patient's history, physical examination, and device interrogation as most problems can be solved by simple ICD reprogramming and/or a change in medical therapy.

Author details

Baris Bugan
Malatya Military Hospital, Cardiology Service, Malatya, Turkey

7. References

[1] Mirowski M, Reid PR, Mower MM et al. (1980) Termination of malignant ventricular arrhythmias with an implanted automatic defibrillator in human beings. The New England journal of medicine. 303:322-4.

[2] van Erven L, Schalij MJ. (2008) Troubleshooting implantable cardioverter-defibrillator related problems. Heart. 94:649-60.

[3] Banker R, Mitchell R, Badhwar N, Goldschlager N. (2010) Pacemaker and Implantable Cardioverter-Defibrillator Emergencies. In: Jeremias A, Brown DL, editors. Cardiac Intensive Care. 2 ed, Saunders: Elsevier. pp 310-338.

[4] Wathen M. (2007) Implantable cardioverter defibrillator shock reduction using new antitachycardia pacing therapies. American heart journal. 153:44-52.

[5] Connolly SJ, Hallstrom AP, Cappato R et al. (2000) Meta-analysis of the implantable cardioverter defibrillator secondary prevention trials. AVID, CASH and CIDS studies. Antiarrhythmics vs Implantable Defibrillator study. Cardiac Arrest Study Hamburg . Canadian Implantable Defibrillator Study. European heart journal. 21:2071-8.

[6] Link MS, Costeas XF, Griffith JL, Colburn CD, Estes NA, Wang PJ. (1997) High incidence of appropriate implantable cardioverter-defibrillator therapy in patients with syncope of unknown etiology and inducible ventricular arrhythmias. Journal of the American College of Cardiology. 29:370-5.

[7] Moss AJ, Hall WJ, Cannom DS et al. (1996) Improved survival with an implanted defibrillator in patients with coronary disease at high risk for ventricular arrhythmia. Multicenter Automatic Defibrillator Implantation Trial Investigators. The New England journal of medicine. 335:1933-40.

[8] Buxton AE, Lee KL, Fisher JD, Josephson ME, Prystowsky EN, Hafley G. (1999) A randomized study of the prevention of sudden death in patients with coronary artery disease. Multicenter Unsustained Tachycardia Trial Investigators. The New England journal of medicine. 341:1882-90.

[9] Moss AJ, Zareba W, Hall WJ et al (2002). Prophylactic implantation of a defibrillator in patients with myocardial infarction and reduced ejection fraction. The New England journal of medicine. 346:877-83.

[10] Gasparini M, Nisam S. (2012) Implantable cardioverter defibrillator harm? Europace : European pacing, arrhythmias, and cardiac electrophysiology : journal of the working groups on cardiac pacing, arrhythmias, and cardiac cellular electrophysiology of the European Society of Cardiology. Epub ahead of print.

[11] Gregoratos G, Abrams J, Epstein AE et al. (2002) ACC/AHA/NASPE 2002 guideline update for implantation of cardiac pacemakers and antiarrhythmia devices: summary article: a report of the American College of Cardiology/American Heart Association Task Force on Practice Guidelines (ACC/AHA/NASPE Committee to Update the 1998 Pacemaker Guidelines). Circulation. 106:2145-61.

[12] Epstein AE, Dimarco JP, Ellenbogen KA et al. (2008) ACC/AHA/HRS 2008 Guidelines for device-based therapy of cardiac rhythm abnormalities. a report of the American College of Cardiology/American Heart Association task force on practice guidelines (Writing Committee to Revise the ACC/AHA/NASPE 2002 Guideline Update for

Implantation of Cardiac Pacemakers and Antiarrhythmia Devices) Journal of the American College of Cardiology. 51: e1-e62.
[13] van Rees JB, de Bie MK, Thijssen J, Borleffs CJ, Schalij MJ, van Erven L. (2011) Implantation-related complications of implantable cardioverter-defibrillators and cardiac resynchronization therapy devices: a systematic review of randomized clinical trials. Journal of the American College of Cardiology. 58:995-1000.
[14] Celik T, Kose S, Bugan B, Iyisoy A, Akgun V, Cingoz F. (2009) Hiccup as a result of late lead perforation: report of two cases and review of the literature. Europace : European pacing, arrhythmias, and cardiac electrophysiology : journal of the working groups on cardiac pacing, arrhythmias, and cardiac cellular electrophysiology of the European Society of Cardiology. 11:963-5.
[15] Klug D, Balde M, Pavin D et al. (2007) Risk factors related to infections of implanted pacemakers and cardioverter-defibrillators: results of a large prospective study. Circulation. 116:1349-55.
[16] Klug D, Lacroix D, Savoye C et al. (1997) Systemic infection related to endocarditis on pacemaker leads: clinical presentation and management. Circulation. 95:2098-107.
[17] Da Costa A, Kirkorian G, Cucherat M et al. (1998) Antibiotic prophylaxis for permanent pacemaker implantation: a meta-analysis. Circulation. 97:1796-801.
[18] Spittell PC, Vlietstra RE, Hayes DL, Higano ST. (1990) Venous obstruction due to permanent transvenous pacemaker electrodes: treatment with percutaneous transluminal balloon venoplasty. Pacing and clinical electrophysiology : PACE. 13:271-4.
[19] Saeed M. (2011) Troubleshooting implantable cardioverter-defibrillators: an overview for physicians who are not electrophysiologists. Texas Heart Institute journal / from the Texas Heart Institute of St Luke's Episcopal Hospital, Texas Children's Hospital. 38:355-7.
[20] Irvine J, Dorian P, Baker B et al. (2002) Quality of life in the Canadian Implantable Defibrillator Study (CIDS). American heart journal. 144:282-9.
[21] van Rees JB, Borleffs CJ, de Bie MK et al. (2011) Inappropriate implantable cardioverter-defibrillator shocks: incidence, predictors, and impact on mortality. Journal of the American College of Cardiology. 57:556-62.
[22] Mishkin JD, Saxonhouse SJ, Woo GW et al. (2009) Appropriate evaluation and treatment of heart failure patients after implantable cardioverter-defibrillator discharge: time to go beyond the initial shock. Journal of the American College of Cardiology. 54(22):1993-2000.
[23] Grimm W, Flores BT, Marchlinski FE. (1993) Shock occurrence and survival in 241 patients with implantable cardioverter-defibrillator therapy. Circulation. 87:1880-8.
[24] Nunain SO, Roelke M, Trouton T et al. (1995) Limitations and late complications of third-generation automatic cardioverter-defibrillators. Circulation. 91:2204-13.
[25] Jodko L, Kornacewicz-Jach Z, Kazmierczak J et al. (2009) Inappropriate cardioverter-defibrillator discharge continues to be a major problem in clinical practice. Cardiology journal. 16:432-9.
[26] Weber M, Block M, Brunn J et al. (1996) [Inadequate therapies with implantable cardioverter-defibrillators--incidence, etiology, predictive factors and preventive strategies]. Zeitschrift fur Kardiologie. 85:809-19.

[27] Klein GJ, Gillberg JM, Tang A et al. (2006) Improving SVT discrimination in single-chamber ICDs: a new electrogram morphology-based algorithm. Journal of cardiovascular electrophysiology. 17:1310-9.
[28] Schaumann A, von zur Muhlen F, Gonska BD, Kreuzer H. (1996) Enhanced detection criteria in implantable cardioverter-defibrillators to avoid inappropriate therapy. The American journal of cardiology. 78:42-50.
[29] Ferreira-Gonzalez I, Dos-Subira L, Guyatt GH. (2007) Adjunctive antiarrhythmic drug therapy in patients with implantable cardioverter defibrillators: a systematic review. European heart journal. 28:469-77.
[30] Rauwolf T, Guenther M, Hass N et al. (2007) Ventricular oversensing in 518 patients with implanted cardiac defibrillators: incidence, complications, and solutions. Europace: European pacing, arrhythmias, and cardiac electrophysiology : journal of the working groups on cardiac pacing, arrhythmias, and cardiac cellular electrophysiology of the European Society of Cardiology. 9:1041-7.
[31] Kolb C, Zrenner B, Schmitt C. (2001) Incidence of electromagnetic interference in implantable cardioverter defibrillators. Pacing and clinical electrophysiology : PACE. 24:465-8.
[32] Eifling M, Razavi M, Massumi A. (2011) The evaluation and management of electrical storm. Texas Heart Institute journal / from the Texas Heart Institute of St Luke's Episcopal Hospital, Texas Children's Hospital. 38:111-21.
[33] Nademanee K, Taylor R, Bailey WE, Rieders DE, Kosar EM. (2000) Treating electrical storm : sympathetic blockade versus advanced cardiac life support-guided therapy. Circulation. 102:742-7.
[34] Hauser RG, Kallinen L. (2004) Deaths associated with implantable cardioverter defibrillator failure and deactivation reported in the United States Food and Drug Administration Manufacturer and User Facility Device Experience Database. Heart rhythm : the official journal of the Heart Rhythm Society. 1:399-405.
[35] Wilkoff BL, Auricchio A, Brugada J et al. (2008) HRS/EHRA expert consensus on the monitoring of cardiovascular implantable electronic devices (CIEDs): description of techniques, indications, personnel, frequency and ethical considerations. Heart Rhythm. 5(6):907-25.
[36] Page RL. (2000) Effects of antiarrhythmic medication on implantable cardioverter-defibrillator function. The American journal of cardiology. 85:1481-5.
[37] Goldschlager N, Epstein A, Friedman P, Gang E, Krol R, Olshansky B. (2001) Environmental and drug effects on patients with pacemakers and implantable cardioverter/defibrillators: a practical guide to patient treatment. Archives of internal medicine. 161:649-55.
[38] Greene HL. (1996) Interactions between pharmacologic and nonpharmacologic antiarrhythmic therapy. The American journal of cardiology. 78:61-6.
[39] Echt DS, Gremillion ST, Lee JT et al. (1994) Effects of procainamide and lidocaine on defibrillation energy requirements in patients receiving implantable cardioverter defibrillator devices. Journal of cardiovascular electrophysiology. 5:752-60.
[40] Brode SE, Schwartzman D, Callans DJ, Gottlieb CD, Marchlinski FE. (1997) ICD-antiarrhythmic drug and ICD-pacemaker interactions. Journal of cardiovascular electrophysiology. 8:830-42.

Section 4

Frontiers of Pacemaker Technology

Chapter 11

Nonlinear Cardiac Dynamics

Charles L. Webber, Jr.

Additional information is available at the end of the chapter

http://dx.doi.org/10.5772/48753

1. Introduction

1.1. The pulse as window into the heart

The beating heart has attracted attention since antiquity and probably before recorded history [1]. Some cultures have centered the human soul within the heart because of its vivacious and incessant actions. Careful reading of the Hebraic Psalms, for example, attributes thinking, feeling and soulish behaviors to this remarkable organ. Consider King David's anguish: "I am benumbed and badly crushed; / I groan because of the agitation of my heart. / Lord, all my desire is before You;/ And my sighing is not hidden from You. / My heart throbs, my strength fails me; / And the light of my eyes, even that has gone from me" [2]. Since time immemorial the cardiac pulse has been viewed as a window into the heart [1].

To the modern observer, the vigorous motions of the heart are a strong reminder that living physiological systems are dynamical in nature. Over the last century the dynamics of the heart have been refined and redefined by analogy to naturally rhythmical systems of nature extending to mathematical modeling and simulations. Indeed, the whole concept of homeostasis, a foundational so-called law of physiology, is even under revision. If homeostasis implies that a system is static with no motion, maybe the prime exemplar of homeostasis is the cadaver state! Possibly a simplistic but meaningful redefinition of physiology is "If it wiggles, it's physiology; if it stops wiggling it's anatomy" [3]. In this sense and beyond homeostasis, homeodynamics is being promoted as a better descriptor of living systems [4]. In terms of the heart, there are a variety of pressures fluctuations and heart rates that are permitted and even necessitated by the extant dynamical state (sleeping, sitting, running, etc.).

2. The sinusoidal cardiac pulse

The ubiquitous sine wave holds a unique position in the history of linear motions from sea-wave patterns to planetary revolutions around the solar mass. As shown in Figure 1, the sine wave may be considered a good first approximation to the waxing and waning of ventricular and aortic pressure traces, both of which are attributed to alternations between ventricular muscle contractions (active phase) and relaxations (quiescent phase). The heart beats through the lifespan of the individual, but this does not infer that the heart gets no rest. It is good to remember that the "wake/sleep" cycle of this automatic organ is measured in terms of milliseconds, not hours or days. Rest in this context means that the myocardium is electrically silent, but the heart still continues to consume energy throughout both systolic and diastolic phases.

On closer inspection, however, the mechanical motions of the heart are highly complex and ventricular pressure waves and arterial pressure pulses are not well-fit by the simple sine wave. A single sine wave has a characteristic amplitude and period that repeats forever (infinite series), and knowing the details of one wave allows one to accurately extrapolate into the future with mathematical confidence. But the heart is not like this. Each beat and each period of the heart is different, unique to the moment and suited for the current environmental challenge. Besides this, the heart is a noisy system (noisy dynamic) simply because it resides within a noisy world. There is dynamical noise arising from within the organ itself, the heart is jostled by breathing and stepping motions, neuronal reflexes are constantly modulating cardiac function, and external noise from the environment shape and

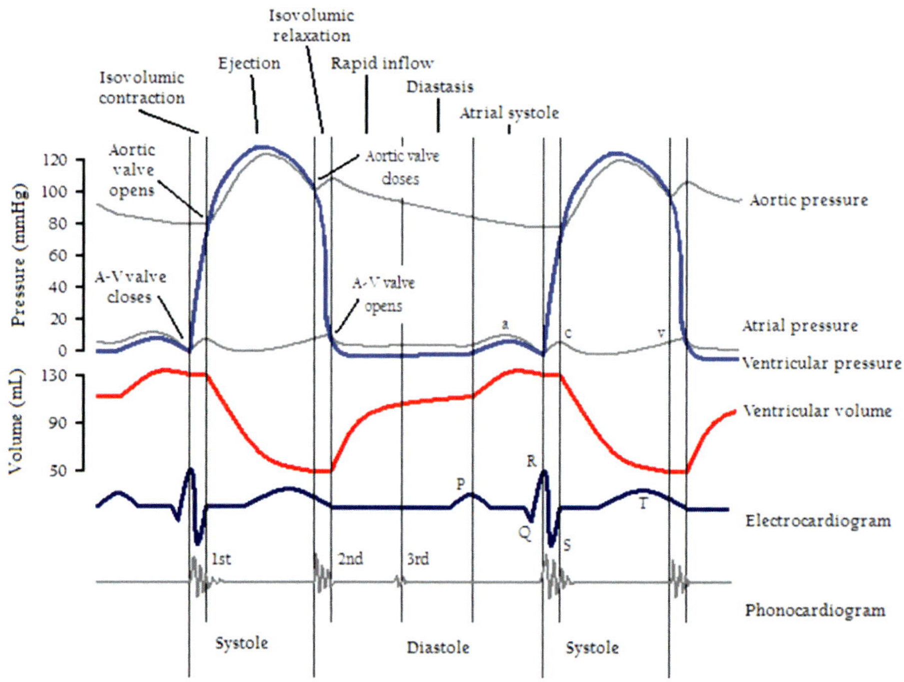

Figure 1. The famous Wiggers diagram displaying the time variations in cardiac electrical and mechanical functions as recorded by a polygraph. Note that the shape of the ventricular and aortic pressure traces can, on first pass, be mimicked by a simple sine wave. (from Wikepedia: http://en.wikipedia.org/wiki/Wiggers_diagram)

mold the activity of the heart. Thus, not only is the heart dynamic in nature, it is also very flexible, perfectly suited to the world in which we live.

3. Electrical underpinnings of the cardiac pulse

Cardiac dynamics go way beyond mechanical pressure generation (which can be sensed by arterial vessel palpitation), but also depends upon electrical activities inherent within the myocardium (which are insensible, save by electronic amplification and display). The heart remains mechanically silent until it is electrically activated. But activation depends upon electro-mechanical coupling which is calcium dependent in cardiac myocytes. The physiological principle (cause → effect) as shown in Figure 2 is this: electrical activity (phase 0) → calcium induced calcium release (CICR of phase 2) → mechanical contraction of atrial and ventricular muscle cells [5]. In one study, the median left ventricular electromechanical delay (EMD) of 103 control subjects was 17 ms, with calcium release preceding mechanical force generation [6]. The summation of electrical depolarizations of ventricular action potentials (phase 0 in Fig. 2) are registered as the QRS waves in the ECG (electrocardiogram in Fig 1). Likewise, the summation of electrical repolarizations of ventricular action (Phase 3 in Fig. 2) are registered as T waves in the ECG (electrocardiogram in Fig 1). Note that because of the long phase 2 plateau of the ventricular action potential, there is an isopotential phase between the Q and T waves, the QT interval.

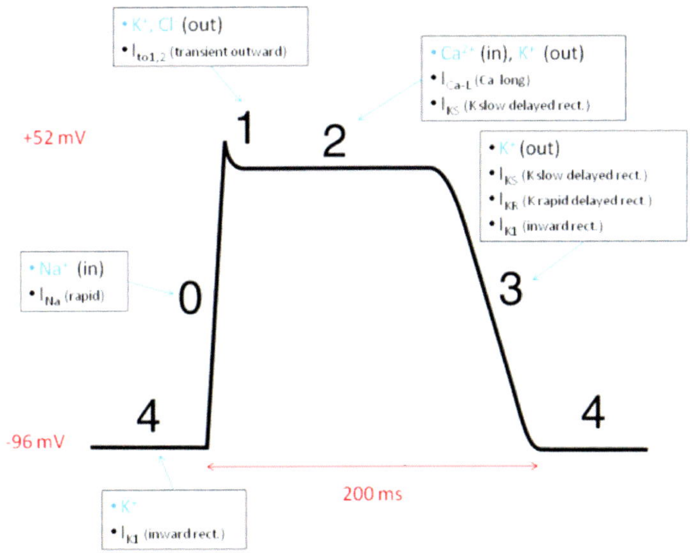

Figure 2. The five phases of the ventricular muscle action potential. (from Wikepedia: http://en.wikipedia.org/wiki/Cardiac_action_potential)

What all this means is that there are different levels or different dimensions of cardiac rhythmicity. One could study cardiac mechanics and blood pressures, one could examine electrocardiological signals of the whole organ or isolated cardiac myocytes, or one might delve into the dynamics of calcium fluxes within single heart cells. Dynamical details abound for the clever investigator to mine, interpret and hopefully apply to cardiac patients with abnormal dynamics for a myriad of different, sometimes subtle, reasons. But before one can discuss abnormalities in cardiac functioning, normal rhythms, beatings and cyclings of the heart must first be comprehended as best as possible. What is normal in this respect must cover a wide territory or legal (healthy) dynamical possibilities (homeodynamics). Because so many demands are placed on the heart, the normal heart must be flexible enough to survive environmental challenges and heavy workloads. It is.

4. The rate of the heart

Starting off most simply, cardiac dynamics can be captured in the variable heart rate. As an aside, some reports in the literature erroneously label as adjustable fixed parameters those observables which are in reality fluctuating physiological variables [7]. Heart rate can be detected manually by palpitation of the radial systolic pulse or automatically measured from an intravascular catheter (beats per minute). Heart rate of a different flavor can be recorded from surface electrocardiograms or cardiac muscle electrograms (electrical pulses per minute). These two heart rates are similar but not identical. Notably, in some diseased hearts it is possible for the developed ventricular pressure to be so weak that cardiac ejections occur only on every other contraction cycle. In this case the radial pulse rate would be half that of the ECG rate. Since artificial pacemakers take their cues not from hemodynamic feedbacks, but from non-physiological indicators, their clinical effectiveness can be compromised in certain situations.

However measured, the fundamental problem with heart rate is that it represents an average over several beats in which case beat-to-beat periods (instantaneous rates) are not identical. Here the variability of the dynamic can be captured in the standard deviation. Still, this is not a fool-proof definition of variability since these deviations from the mean may not be normally distributed (non-Gaussian). To the extent that these physiology-math mismatches are real, attempting to capture natural variability in terms of homestatic and Gaussian statistics is a huge error both conceptually and practically [8]. Means and standard deviations are linear descriptors fully appropriate for linear systems. But what if, in fact, cardiac dynamics are actually non-linear? The truth is that it is now widely recognized that the functions and fluctuations of the heart are highly nonlinear [9]. Might it be concluded that as the sine wave is to the arterial pressure pulse, so are the mean and standard deviation to cardiac dynamics?

As second point to grasp is that taking the mean filters out and minimizes (morphs, contorts or even destroys) dynamical details. Worse yet, taking means create fictive realities that do not exist in nature. For example, it is well known that the heart accelerates as one starts exercising. And even when the heart rate levels off at some plateau correlated to the work load of the exercise regime, it is proper to stay the system is in some kind of "steady-state?" What does steady-state really mean anyway? Again, in the spirit of homeodynamics [4], maybe such states are better comprehended as quasi-steady states or simply dynamic states within a corralled boarder consistent with the status of the individual. And over time, the dynamic state can move in time and space either by following deterministic rules within a narrow regime or by allowing for some stochastic expansion of the perimeter border in which multiple motions are permitted and encouraged.

5. The cardiac period

If the cardiomyocyte is the functional unit of the myocardium, the cardiac period is the fundamental time signature of the heart cycle. This cardiac period can be measured in different ways and yielding different values, yet time intervals are superior to rates since no ratios are encountered. The absolute interval (neither relative nor ratio) could span the time from one systolic beat to another between aortic pressure pulses, or it could be the time lapse from one R wave to the next in the ECG (see Fig. 1). RR intervals must be understood as discrete events weather or not they form random point processes or are connected entities with deterministic structures. Quantitative analyses can distinguish the two possibilities, but the discrete RR interval remains the fundamental marker of cardiac timings.

The second marker of cardiac timing represents the smooth flow of events occurring between beats. In this case (see Fig. 1) the variable could be the continuous ventricular or aortic pressure trace, the simple ECG presented as a time series, or even a cardiac electrogram measured with electrodes embedded in the heart. In either case, mechanical or electrical, the variable of interest is a single continuous function, one that is not discretized into intervals (e.g. analogous to a sine wave). Many models of cardiac function, mechanical or electrical, can take the form of continuous differential equations that are parameterized to captures the contours of the wave being mimicked. High digitization rates are, of course, required to faithfully capture accurate waveforms.

Sequences of discrete cardiac intervals and continuous heart variables can be studied in the time domain (functions of time) as displayed on polygraph recordings. However, another perspective on discrete and continuous events is to transpose the signals into the frequency domain. For example, if one computed the frequency spectra of the ECG, the resultant spectrum would consist of the power of the signal at different frequency bands (not shown). One of the most useful techniques, however, has been computing the frequency spectra of sequenced cardiac periods using the Fast Fourier transform [10]. Three typical peaks emerge from such an approach as shown in Figure 3. High frequency oscillations (HFO. 0.15-0.40 Hz) are typically attributed to ventilation effects on the cardiac cycle due to the waxing (inspiration) and waning (expiration) of vagal efferent inputs to the sinoatrial node. This is known as the classic respiratory sinus arrhythmia (SA) [12]. The HFO peak (hatched area) near 0.3 Hz represents a breathing frequency of 18 breaths per minute. Low frequency oscillations (LFO, 0.04-0.15 Hz) are associated with sympathetic activity with some parasympathetic contamination as it were. Nevertheless, the LFO/HFO ratio is commonly computed as a measure of autonomic imbalance with high ratios favoring sympathetic tone and low ratios favoring parasympathetic tone. Lastly, the origination of very low frequency oscillations (VLFO, 0.01-0.04 Hz) is very controversial but may be related to heart period changes driven by the very slow oscillation in the renin-angiotensin-aldosterone system or thermoregulation [13]. One major clinical investigation has produced standards of RR spectral measurements, physiological interpretation, and clinical utilization [14].

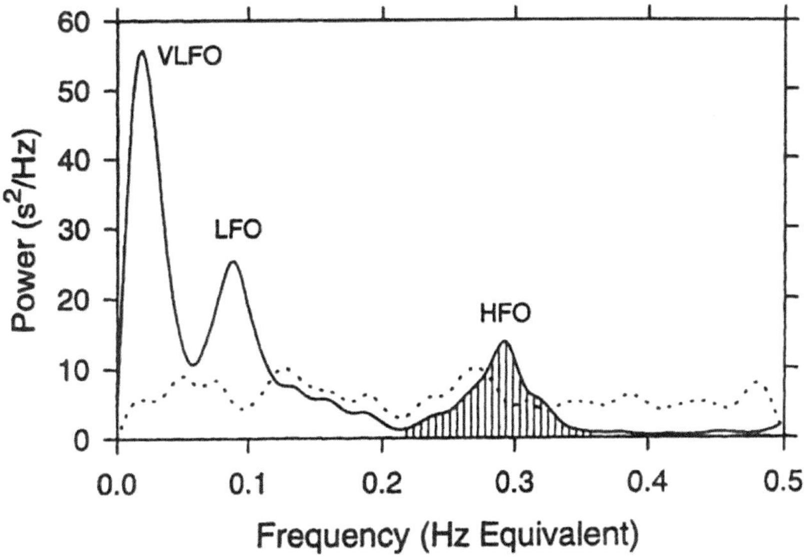

Figure 3. Power spectrum of human PP intervals before (solid line) and after random shuffling (dotted line) of intervals. Reproduced from reference [11] with permission.

The spectral analysis of RR intervals is commonly known as heart rate variability (HRV). The name is kind of a misnomer, because the spectral analyses are performed on heart periods not heart rates (a ratio). Nevertheless, all such computations are classified as linear and one dimensional. That is, the Fourier spectrum consists of the linear sums of sine and cosine waves which reconstruct the time domain signals (even square waves can be approximated with an infinite number of summations of wide ranging frequencies). With the growing appreciation that physiological signals are, among other things, highly nonlinear, another popular methodology has come to the forefront, approximate entropy (ApEn) [15]. This technique uses RR intervals as the input and treats then as chains of information. Low values of ApEn indicate that the cardiac signals have a deterministic structuring, whereas high ApEn values signal that the signals are more random or stochastic. There are technical problems associate with ApEn measures of complexity [3], but the utility of the approach cannot be denied.

6. The cardiac period in recurrence space

Physiological systems, including the cardiovascular system, are not only nonlinear, but they can be nonstationary, high-dimensional, and noisy. Such "miss-behaved" dynamics are characteristic of real-world systems. To tame the signals rendering them suitable for classical analyses often requires filtering, smoothing, clipping of outliers, detrending, interval replacements, etcetera, all of which contort the original signals. For this reason the first introduction of recurrence plots in the physics literature [16] became highly attractive to physiologists [17, 18]. Recurrence plot can be generated from any time-varying (or space-varying) signals consisting of either discrete intervals or continuous flows. The attraction of recurrence plots is that they are distribution-free, model-free, and have utility in dissecting out meaningful information from signals living on a dynamical transient and buffeted by noise. Higher dimensions are captured in surrogate variables by employing the principles of the embedding theorem of Takens [19]. What this means is that the windowed signal is divided up into short vectors of length EMBED and compared with each other exhaustively. If two vectors "match" by falling beneath a threshold radius value, then the leading points of the paired vectors are said to be recurrent. To render the data visible, a point is placed at the intersection of each and every vector i and vector j (e.g. for i = 1 to 500 and j = 1 to 500) falling within the allowed radius.

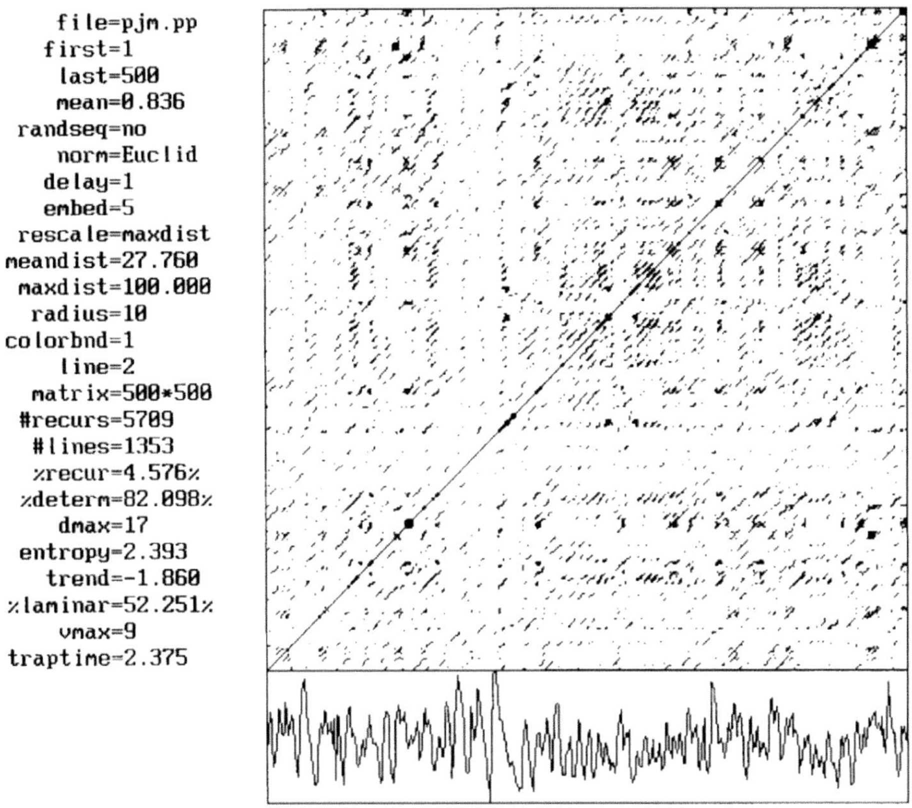

Figure 4. PP time series (bottom) and RR recurrence plot (top) along with recurrence parameters and quantifications (left). The plot is symmetrical on either side of the line-of-identity. The PP time series has 500 points displayed (417.9s) with HRV fluctuations centered on mean of 71.8 beats per min.

The recurrence plot of a 500 sequential PP intervals from a disease-free human is shown in Figure 4. In this case the embedding dimension was set to 5 such that all possible vectors of 5 points were compared with each other. The plot presents with lacelike delicacy revealing hidden patterns that are not seen in the one-dimensional time series beneath the plot. For quantitation, however, eight recurrence variables are extracted from the plot (%recur, %determ, dmax, entropy, trend, %laminar, vmax, traptime). Each variable has a critical, non-biased definition [20, 21] which report eight unique perspectives on the data derived from the time series. In the example shown, the density of points in the plot (%recur) is 4.576% and the probability of diagonal lines in the plot (%determ) is 82.098%. However, after randomly shuffling the PP intervals into a "nonsense" sequence (destroying the dynamical structure), %recur fell to 0.162% and %determ fell to 46.535% (not shown). These shuffling changes indicate that the original time series had deterministic structures attributed to physiological laws of the heart.

Proper implementation and interpretation of recurrence strategies requires careful selection of recurrence parameters for which a tutorial primer has been written [22] and freeware developed [23]. Recurrence windows can also move through very long time series, converting the eight unique recurrence variables into separate time series for further analysis. Little to no changes in these variables after random shuffling indicates rule-free signals. But such pure stochasticities are very rare in the world of structured physiological systems.

7. Partitioning the cardiac period as a terminal dynamic

Most modern quantifications of the cardiac dynamics, either linear or nonlinear, revert back to the fundamental RR or PP interval. Electrically speaking, during this time period two specific and alternating dynamics are occurring, electrical depolarization/repolarization during the beat and electrical isopotential between beats. Clean separation of these two phases can be realized by simply dividing the PP interval into two parts: the PT interval (the dynamic trajectory) and the TP interval (the stochastic pause) as shown in Figure 5A. Most interesting is Figure 5B in which the PP interval, the PT interval and the PT interval are all plotted as functions of time (or cardiac cycle number). The PP interval shows the typical respiratory sinus arrhythmia as expected. However, most of the variability is carried by the TP intervals when the heart is at isopotential rest, not the PT intervals when the heart is self-excited, actively contracting, and repolarizing. This arrangement forms what is called a terminal dynamic [24].

What is a terminal dynamic? Simply stated, a terminal dynamic is a dynamic the reaches its terminus [25]. It comes to its end and simply stops. The incoming plane (active) is not asymptotic to the runway, but it actually lands and comes to a standstill at the gate (resting). The ant that runs (active) makes intermittent pauses along its path (resting). In the same way the heart follows an almost stereotypic trajectory while being electrically depolarized and repolarized (active) before it come to its rest during the inter-beat isopotential of the ECG (resting). The key here is that while the dynamic is "living" on the transient trajectory, it is robust against noise. On the other hand, once the dynamic has ended and the dynamic is paused, it is at this point (technically, its singularity) when it becomes most vulnerable to external noise. This is why cardiac pacemakers can only pace the myocardium (e.g. select the next active trajectory) between beats during quiescent phases of the electrical cycle. The complex interplay of ion channel activation and inactivation during the active phase generates a refractory period for external stimuli.

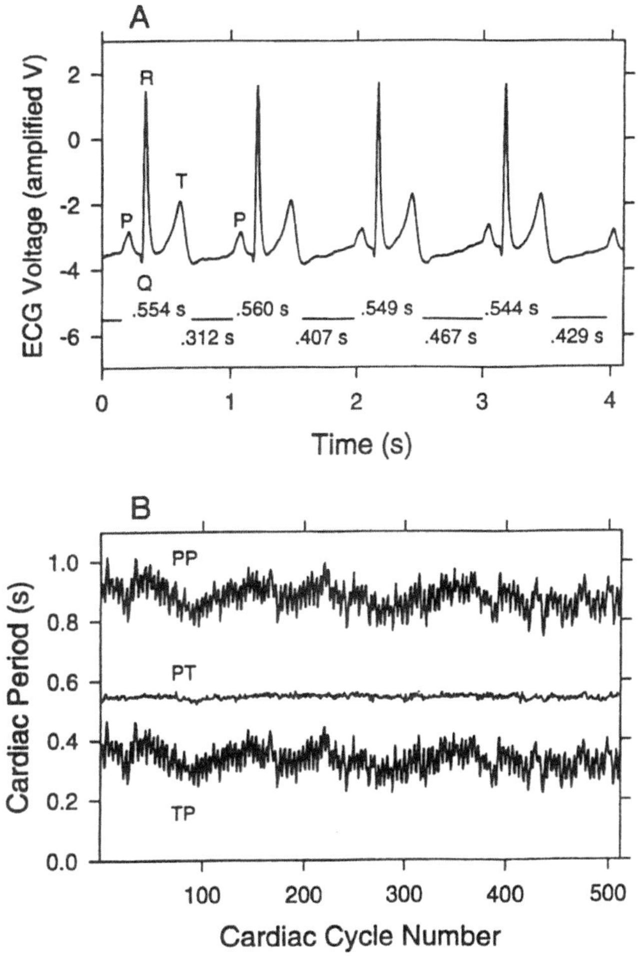

Figure 5. (A) Partitioning of PP intervals into PT and TP intervals for 512 beats. (B) HRV in PP intervals is carried almost exclusively in the TP intervals, not the PT intervals. Reproduced from reference [11] with permission.

How can a terminal dynamic be modeled? Well, instead of devising some fancy differential equation depicting beat after ECG beat, a better approach would be to write a single equation for the active phase of the heart which starts and comes to its end [26]. Then a pause or varying duration can be interposed before initiating the next beat. To impart more reality to the picture, the trajectory selection could come randomly, say, from a dozen slightly different differential equations (imparting a realistic wobbling in the active trajectory path). Likewise, the pause period could be randomly selected from a collection of actual cardiac isopotential times.

Thus the cardiac dynamic recorded in the ECG is really an alternation between a deterministic trajectory (which can be modeled by a differential equation) and a stochastic pause (which can only be randomly sampled from a collection of measure real-time pauses). This pause is termed the cardiac singularity, from which one of many trajectories can be selected for the next beat. The dynamic is also called a terminal dynamic, because the active heart actually stops (rests) at a terminus each and every beat. When one thinks about it, this type of modeling constitutes a piecewise deterministic system. The trajectory is the deterministic piece and the pause is the stochastic piece. Thus during the PP interval the heart alternates between determinism (PT interval) and stochasticity (TP interval).

8. Atrial fibrillation

One of the most common arrhythmias in human medicine is atrial fibrillation due to ectopic foci with possible spiral wave reentries [27]. Modeling of these three-dimensional patterns is very difficult, and control of atrial fibrillation is not fool-proof [28]. The thesis of a recent report is that atrial fibrillation may arise from unstable cardiac singularities [21]. As hinted at in the previous section, a singularity can be understood as the disruption or termination of an otherwise continuous event. For example, a sine wave has two singularities, one at its peak and another at its nadir. Under the influence of gravity, a ball tossed up into the air reaches its first unstable singularity at its peak. Then falling back to earth (the trajectory) again, the ball experiences a few bouncing cycles (unstable singularity-trajectory alternations) before finally coming to rest on the ground (stable singularity). Balancing a pencil on it stub end is easy (stable singularity), but balancing the same pencil on its point is very difficult (unstable singularity).

Beyond sine waves, bouncing balls and balancing pencils, how can singularities be identified in the cardiac electrogram and what might they have to do with the detection of electrical patterns that may precipitate out as full atrial fibrillation? In the bottom panels of Figure 6, two atrial electrograms are shown as recorded from roving bipolar electrodes in human patients [21]. Each window consists of 2048 points spanning 2.10 seconds in time (digitization frequency 977 Hz). The first recording shows a spike pattern at 254 pulses per minute (4.2 Hz, Fig. 6A) and the second recording shows a spike pattern at 881 pulses per min (14.7 Hz, Fig. 6B). Although these rates are much too fast for each depolarization to be conducted through the atrioventricular node, the can still wreak havoc with arrhythmias in the main pumping chambers of the heart.

Recurrence plots of these two atrial signals clearly display singularities as square blocks stair-casing upward along the central diagonal line (line of identity, Fig. 6A and Fig. 6B). These singularities are coincident with the quasi-isopotentials periods in the electrograms. Off-central recurrences form rectangular boxes due to variability in isopotential durations among the windowed beats (analogous to the TP variability discussed above). Clearly, the faster the arrhythmia, the smaller the singularity that is inscribed. The postulate is that as atrial singularities become vanishingly small, then unrestrained atrial fibrillation is unleashed. Somewhere along the continuum to oblivion, the singularities become unstable, triggering fibrillation. The clinical application of this methodology may evolve such that mapped regions in the atria lacking singularities may be candidate sites for ablation in halting the dysrhythmia expressed within the larger tissue [29].

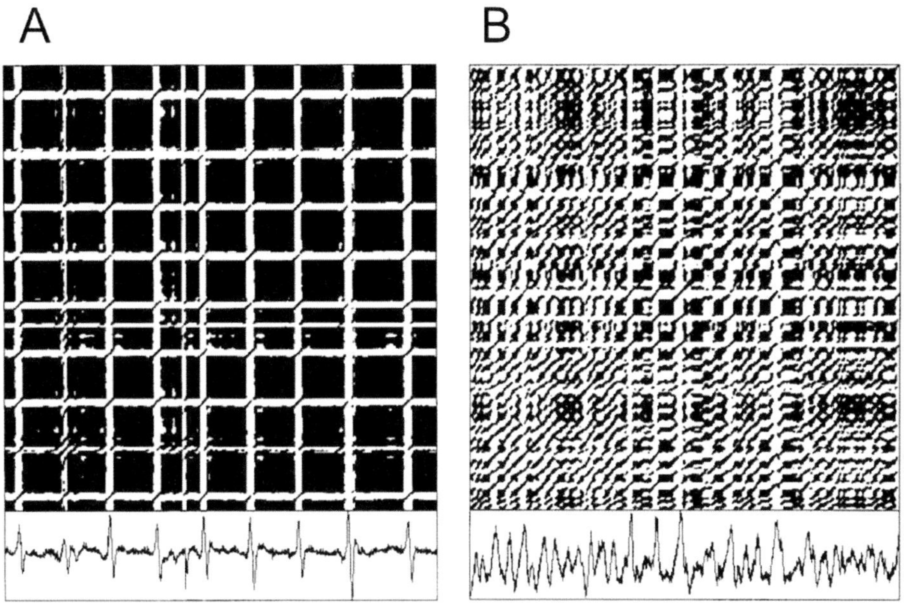

Figure 6. Singularities in atrial electrograms. (A) Fast atrial waves (4.2 Hz) with relatively long singularities. (B) Very fast atrial waves (14.7 Hz) with relatively short singularities. Recurrence parameters: delay = 1, embedding dimension = 15, norm = Euclidean, radius = 15% of maximum distance, line = 2. Data from reference [21].

9. Conclusions

The heart is a homeodynamic organ with automatic rhythms expressed in both mechanical electrical domains. Mechanical activities presume electrical underpinnings, but the reverse is not necessarily true except for possible stretch-activated electrical channels [30]. To get a window into cardiac dynamics, this chapter has majored on linear and nonlinear analyses that tease apart the cardiac cycle as defined as the R-R (or P-P) interval. For clinical medicine, the quest has been to define cardiovascular dynamics that may forecast unstable patterns (arrhythmias) or fatal events (asystole). Can it be that dis-homeodynamics is a kind of dynamical disease [31]?

Numerous studies have examined heart rate variability (HRV) and concluded that high HRV is good (how high?) and low HRV is bad (how low?). There are methodological problems associated with the measurement of HRV restricted to linear the perspective (spectral analysis) and low-dimensionality perspective (approximate entropy). One thing is for sure – autonomic imbalance and heart rate variability are important risk factors for cardiovascular disease [32]. Importantly, the reciprocity or co-activation of the sympathetic and parasympathetic branches of the autonomic nervous system is decidedly non-linear [33] and non-Gaussian [34]. This being true, it becomes apparent and necessary to apply the proper nonlinear tools to assess the signals. One proven too is recurrence quantification analysis (RQA) which has a demonstrated utility in diagnosing nonstationary cardiac dynamics [35].

As can be seen, the normal cardiac dynamic (mechanical or electrical) has a wealth of descriptors. With these in hand, it becomes easier to detect and possibly predict heart dysfunction and failure. Returning to the concept of homeodynamics, as people age or become ill, the dynamic range of cardiac functionality becomes limited. The loss of complexity and high-dimensional dynamics become markers for dysrhythmias, fibrillations and possibly even death [36].

Although current implanted artificial pacemakers are limited in their computational capacity, advances in nonlinear dynamics are being investigated to augment signal filtering and facilitate event detection [37-38].

Author details

Charles L. Webber, Jr.
Department of Cell & Molecular Physiology, Loyola University Chicago,
Stritch School of Medicine, Maywood, IL, USA

10. References

[1] Hajar R (1999) The Pulse in Antiquity. Heart Views 1: 89-94.
[2] King David (1995) Psalm 38:8-10. New American Standard Bible. Zondervan Publishing pp. 808-809.
[3] Webber CL Jr (2005) The Meaning and Measurement of Physiologic Variability? Crit. Care Med 33: 677-678.
[4] Rose S (1997) - Lifelines: Biology, Freedom, Determinism. Oxford University Press, 334 pp.
[5] Bers DM (2002) - Excitation-Contraction Coupling and Cardiac Contractile Force. Kluwer Academic Publishers, 452 pp.

[6] Badano LP, Gaddi O, Peraldo C, Lupi G, Sitges M, Parthenakis F, Molteni S, Pagliuca MR, Sassone B, Di Stefano P, De Santo T, Menozzi C, Brignole M. (2007) Left Ventricular Electromechanical Delay in Patients with Heart Failure and Normal QRS Duration and in Patients with Right and Left Bundle Branch Block. Europace 9: 41–47.

[7] Ferrer R, Artigas A (2011) Physiologic Parameters as Biomarkers: What Can we Learn from Physiologic Variables and Variation? Crit Care Clin 27: 229-240.

[8] West, B.J. (2010). Homeostasis and Gauss statistics: Barriers to Understanding natural Variability. J Eval Clin Pract 16: 403-408.

[9] González, J.J., Cordero, J.J., Feria, M., Pereda, E. (2000). Detection and Sources of Nonlinearity in the variability of Cardiac R-R Intervals and Blood Pressure in Rats. Am. J. Physiol. Heart Circ. Physiol. 279: H3040-H3046.

[10] Grafakos L (2003) - Classical and Modern Fourier Analysis. Prentice Hall, 931 pp.

[11] Webber CL Jr, Zbilut JP (1998) Recurrent Structuring of Dynamical and Spatial Systems. In: Complexity in the Living: A Modelistic Approach. Colosimo A, ed, Proc Int Meet, Feb. 1997, University of Rome "La Sapienza," pp. 101-133.

[12] Mazzeo, A.T., La Monaca, E., Dileo, R., Vita, G., Santamaria, L.B. (2011). Heart Rate Variability: A Diagnostic and Prognostic Tool in Anesthesia and Intensive Care. Acta Anaesthesiol Scand 55: 797-811.

[13] Taylor JA, Carr DL, Myers CW, Eckberg DL (1998) Mechanisms Underlying Very-Low-Frequency RR-Interval Oscillations in Humans. Circ 98: 547-555.

[14] MalikM (1996) Heart Rate Variability: Standards of Measurement, Physiological Interpretation, and Clinical Use. Circ 93: 1043-1065.

[15] Pincus, S.M. (1991). Approximate Entropy as a Measure of System Complexity. Proc. Natl Acad Sci 88: 2297-2301.

[16] Eckmann, J.-P., Kamphorst, S. O., & Ruelle, D. (1987). Recurrence Plots of Dynamical Systems. Europhys Lett, 4, 973-977.

[17] Zbilut, J.P., Webber, C.L., Jr. (1992). Embeddings and Delays as Derived from Quantification of Recurrence Plots. Phys Let A 171: 199-203.

[18] Webber, C.L., Jr., Zbilut, J.P. (1994) Dynamical Assessment of Physiological Systems and States using Recurrence Plot Strategies. J Appl Physiol 76: 965-973.

[19] Takens F (1981) Detecting Strange Attractors in Turbulence. In: Rand D & Young L-S, Lecture Notes in Mathematics, Vol. 898, Dynamical Systems and Turbulence, Warwick 1980. Springer-Verlag, pp. 366-381.

[20] Webber, CL Jr, Zbilut, JP (2007) Recurrence Quantifications: Feature Extractions from Recurrence Plots. Int J Bifurcation Chaos 17: 3467-3475.

[21] Webber CL Jr, Hu Z, Akar J (2011) Unstable Cardiac Singularities May Lead to Atrial Fibrillation. Int J Bifurcation Chaos 21: 1141-1151.

[22] Webber, C.L., Jr., Zbilut, J.P. (2005) Recurrence Quantification Analysis of Nonlinear Dynamical systems. In: Tutorials in Contemporary Nonlinear Methods for the Behavioral Sciences, (Chapter 2, pp. 26-94), Riley MA, Van Orden G, eds. Retrieved December 1, 2004 http://www.nsf.gov/sbe/bcs/pac/nmbs/nmbs.jsp

[23] Webber, C.L., Jr. (2012) Introduction to Recurrence Quantification Analysis. RQA Version 14.1 README.PDF: http://homepages.luc.edu/~cwebber/

[24] Zbilut JP, Webber CL Jr, Zak M (1998) Quantification of Heart Rate Variability using Methods Derived from nonlinear Dynamics. In: Analysis and Assessment of Cardiovascular Function. Drzewiecki G and Li JK-J, eds. Springer Verlag, New York, Chapter 19, pp. 324-334.
[25] Giuliani A, Giudice PL, Mancini AM, Quatrini G., Pacifici L., Webber CL Jr, Zak M, Zbilut JP (1996) A Markovian Formalization of Heart Rate Dynamics Evinces a Quantum-like Hypothesis. Biol Cyber 74: 181-187.
[26] Zbilut JP, Hübler A, Webber CL Jr. (1996) Physiological Singularities Modeled by Nondeterministic Equations of Motion and the Effect of Noise. In: Fluctuations and Order: The New Synthesis. Millonas MM, ed, Springer-Verlag, Chapter 24, pp. 397-417.
[27] Nattel S (2002) New Ideas about AtrilaFibrillation 50 Years On. Nature 414: 219-226.
[28] Garfinkel A, Chen PS, Walter DO, Karagueuzian HS, Kogan B, Evans SJ, Karpoukhin M, Hwang C, Uchida T, Gotoh M, Nwasokwa O, Sager P, Weiss JN (1997) Quasiperiodicity and Chaos in Cardiac Fibrillation. J Clin Inv 99: 305-314.
[29] Wilber DJ, Pappone C, Neuzil P, De Paola A, Marchlinski F, Natale A, Macle L, Daoud EG, Calkins H, Hall B, Reddy V, Augello G, Reynolds MR, Vinekar C, Liu CY, MPH; Berry SM, Berry DA (2010) Comparison of Antiarrhythmic Drug Therapy and Radiofrequency Catheter Ablation in Patients With Paroxysmal Atrial Fibrillation - A Randomized Controlled Trial. J Am Med Assoc 303: 333-340.
[30] Kohl P, Sachs F, Franz MR (2011) Cardiac Mechano-Electric Coupling and Arrhythmias. Oxford Univesity Press 477 pp.
[31] Beliar J, Glass L, Heiden UAD, Milton J (1995) Dynamical Disease: Mathematical Analysis of Human Illness. Am Inst Physics 220 pp.
[32] Thayer JF, Yamamoto SS, Brosschot JF (2010) The Relationship of Autonomic Imbalance, Heart Rate Variability and Cardiovascular Disease Risk Factors. Int J Cardiol 141: 122–131.
[33] Mourot L, Bouhaddi M, Gandelin E, Cappelle S, Nguyen NU, Wolf J-P, Rouillon JD, Hughson R, Regnard J. (2007) Conditions of Autonomic Reciprocal Interplay versus Autonomic Co-activation: Effects on Non-linear Heart Rate Dynamics. Autonomic Neuroscience: Basic and Clinical 137: 27–36.
[34] Kiyono K, Hayano J, Watanabe E, Struzik ZR, Yamamoto Y (2008) Non-Gaussian Heart Rate as an Independent Predictor of Mortality in Patients with Chronic Heart Failure. Heart Rhythm 5:261–268.
[35] Zbilut JP, Thomasson N, Webber CL Jr (2002) Recurrence Quantification Analysis as a Tool for Nonlinear Exploration of Nonstationary Cardiac Signals. Med Engin Physics 24: 53-60.
[36] Beckers F, Verheyden B, Aubert AE (2006) Aging and Nonlinear Heart Rate Control in a Healthy Population. Am J Physiol – Heart 290: H2560-H2570.
[37] Polpetta A, Banelli P)2008) Fully digital pacemaker detection in ECG signals using a non-linear filtering approach. Conf Proc IEEE Eng Med Biol Soc. 2008:5406-5410.
[38] Aström M, Olmos S, Sörnmo L (2006) Wavelet-based event detection in implantable cardiac rhythm management devices. IEEE Trans Biomed Eng. 53: 478-484.

Chapter 12

Mobile and Wireless Technologies on Sphygmomanometers and Pulsimeters for Patients with Pacemakers and Those with Other Cardiovascular Diseases

Ching-Sung Wang and Teng-Wei Wang

Additional information is available at the end of the chapter

http://dx.doi.org/10.5772/48565

1. Introduction

The population with pacemaker implants varies by age, sex or race. Over 100,000 pacemakers are implanted every year in the United States with approximately 500,000 Americans having an implanted permanent pacemaker device [1]. Pacemakers can be affected by electromagnetic interference in several different ways, including temporary inhibition of the pacemaker, temporary function at the fixed noise rate, temporary function at the fixed magnet rate, permanent inhibition or malfunction and random reprogramming. For any of these results to occur, the E field strength must be greater than 200V/m or the magnetic field strength must be greater than 10 Gauss [2].

Mobile tele-medicine is a future development trend. There is much research on it, but most of them discuss GSM, GPRS, 3G, WiMax or LTE. Another key point of mobile tele-medicine is variable electronic medical instrumentation. Our research is expected to integrate embedded system design, wireless communication and medical know-how to implement remote medical care. Long-term blood pressure management is very important for patients who are at risk of stroke or heart attack, therefore, monitoring blood pressure and the ability to immediately call for help are both important. This research will use a portable manometer combined a Bluetooth and GSM cell phone. It can monitor BP and transmit emergency information from wherever people live and wherever they go.

Cellular telephones can interfere with the function of implanted cardiac pacemakers [3,4,5]. However, when telephones are placed over the ear, the normal position, this interference does not pose a health risk [5]. Barbaro V, et al.'s research indicated influence between a

GSM mobile phone and an implanted pacemaker. Electromagnetic interference effects were detected at a maximum distance of 10 cm with the pacemaker programmed at its minimum sensing threshold. When the phone antenna was in direct contact with the patient's skin over the implant, electromagnetic interference effects occurred at the maximum ventricular and atrial sensing thresholds of 4 mV and 2.5 mV, respectively [6]. Therefore, decreasing wireless emission power and increasing pacemaker emission distance are the most useful methods of lowering the magnetic interference to the pacemaker. In order not to affect users' habits of using mobiles and to avoid the electromagnetic interference effects to a pacemaker, we have designed a wristable sphygmomanometer and pulsimeter which uses Bluetooth power class II [7,8] as the device for short-distance transmission. Furthermore, by combing with a cellular phone, we can do prolonged, distant observation and treatment immediately for patients who require adjustments to pacemaker settings or those with other cardiovascular diseases.

2. System architecture

This research aims at designing a wristable sphygmomanometer and pulsimeter. We designed a non-invasive sphygmomanometer [9] to remind the user to measure blood pressure every hour. A pulsimeter is an electronic device which is based on a pressure sensor and can observe pulse continuously. In order to avoid the influence of electromagnetic waves on the pacemaker, this research uses the Bluetooth power class II equipment for short-distance wireless data transmission from the sphygmomanometer to the client-end cellular phone, then uses the GPRS (General Packet Radio Service) [10,11] to do the long distance data transmission. This can transmit blood pressure and pulse rate to a Remote Medical Server and then provide them to specialist doctors for reference data.

2.1. Client-side hardware architecture

Because of the connecting method of GPRS is a packet switch [10,11], it does not connect with the Remote Medical Server continuously. Therefore, this research utilized a GSM (Global System for Mobile Communications) circuit connection (voice connection) [10,11,12] for the Remote Medical Server to inform the wristable sphygmomanometer and pulsimeter, and to drive the sphygmomanometer to measure blood pressure immediately. Then, the sphygmomanometer will send the results of blood pressure measurements to the Remote Medical Server by GPRS [10,11]. **Figure 1** details the block diagram of the client-side hardware architecture.

2.2. Server-side hardware architecture

Figure 2 details the block diagram of the server-side hardware architecture [13]. Server-side includes a PSTN (Public Switched Telephone Network) phone controller and a monitoring terminal. Furthermore, the PSTN phone controller is constructed by an ATA (Analogue Telephone Adapter), microcontroller and the accessories, which takes the incoming call from the client. W681388 [14] is used as the baseband IC of ATA for ring detection and coding of voice signals. PIC24FJ64 [15] is used as a microcontroller, which receives the command of the monitoring terminal through the UART interface and controls the W681388 Hook ON/OFF and voice output through the SPI (Serial Peripheral Interface) interface. W681388 is made by Winbond. PIC24FJ64 is made by Microchip.

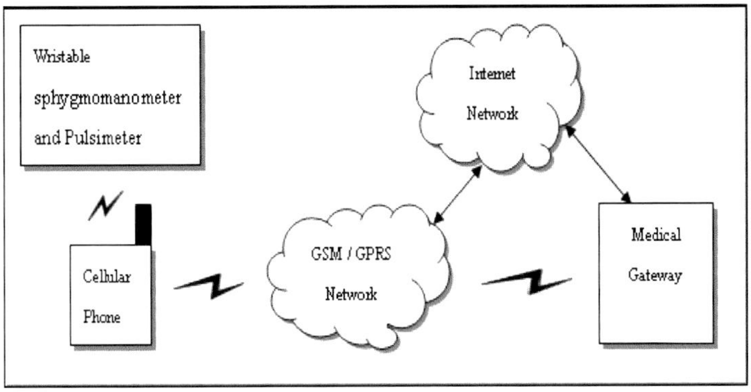

Figure 1. Client-side hardware architecture

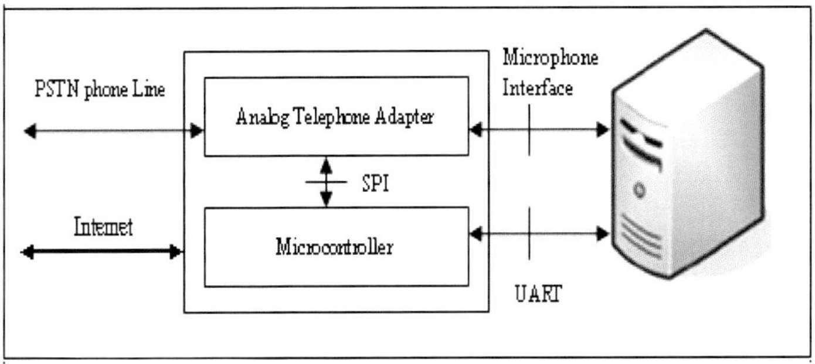

Figure 2. Server-side hardware architecture

2.3. Client-end cellular phone hardware architecture

Figure 3 details the block diagram of client-end cellular phone hardware architecture, which includes two main parts, Bluetooth and GSM/GPRS.

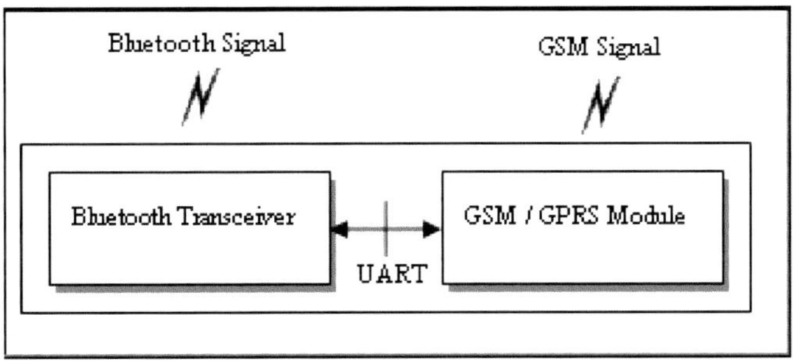

Figure 3. Client-end Cellular Phone Hardware Architecture

1. Bluetooth transceiver [16,17,18]: the hardware framework is similar to the Bluetooth transceiver of wristable sphygmomanometer and pulsimeter. It communicates with GSM/GPRS module by UART interface.
2. GSM Module [18]: includes Baseband part and RF part. The main components are Baseband IC (including DSP), TFT-LCD, NOR Flash, SRAM, Power Management IC and RF IC. We use MT6219 made by MediaTek as the platform for the GSM/GPRS system.

2.4. Tele-care system architecture

Figure 4 details the block diagram of the tele-care system architecture. The data is acquired from the wristable sphygmomanometer which transmits to the client-end cellular phone by the Bluetooth device. IMEI (International Mobile Equipment Identity) [19] measure the time and blood pressure data which were transmitted to the server-end cellular phone and all the data are classified, saved then applied.

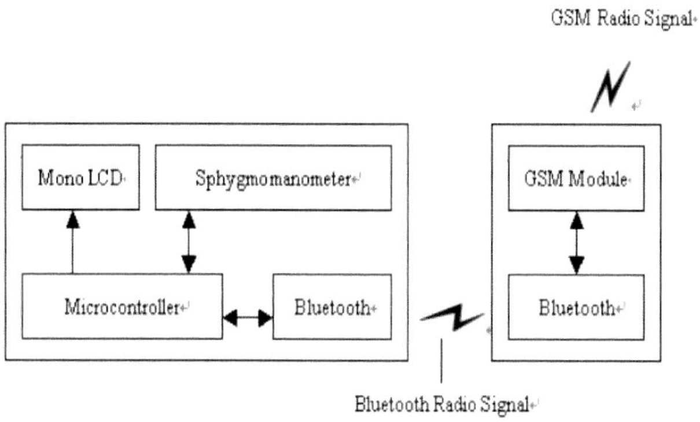

Figure 4. Tele-care system architecture

2.5. Tele-emergency announcement system architecture

Figure 5 details the block diagram of the tele-emergency announcement system architecture. When the data exported by the motion sensor is fixed for a period of time, the microcontroller goes into emergency mode. Then the client-end cellular phone establishes a voice connection with the server-end cellular phone. After the connection is established, it transmits IMEI [20], location, time, and blood pressure in DTMF (Dual-tone multi-frequency) format.

3. Hardware architecture

The hardware system of this research is divided into two parts, one is a wristable sphygmomanometer and pulsimeter; the other one is a client-end cellular phone. Details are discussed below.

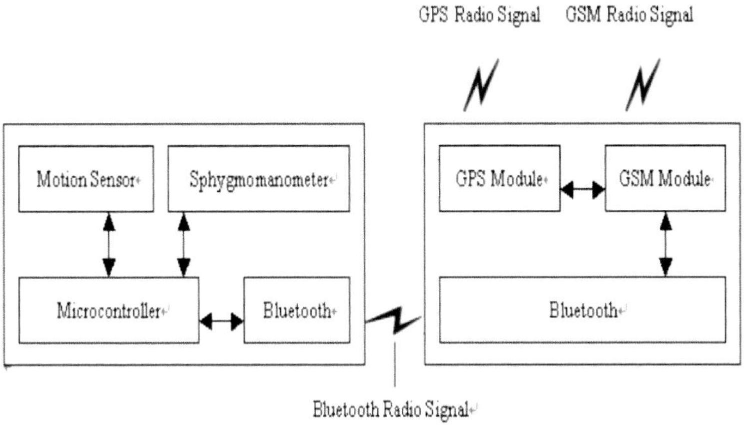

Figure 5. Tele-emergency announcement system architecture

3.1. Wristable sphygmomanometer and pulsimeter

Figure 6 details the block diagram of the wristable sphygmomanometer and pulsimeter hardware architecture. The Controller unit of the wristable sphygmomanometer and pulsimeter is the microcontroller [16], which controls and reads the peripheral units. Here is the description of each unit.

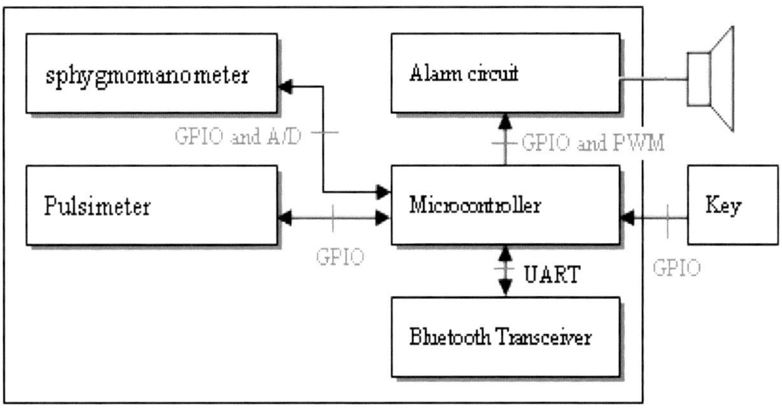

Figure 6. Wristable sphygmomanometer and pulsimeter hardware architecture

1. Sphygmomanometer [9, 16, 17, 18]: **Figure 7** details the block diagram of the wristable sphygmomanometer hardware architecture. The wristable sphygmomanometer consists of a 16 bit RISC microcontroller, Bluetooth transceiver, mono LCD, motion sensor and accessories. The microcontroller controls the other components. This is an electronic medical instrument; the microcontroller communicates with the device by the

UART interface of 8051. Bluetooth module [16,18]: the project uses BC3 made by CSR as the Bluetooth transceiver. The microcontroller communicates with the Bluetooth by UART interface and controls all the process by software. Mono LCD[16,21]: mono LCD displays all information in the system. The mono LCD was driven by the microcontroller and communicated to by the parallel LCD interface. Motion sensor [16,22]: we use the MXC6202 chip made by MEMSIC as the motion sensor. It detects the movements of the object and gives all kinds of information for the microcontroller to classify every situation. It uses I2C as the interface.

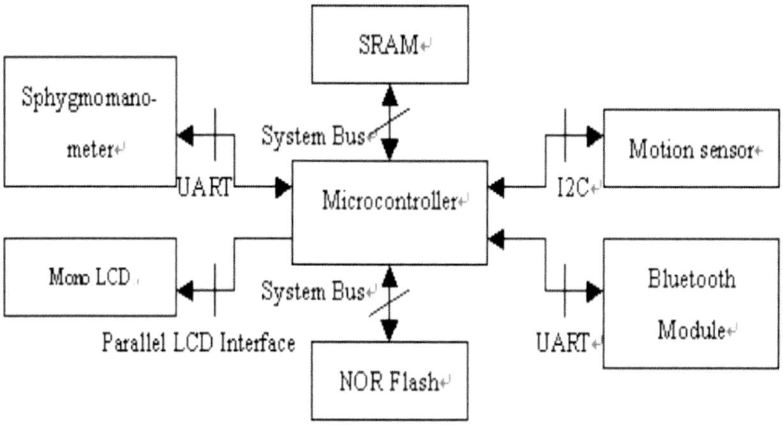

Figure 7. Wristable sphygmomanometer hardware architecture

Details of the sphygmomanometer include the LDO (Low Dropout Regulators) as power controller, pressure sensor, filter, amplifier circuit and accessories. The project is using the pressure sensor of the SCC series which is manufactured by HoneyWell's company. The pressure sensor will transmit different messages according to the changing pressure. The messages pass through the procedures of magnifying (magnify the micro-message form sensor), and filtering (noise removal), and then all the analogue messages are sent to the microcontroller via A/D (Analogue/Digital) interface. **Figure 8** shows the implementation of the sphygmomanometer device architecture.

2. Pulsimeter [9,16,17,18] : the pulsimeter includes LDO, pressure sensor, filter, amplifier circuit and accessories. The circuit is using the SCC series made by HoneyWell, but it has a different sensitivity pressure sensor. Putting the sensor pad over the radial pulse, the pressure sensor will convert the normal pulse to a larger voltage output by magnifying, filtering and then converting (transforming to digital signal), and finally inputs it into the microcontroller. **Figure 9** shows the block diagram of the pulsimeter.
3. Bluetooth transceiver [16, 23]: the project uses BC3 made by CSR as the Bluetooth transceiver. The microcontroller communicates with the Bluetooth by UART (Universal asynchronous receiver/transmitter) interface and controls all the processes using the software.

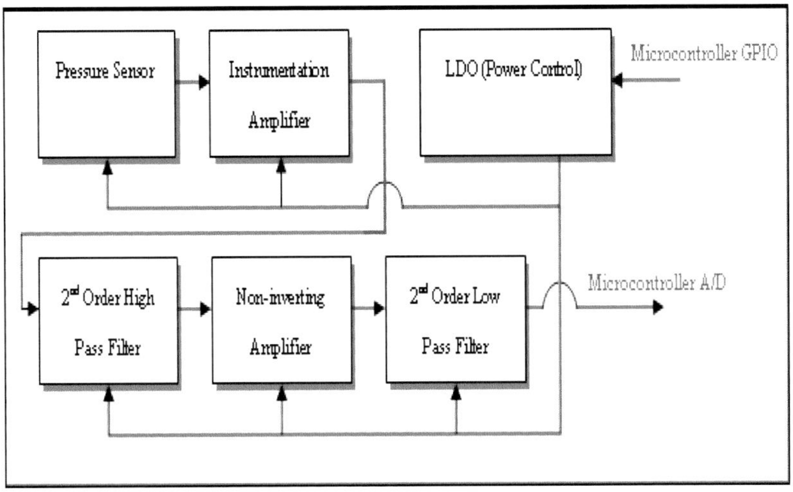

Figure 8. Sphygmomanometer device

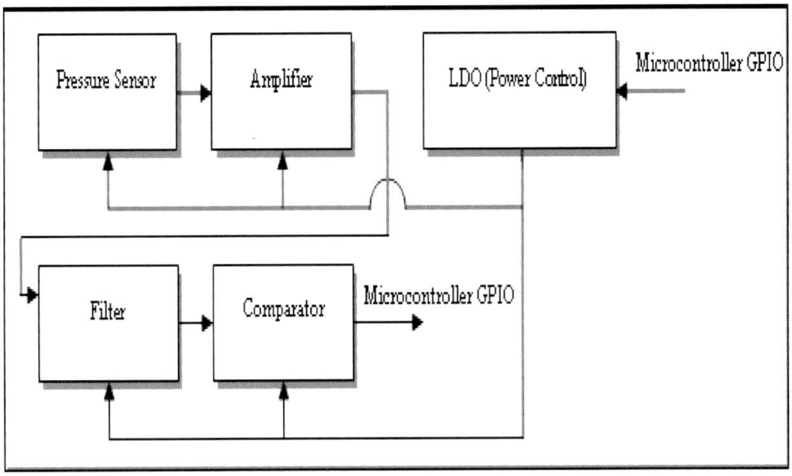

Figure 9. Pulsimeter device

4. Alarm circuit: the main purpose of this part is to send a notice to the users and then to perform blood pressure measurement. The microcontroller can activate the alarm circuit every hour. At the other end, the Remote Medical Server can also order a blood pressure measurement, so that the users can measure their blood pressure when required.

3.2. Wireless personal area network base on Bluetooth

Bluetooth provides point to point and multipoint wireless connection according to the Internet concept. Within any active communication scope, all devices are treated the same. The first one requesting communication is called master and the passive one accepting the signal is called slave. A master and one or more salves construct the Pico-net of Bluetooth [24], [25]. Because not all mobile phones with Bluetooth function in the current market support Serial Port Profile, the GPS device used in this research cannot connect with all the mobile phones with Bluetooth via the Bluetooth function. In order to cover most mobile phones with Bluetooth in the market in this research and make an active Pico-net, we used the Bluetooth device of BAD (Body Activity Detector) as master, and the Bluetooth devices of the mobile phone and GPS as slave. The Bluetooth of BAD connects with the Bluetooth of the mobile phone and GPS, and forms a PAN (Personal Area Network) upon Bluetooth. **Figure 10** indicates the Bluetooth Pico-net in this system.

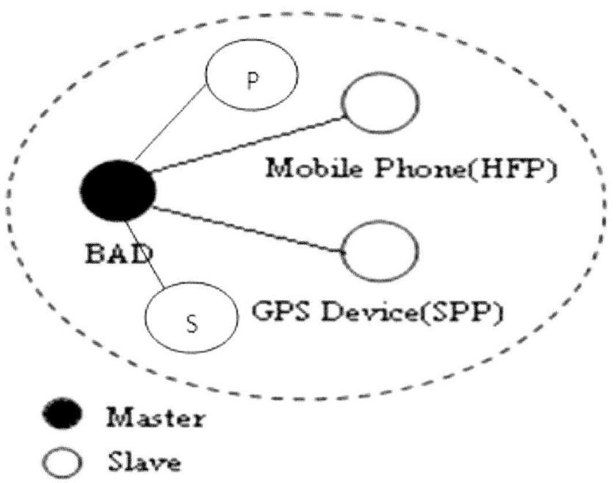

Figure 10. Bluetooth Pico-net

4. Software algorithm

4.1. Continuous pulse and blood pressure measurement, and the monitoring procedure

Pulse monitor procedure [16, 17, 18, 21]: the microcontroller reads the pulsimeter every minute, then transmits the results to the client-end cellular phone by the Bluetooth SPP (Serial Port Profile). Blood pressure measure procedures [9, 16, 17, 18, 21]: the microcontroller enables an alarm system to remind the user every hour to measure blood pressure. Users need to put their hand in the proper position so that the sphygmomanometer can better detect the pulse. When the users put their hand in the proper position and push the trigger button, the microcontroller controls the pulsimeter's LDO to stop the action and start measuring the blood pressure. After that, the microcontroller transmits the blood pressure to the cellular phone by Bluetooth SPP, and activates the pulsimeter. If the user doesn't perform the blood pressure measurement, the microcontroller would re-activate the pulsimeter after a while. The software algorithm of continuous pulse and blood measurement, and the monitoring procedure is shown in **Figure 11** and **Figure 12**.

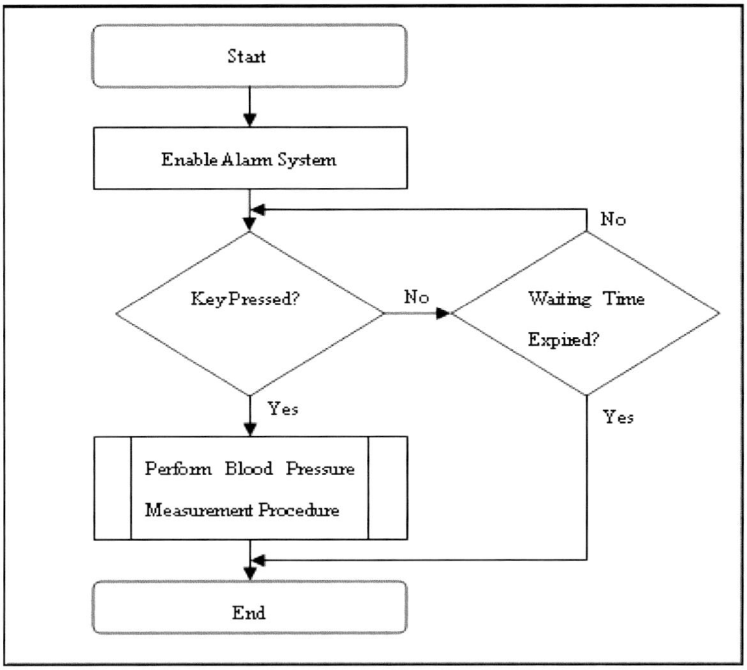

Figure 11. The software algorithm of continuous pulse and blood measuring, and the monitoring procedure

4.2. Client-end cellular phone data handling procedure

When the Bluetooth of the mobile receives the data from the Bluetooth of the wristable sphygmomanometer and pulsimeter, it analyses blood pressure or pulse data and stores (including the measurement time) locally first. Finally, it establishes a GPRS connection. After successful connection, the mobile scans the stored blood pressure and pulse data, and then transmits them to the Remote Medical Server if the data has not yet been sent. The software algorithm of the mobile data handling procedure is shown on **Figure 13** [13, 21, 22,25].

4.3. Remote Medical Server claim for measuring blood pressure

If the physician considers that it is necessary to get the patient's current blood pressure immediately, he/she can call the client-end cellular phone using the GSM module on the Remote Medical Server. While the client-end cellular phone receives the incoming call from the server-end, the Bluetooth SPP transmits the command of measuring blood pressure to the wristable sphygmomanometer and pulsimeter. While the wristable sphygmomanometer and pulsimeter receive the command from the Remote Medical Server, they activate blood pressure measurements and transmit procedures. The software algorithm of the Remote Medical Gateway claims for measuring blood pressure are shown in **Figure 14** [13, 21, 22, 25].

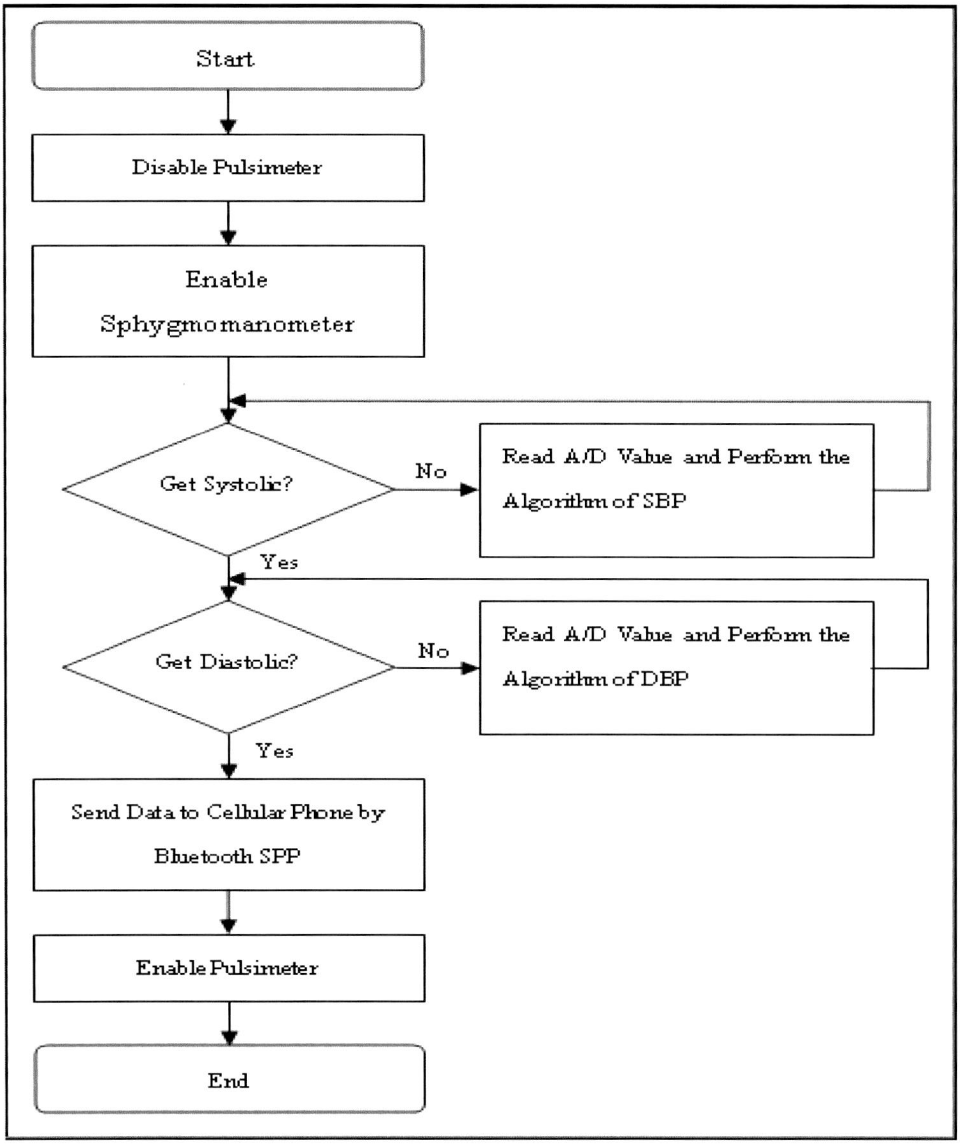

Figure 12. The software algorithm of the blood pressure measurement procedure

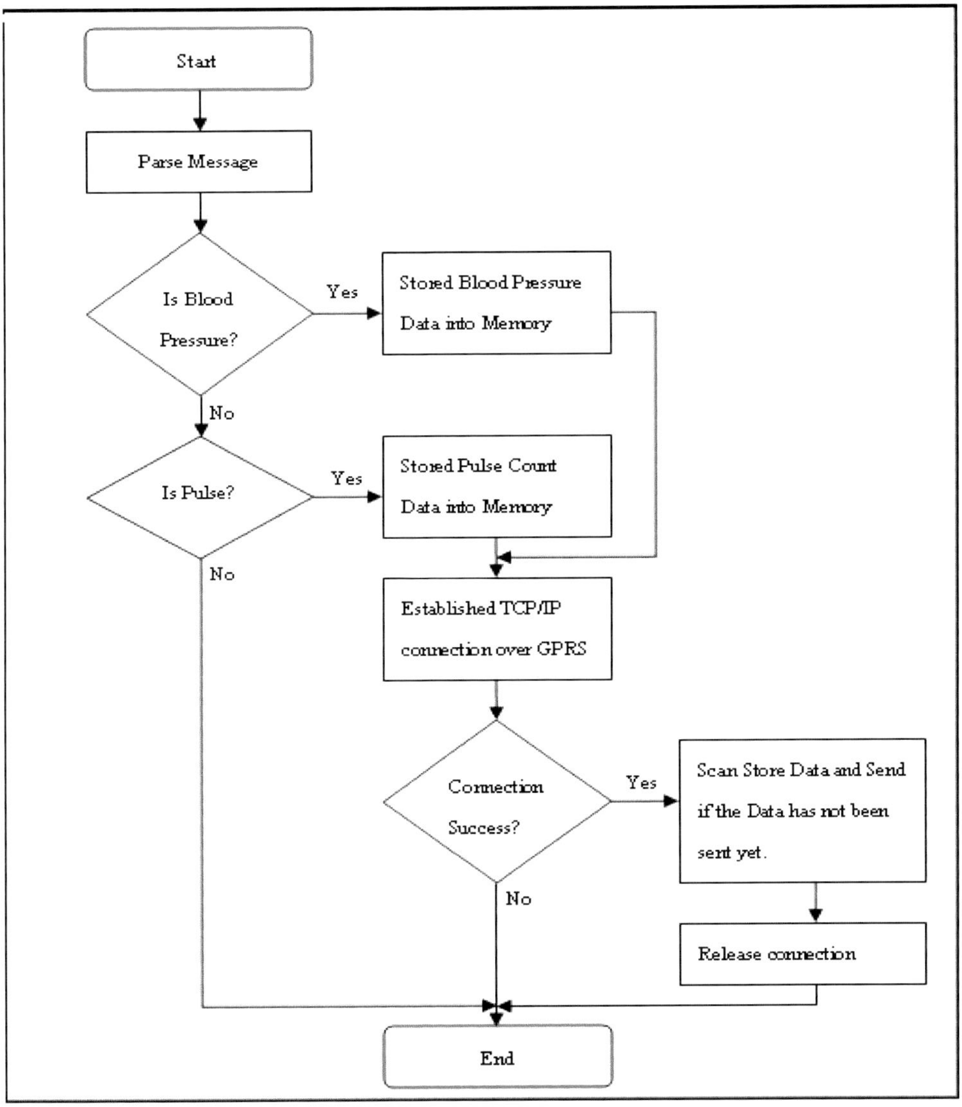

Figure 13. The software algorithm of client-end cellular phone data handling procedure

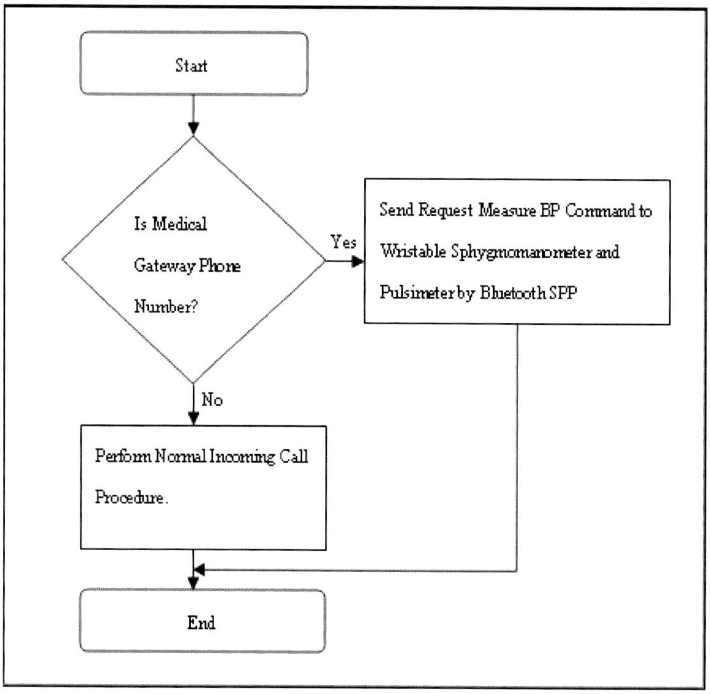

Figure 14. The software algorithm of remote medical server claim for measuring blood pressure

4.4. The whole system operation procedure

1. The procedure of measuring blood pressure by the wristable sphygmomanometer of the tele-care system is shown in **Figure 15** [16,21,27,28,29]. The measurement was triggered by the user. When the microcontroller receives the trigger, it starts the procedure. First, the sphygmomanometer measures the pressure and sends back the data. The data are shown on the mono LCD and transmitted to the client-end cellular phone by Bluetooth SPP (Serial Port Profile).
2. The procedure of measuring blood pressure using the client-end cellular phone of tele-care system is shown in **Figure 16** [20,28,29,30,31,32]. When the Bluetooth of the client-end cellular phone receives signals, it checks the format and the Checksum of the data. The data is saved and sent to the sever-end cellular phone by Send Message over SD (Circuit Switched Data) if it is correct.
3. The procedure of measuring blood pressure using the server-end cellular phone of tele-care system is shown in **Figure 17** [19,20,29,30,31]. When the server-end cellular phone receives a short message from the client-end cellular phone, it checks the format and the Checksum of the data. If it is correct, the short message is decoded and saved according to IMEI. Then the message is erased.
4. The emergency procedure of the wristable sphygmomanometer of the tele-emergency announcement system is shown in **Figure 18** [16,27,28,32]. The microcontroller reads the

data which was acquired from the motion sensor every second. If the data repeats 30 times, it is called the Emergency Task and Alarm. If the user pushes the button, the Emergency Task will stop. Otherwise it will trigger sphygmomanometer measuring. The microcontroller sends an emergency message to the client-end cellular phone by Bluetooth SPP, once the number which is received from the sphygmomanometer measurement is defined as dangerous.

5. The procedure of emergency of the client-end cellular phone of tele-emergency announcement system is shown in **Figure 19** [19,20,28,29,30,31,32]. When the Bluetooth of the client-end receives signals, it checks the format and the Checksum of the data. If it shows an emergency message, it is called the Emergency Task. In order to transmit a clear DTMF tone, the phone closes the microphone and forces the system to send out a Caller ID. Then the client-end cellular phone establishes voice connection with the server-end cellular phone. After the connection is established, it transmits IMEI, location, time and blood pressure in DTMF format.
6. The procedure of emergency of the server-end cellular phone of tele-emergency announcement system is shown in **Figure 20** [19,20,29,30,31]. When the server-end mobile receives the incoming call from the client-end mobile phone, it will be forced to connect, and turn off the microphone, then switch audio path to the DTMF decoder [33]. After 2 seconds, if the controller receives the correct format and Checksum from the DTMF decoder, the phone will make a specific tone at the loudest setting, start the vibrator, then an emergency message will show on the display. It won't stop the tone and vibrator, even if it is disconnected.

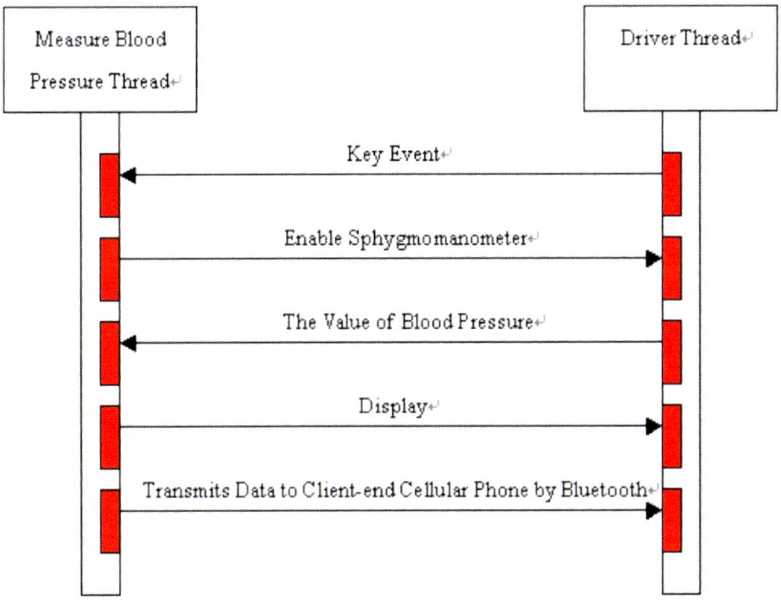

Figure 15. Procedure of measuring blood pressure by the wristable sphygmomanometer of the tele-care system

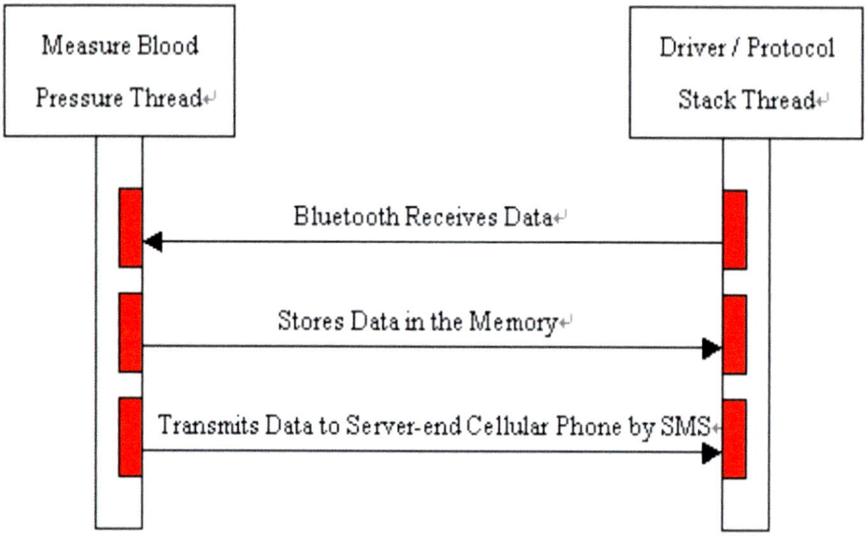

Figure 16. Procedure of measuring blood pressure using the client-end cellular phone of the tele-care system

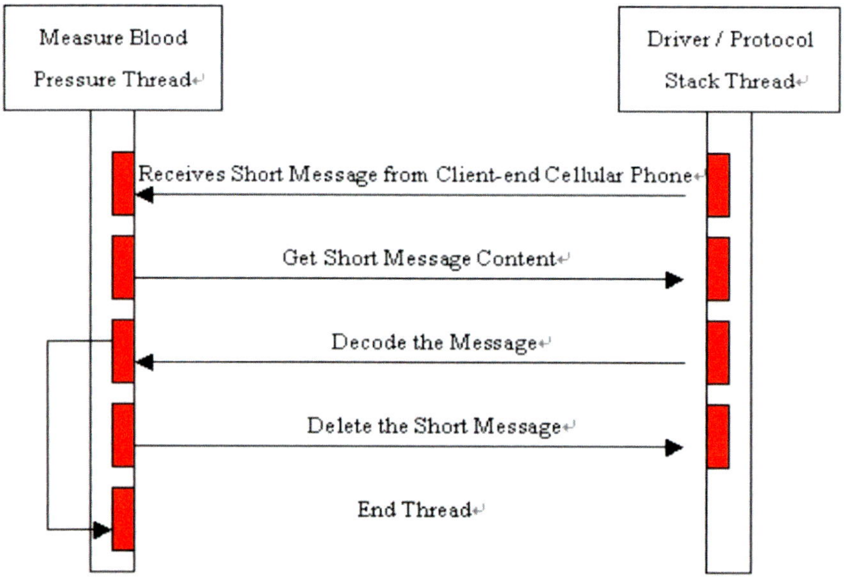

Figure 17. Procedure of measuring blood pressure of the server-end cellular phone of tele-care system

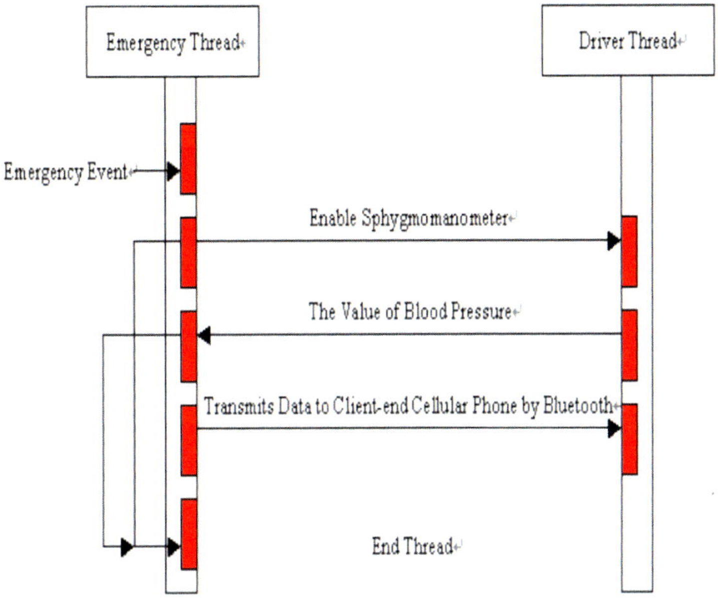

Figure 18. Emergency procedure of the wristable sphygmomanometer of the tele-emergency announcement

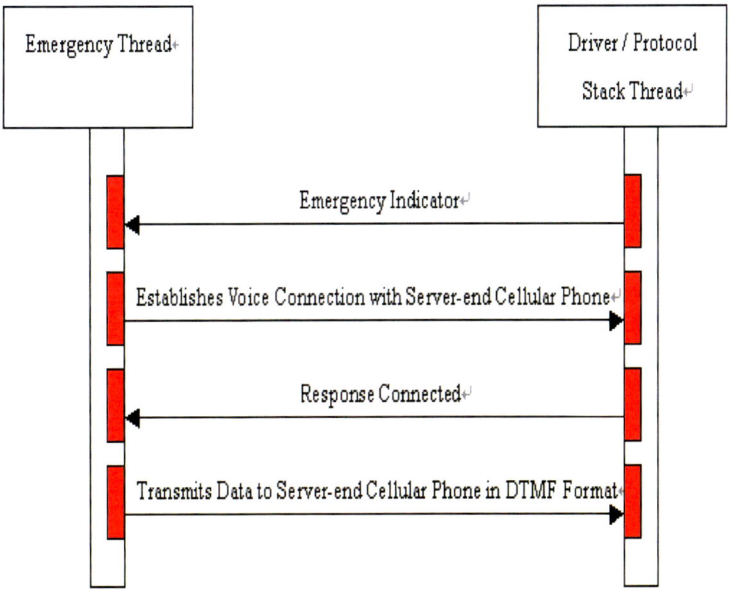

Figure 19. Emergency procedure of the wristable sphygmomanometer of the tele-emergency announcement system

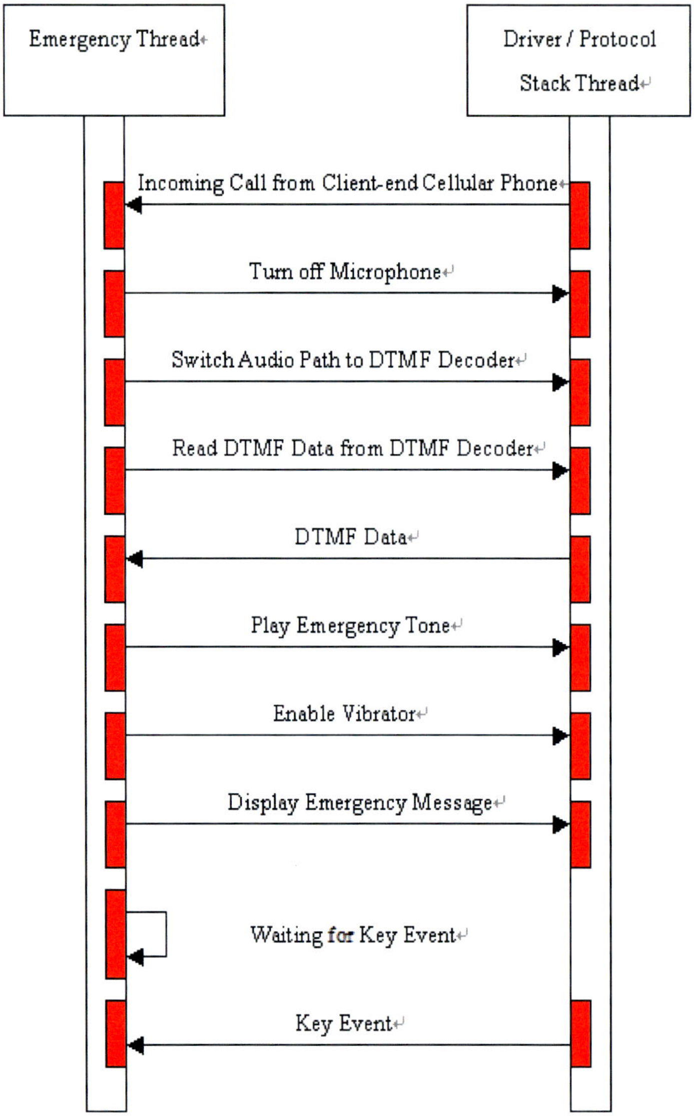

Figure 20. Emergency procedure of the server-end cellular phone of tele-emergency announcement system

5. Remote monitoring measurement example

We conducted an experiment using SpO2 and ECG using the GPS device and the 3G system of an Android smart phone to form a remote monitoring system, which can be used in the daily care of patients with implanted pacemakers.

This system is categorized into three main structures, client, server and first aid unit. The client includes BAD, a biomedical signal monitoring device (including ECG and SpO_2 monitoring devices) and an Android mobile phone with Bluetooth communication ability. When BAD detects an abnormal health response from the user, it will give the mobile a report by means of the Bluetooth. In the meantime, the operating biomedical device, with sending signals back, allows GPS coordination to take place. These messages would be sent back to the server through the mobile phone's Internet system. The server-end is predominantly used to save the data, to analyse it and to communicate with others as shown in Figure 21.

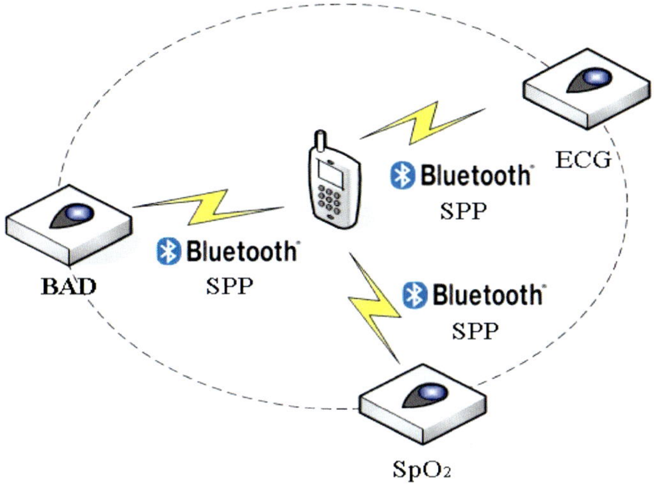

Figure 21. Bluetooth Pico-net

5.1. System communication

Figure 22 is the system communication plot. BAD, ECG and SpO2 will shut down the system into their power save mode after Bluetooth and cell phone pairing. When the BAD detects an emergency, it will resume normal power and contact the cell phone to call out ECG and SpO_2 processing.

5.2. Emergency procedure

After receiving a BAD emergency signal, the system will enter the emergency procedure mode as shown in **Figure 23.** First it will check the signal again. If it is still an emergency signal, it will start the GPS to find out where the user is and identify whether the target moves. If the target stays put, it will start ECG and SpO_2 Bluetooth devices. After receiving the data, it ativates the cell phone monitoring and displaying, and alerts nearby people for further assistance. At the same time, the data is sent back to the server and informs First Aid Units of the need for further help. **Figure 24** shows the biomedical signals of ECG and SpO_2 on the Android smart phone.

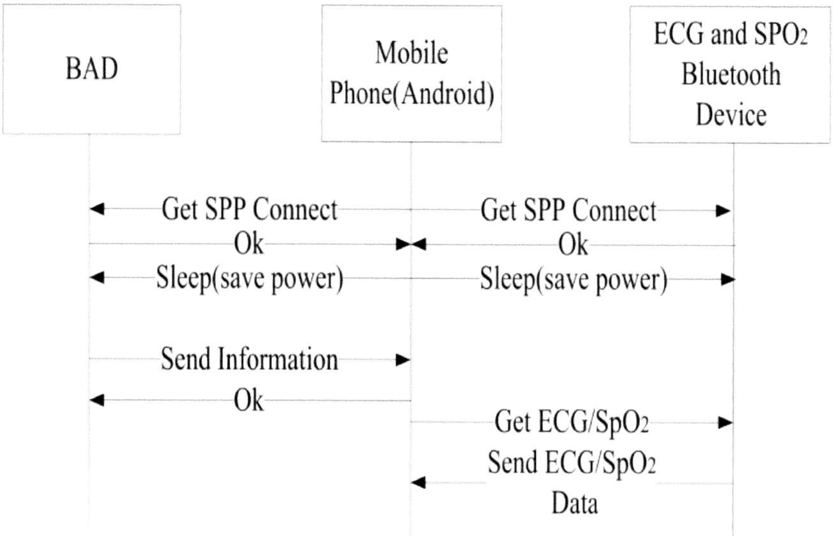

Figure 22. System communication

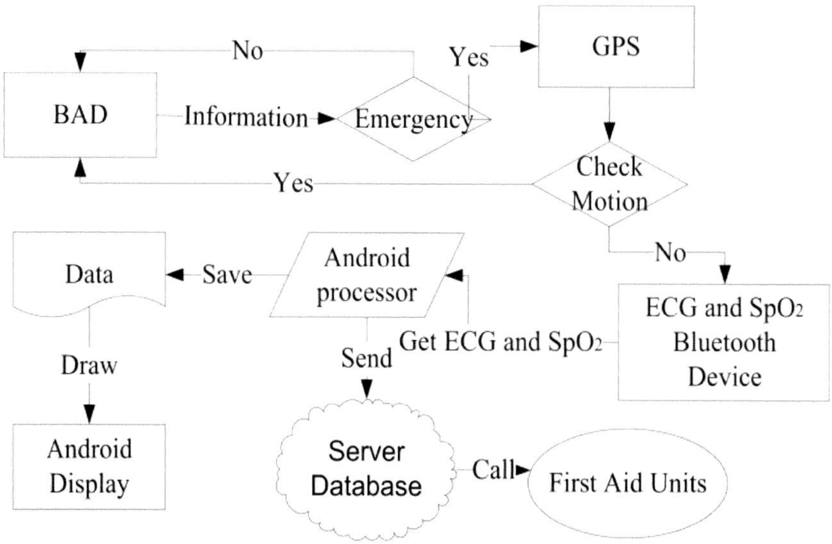

Figure 23. Emergency procedure

5.3. Web-end

The remote monitoring personnel confirm the biomedical information through the WEB interface, such as the ECG shown in **Figure 25**, and receive the signal when the patient needs help. At the same time, it uses GPS to confirm the client position to assist the ambulance to arrive at the right place (see **Figure 26**).

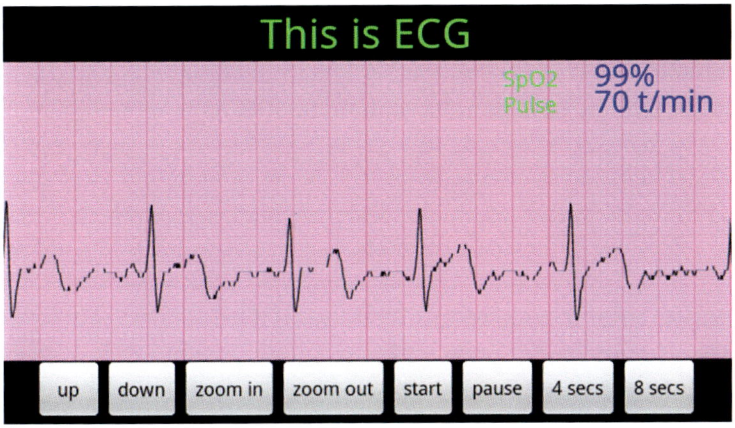

Figure 24. The biomedical signals ECG and SpO_2 on the Android smart phone

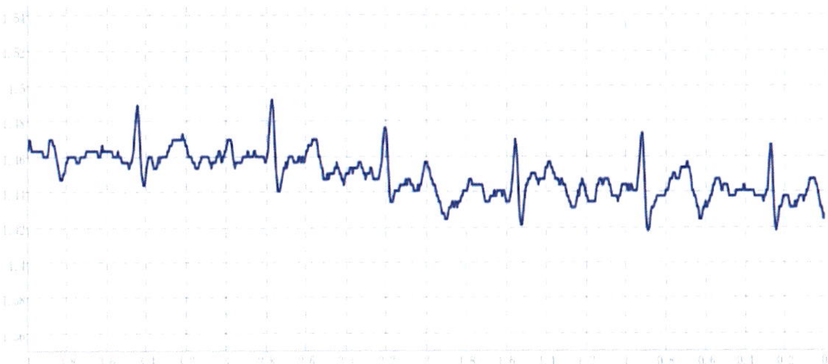

Figure 25. Server Web-end

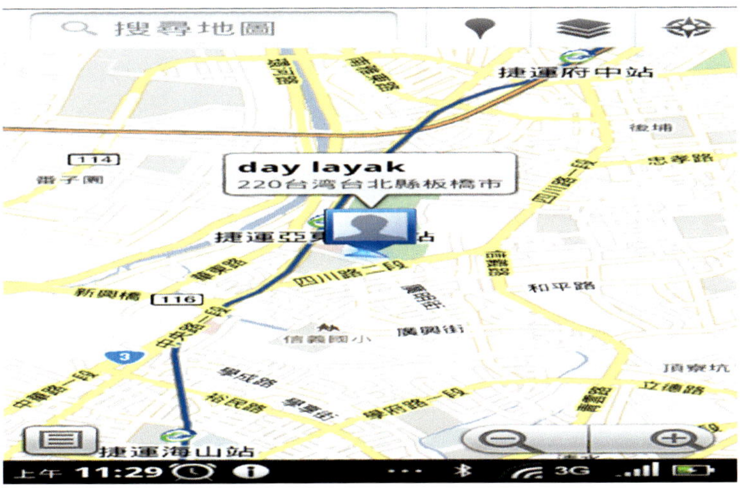

Figure 26. GPS location

6. Conclusion

It may be dangerous to have continuously operating mobile connection close to the heart for patients with artificial pacemakers as it may consider the electromagnetic wave from the mobile to be a cardiac signal, leading to oversensing. However, frequent pulse and blood pressure measurement may be necessary for certain patient groups, such as those with high arrhythmia risk, hypertension, coronary artery disease or heart failure. As Bluetooth technology is safe to use in proximity of pacemakers, we have designed a portable medium based on the Bluetooth power class II RF test specification. We expect that this system will benefit these patients without causing inconvenience to their daily activities or risking adverse interaction with the pacemaker.

Author details

Ching-Sung Wang
Department of Electronic Engineering, Oriental Institute of Technology, Taipei, Taiwan

Teng-Wei Wang
The Third Department of Clinical Research Institute, Peking University, Peking, China

7. References

[1] http://www.surgeryencyclopedia.com/La-Pa/Pacemakers.html
[2] Tacey S, Ronald A, "The Effects of Electromagnetic Fields on Cardiac Pacemakers" IEEE Transactions on Broadcasting, Vol.38,No.2,June 1992
[3] Barbaro V, Bartolini P, Donato A, et al. "Do European GSM mobile cellular phones pose a potential risk to pacemaker patients?" PACE 1995; 18: 1218-24
[4] Okan Erdogan, MD, "Electromagnetic Interference on Pacemakers", Indian Pacing Electrophysiol J. 2002 Jul–Sep; 2(3): 74–78
[5] Hayes DL, Wang PJ, Reynolds DW, et al. "Interference with cardiac pacemakers by cellular telephones". N Eng J Med 1997; 336: 1473-9
[6] Bluetooth, Specification of the Bluetooth System Core, Version 2.0, 2004
[7] Bluetooth, Radio Frequency Test Suite Structure (TSS) and Test Purposes (TP) Specification 1.2, Revision 1.2.3, 2004-08-24
[8] Nissila, S, Sorvisto, M, Sorvoja, H, Vieri-Gashi, E, Myllyla, R, "Non-invasive blood pressure measurement based on the electronic palpation method", Engineering in Medicine and Biology Society, 1998. Proceedings of the 20th Annual International Conference of the IEEE, Volume 4, 29 Oct.-1 Nov. 1998 Page(s):1723 - 1726 vol.4
[9] Yi-Bing Lin, Imrich Chlamtac, "Wireless and Mobile Network Architectures", Wiley Computer Publishing, 1 edition (October 2, 2000)
[10] Mouly, M, Pautet, M-B, "The GSM System for Mobile Communications", Telecom Publishing (June 1992)

[11] Ching-Sung Wang, Jung-Hunag Lee, Yiu-Tong Chu, "Mobile Telemedicine Application and Technologies on GSM", Bioinformatics and Biomedical Engineering, 2007. ICBBE 2007. The 1st International Conference on 6-8 July 2007 Page(s):1125 – 1128
[12] MediaTek "AT Command Set", Revision: 0.03, Sep. 1. 2004
[13] Ching-Sung Wang, Chien-Wei Liu, Teng-Wei Wang, "Tele-care for emergency announcements" Journal of Biomedical Science and Engineering, pp.822-827, Aug.,2010
[14] Winbond Inc., "W681388 Single Programmable Extended CODEC/SLIC", ver1.0, 2006.
[15] Microchip Inc., "PIC24FJ64GA004 Family Data Sheet", 2007.
[16] National Semiconductor "SC14440/431/432, SC14435, SC14436/437/438. Baseband Processor for PP/FP DECT and WDCT", V1.1, June 16, 2005
[17] Champion "CM2838, 300mA Low Esr CMOS LDO With Enable", Rev 1.1, 2004/0501
[18] HoneyWell , "SSC Series Pressure Sensors 0 – 5 psi Through 0 – 300 psi" , 2002
[19] ETSI "Digital cellular telecommunications system (Phase 2+); International Mobile station Equipment Identities (IMEI); (GSM 02.16 version 6.2.0 Release 1997)", 2000-07
[20] ETSI "Digital cellular telecommunications system (Phase 2+); Technical realization of the Short Message Service (SMS); (GSM 03.40 version 7.4.0 Release 1998)", 1999-12
[21] ELAN "EM62100 65 COM/ 132 SEG STN LCD Driver Product Specification", version 1.5, September 2006
[22] MEMSIC "MXC6202xJ/K Data Sheet", Rev A, 2006
[23] CSR, "BlueCore3-ROM CSP Product Data Book", Nov 2006
[24] Specification of the Bluetooth System Core, Version 2.0, 2004
[25] Pravin Bhagwat Reefedge Inc., "Bluetooth: technology for short-range wireless apps", IEEE Internet Computing, Volume 5, Issue 3, May-June 2001 Page(s): 96 – 103.
[26] MediaTek "MT6219 GSM/GPRS Baseband Processor Data Sheet", Revision 1.00, Feb 02, 2004.
[27] ATMEL "AT89C2051 8-bit Microcontroller with 2K Bytes Flash Data Sheet", 6/05.
[28] Bluetooth SIG, "Specification of the Bluetooth System Profile, Part K:5 Serial Port Profile", version 1.1, 2001
[29] MediaTek "Customer Device Driver Document", Revision: 0.1, Nov 03, 2003
[30] PixTel "Writing Applications Using PixTel MMI Platform", version: 1.3, July 10, 2004
[31] ETSI "Digital cellular telecommunications system (Phase 2+); AT command set for GSM Mobile Equipment(ME);(GSM 07.07 version5.9.1 Release 1996)", December 1999

[32] Bluetooth SIG, Specification of the Bluetooth System Core, version 2.0, 2004
[33] MITEL "MT8870D/MT8870D-1 Data Sheet", May 1995

Chapter 13

Phrenic Nerve Pacing: Current Concepts

Jorge F. Velazco, Shekhar Ghamande and Salim Surani

Additional information is available at the end of the chapter

http://dx.doi.org/10.5772/48808

1. Introduction

Anatomy: The diaphragm is the main inspiratory muscle in mammals, it is a highly active muscle with a duty cycle of 30-40%, and therefore, the diaphragm may be particularly susceptible to inactivity or disuse (1). It is innervated by the phrenic nerves that arise from the nerve roots C3 through C5, and is primarily composed of fatigue-resistant slow-twitch type I and fast-twitch IIa myofibers. As the diaphragm contracts, the abdominal contents are displaced caudally, abdominal pressure increases and the lower ribcage expands (2). The phrenic nerve contains sensory, motor and sympathetic nerve fibers, and it supplies motor supply to the diaphragm and sensory supply to the central tendon (3). Both phrenic nerves run along the anterior scalene muscle deep to the carotid sheath. The right phrenic nerve passes over the brachiocephalic artery and posterior to the subclavian vein and over the right atrium. It enters the diaphragm at the level of T8 vertebrae. The left phrenic nerve also runs posterior to the left subclavian vein and passes over the pericardium of the left ventricle and penetrates the left hemidiaphragm separately (3). See Figures 1 and 2.

Pathophysiology: Diaphragmatic dysfunction can manifest as weakness or paralysis, and is related to different entities. Patients with bilateral diaphragmatic paralysis are more likely to have symptoms like dyspnea or recurrent respiratory failure; other complications include subsegmental atelectasis and infections of lower respiratory tract (2). See Figure 3.

Of the 11,000 new cases of spinal cord injury (SCI), approximately one half (56.4%) are sustained at the cervical level (4). Currently, the average age of injury is 37.6, and about 80% are male (5). Cervical SCI often leads to an interruption of the descending bulbospinal respiratory pathways, resulting in respiratory muscle paresis and/or paralysis. The more rostral the level of injury the greater the likelihood of a major respiratory compromise, however the most caudal segment of the spinal cord with normal motor function defines the motor level of injury. The injuries above the level of the phrenic motoneurons (C3, C4, C5)

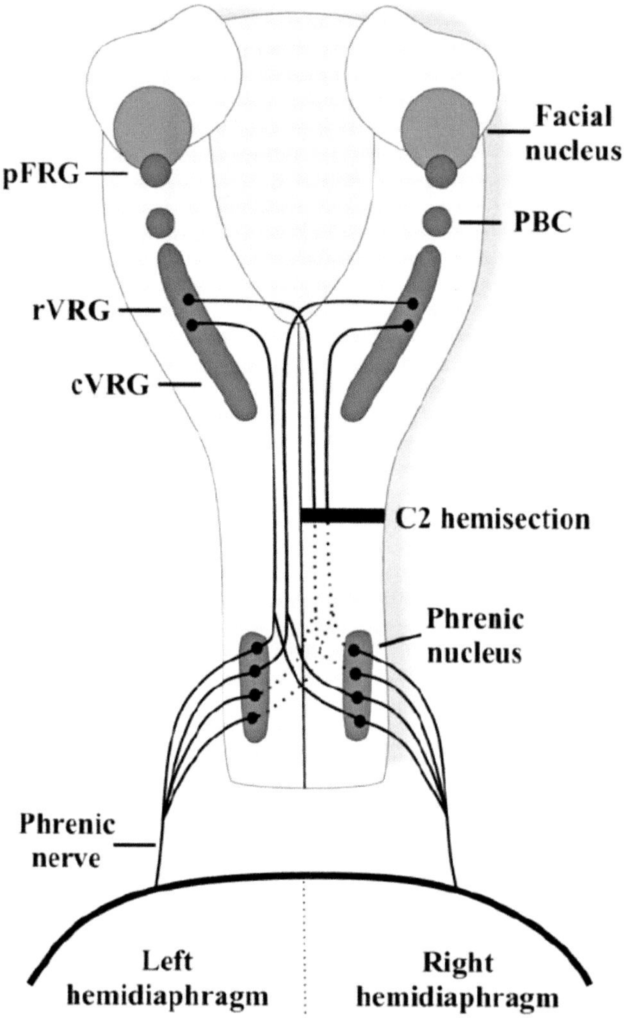

Legend: pFRG: parafacial respiratory group; rVRG: rostral ventral respiratory group; cVRG: caudal ventral respiratory group; PBC: preBotzinger complex.

Reproduced with permission. Effect of Spinal Cord Injury on the Respiratory System: Basic Research and Current Clinical Treatment Options. Beth Zimmer et al. J Spinal Cord Med. 2007; 30:319-330

Figure 1. Schematic drawing of the major respiratory neural centers and pathways in the rat. Respiratory rhythm generation is formed by neurons located within the pFRG and the PBC. Impulses are transmitted to premotor neurons located within the VRG with inspira-tory neurons located predominantly in rVRG and expira-tory neurons localized to cVRG. Premotor neurons project either unilaterally or bilaterally down to phrenic motor neurons located on both sides of the spinal cord (C3—C6). Crossed respiratory axons (arising from VRG neurons bilaterally) have been localized at the level of the phrenic nucleus and contribute to the expression of the crossed phrenic phenomenon. Phrenic axons from each side of the spinal cord form the phrenic nerve, which projects to each half of the diaphragm.

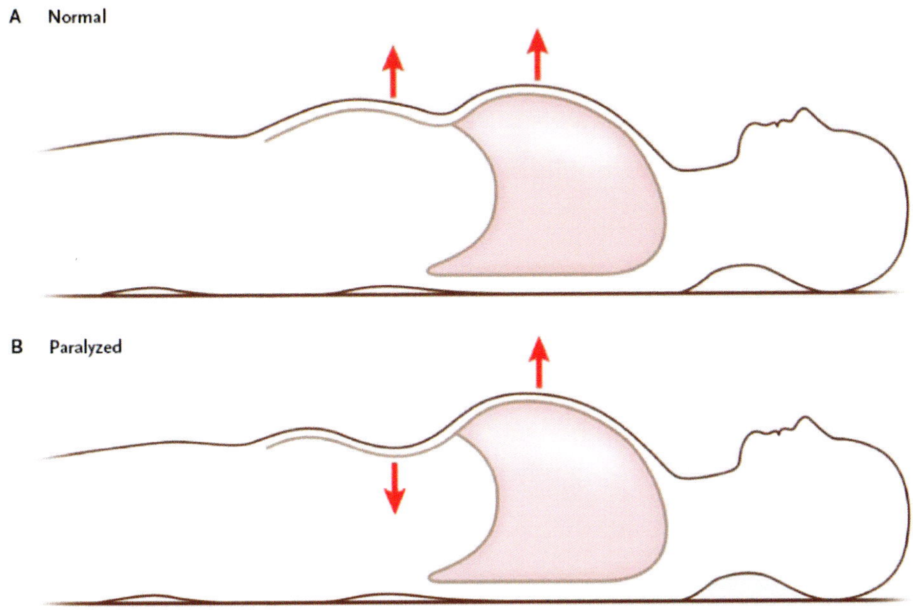

Reproduced with permission. Dysfunction of the Diaphragm. McCool, MD et al. N Engl J Med 2012; 366:932-42

Figure 2. Comparison of Rib-Cage and Abdominal Motion in Normal and Paralyzed Diaphragms. Panel A shows how normal diaphragmatic contraction results in an outward motion of the abdomen and rib cage (arrows). Panel B shows how diaphragmatic paralysis results in a paradoxical inward motion of the abdomen (down-ward-pointing arrow) during inspiration. The accessory inspiratory muscles contract, lifting the rib cage (upward-pointing arrow) and lowering the intrathoracic pressure. This change causes the flaccid diaphragm to move in a cephalad direction and the anterior abdominal wall to move inward.

cause virtually complete paralysis of both the inspiratory and expiratory muscles with mechanical ventilator dependency (5,6). It may be possible to maintain neuromuscular transmission and functional properties of diaphragm muscle fibers after spinal cord injury when motoneurons are not directly injured (1). More than 80% of injuries are traumatic in nature, and up to 1.5% of such injuries are sustained in children. Many of these patients cannot be eventually weaned off mechanical ventilation, and require chronic ventilator support in as much as 4% of the cases (4,6,7,8). In the United States more than 100,000 tracheostomies are performed for patients who are unable to be weaned from ventilator (8,9). In most of these cases the lungs, chest wall, and respiratory muscles are usually physiologically normal (4). Acute SCI is complicated by respiratory complications in 67% of cases with pneumonia being the most common cause of death (6,9,10). The C1-C4 injury group had pneumonia in 63% of cases at a mean interval of 30 days post-injury. Patients with high level lesions associated with bilateral diaphragm paralysis cannot achieve and sustain a vital capacity of 5mL/Kg (10). Controlled mechanical ventilation leads to rapid atrophy of the diaphragm. Within 18 hours of mechanical ventilation there is a decrease in type I muscle fibers with conversion to less functional fast-twitch type IIb muscle fibers (8).

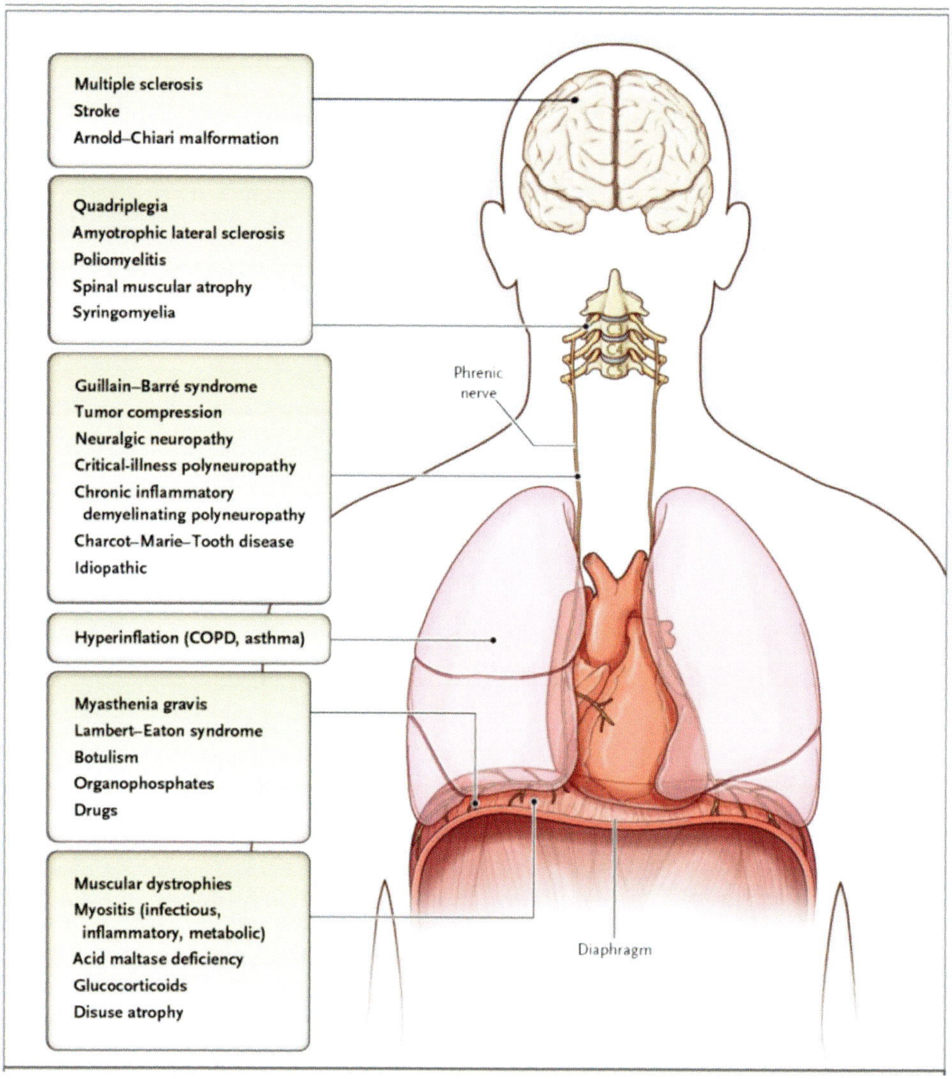

Reproduced with permission. Dysfunction of the Diaphragm. McCool, MD et al. N Engl J Med 2012; 366:932-42

Figure 3. Causes of Diaphragmatic Dysfunction, According to Level of Impairment. Disorders that occur at various regions in the body can lead to diaphragmatic dysfunction. COPD denotes chronic obstructive pulmonary disease.

Beyond one year the chances of recovery of fully independent breathing is probably less than 5% of patients with complete high tetraplegia (10). Loss of diaphragm function reduces survival. It is estimated that a 15 year-old who sustains a high SCI and survives the first 24 hours, the need of mechanical ventilation decreases life expectancy by 21 years (7); in the case of a 40 year-old patient with tetraplegia and ventilator dependence who survives the first 24 hours life expectancy is 7 years. It is dramatically reduced to 1.8 years in a 60 year-old with SCI (8,9).

Mechanical ventilation in tracheostomy patients has several complications such as speech difficulties, reduced mobility, difficulty with transfers, social limitations, loss of sense of smell, equipment malfunction, increased respiratory infections, and increased cost of care approaching $200,000 a year (7,8,10,11).

Central Alveolar Hypoventilation Syndrome (CAHS) or "Ondine's curse" is extremely rare condition that shares the ventilatory failure pattern along with preserved lung functions, normal chest wall mechanics, and physiologically normal respiratory muscles. It is characterized by failure of the autonomic control of breathing during sleep (12). The term originates from a German myth about Ondine, an oceanic nymph who punished her unfaithful lover with the loss of all movements that did not involve his conscious will. Thus, he was condemned to remain awake forever to be able to breathe (12,13). Blunted response of the respiratory center to carbon dioxide leads to hypoventilation and central apneas resulting in hypercarbia and hypoxemia; typically exacerbated during periods of sleep. Pulmonary hypertension and cor pulmonale lead to death (12).

Besides trauma, other causes of phrenic nerve involvement leading to chronic diaphragm dysfunction include vasculitis, neuralgic amyotrophy (14).

Amyotrophic lateral sclerosis is a relentlessly progressive neuromuscular disease of unknown origin that affects both upper and lower motor neurons causing weakness, hyperreflexia and atrophy (15). The incidence is 0.2 to 2.4 cases per 100,000 populations; it is most commonly diagnosed in middle age, affects more men than women. Life expectancy of ALS is 3 to 5 years after diagnosis (15). The major cause of mortality in patients with ALS is respiratory failure because of the progressive decline of 3-5% per month of Forced Vital Capacity (FVC) due to progressive loss of motor neurons leading to respiratory muscle weakness. Phrenic nerve pacing is a novel method being investigated to treat the diaphragm involvement in ALS (11).

Diaphragm pacing is a technique of artificial ventilation using electrical stimulation of the phrenic nerves to produce diaphragm contraction, providing many ventilator-dependent tetraplegic patients with freedom from mechanical ventilation (16,17,18,19). Compared with mechanical ventilation, phrenic pacing provides more natural breathing dynamics, reduces the occurrence of respiratory infection, and improves quality of life. Additionally earlier home discharge and lower infections drive down health care costs (20). Diaphragm muscle pacing, phrenic nerve pacing, and combined intercostal and unilateral diaphragm pacing techniques are currently been used to wean patients from ventilators and reduce the incidence of infection, atelectasis and respiratory failure (6).

Diaphragm pacing is conducted with low frequency electrical stimulation at a slow repetition rate to condition the diaphragm muscle against fatigue (21).

2. History

The use of electricity for therapeutic purposes dates back to 15 AD, when Scribonious Largus, a court physician to the Roman emperor Claudius began using electric shocks from the torpedo ray fish to treat gout pain and headaches (22).

Sophisticated techniques for electrical stimulation of excitable tissue in neuromuscular disorders have been developed over the past three decades. Caldani in 1786 was probably the first to note movement of the diaphragm upon electrical stimulation of the phrenic nerve. In 1818 Ure applied electricity to the phrenic nerve of a recently hung criminal producing "strong and laborious respirations". In 1873, Hufeland proposed stimulating the phrenic nerve to treat asphyxia in neonates. During 19th century attempts were made to apply direct electrical stimulation to the diaphragm or to phrenic nerves in the neck (21,23,24).

By 1878, phrenic nerve stimulation was accepted as a rational procedure. Ziemssen used placement of large well-moistened sponges firmly over phrenic nerves at the outer borders of sternocleidomastoid muscles at the lower end of the scalene muscles to electrically stimulate the nerves (21).

The advent of mechanical ventilation led to abandonment of efforts at diaphragm stimulation as a means of supporting ventilation except for a few case reports. Sarnoff in 1948 that provided adequate ventilation with transcutaneous phrenic nerve stimulation for up to 52 hours in paralyzed patient with cerebral aneurysm. He also demonstrated this in bulbar poliomyelitis (3,4,16,21,25). Sarnoff et al experimented extensively with electrical stimulation of the phrenic nerve and demonstrated that submaximal electrical stimulation of only one phrenic nerve could affect normal oxygen and carbon dioxide exchange; they called this method electrophrenic respiration (EPR) (26). In 1966 Glenn and coworkers first treated a patient with chronic ventilatory failure, using a radiofrequency system with an implantable receiver and electrode but an external power source. This technique was adopted as the gold standard of clinical application for more than 20 years. The surgery involved placement of electrodes on the phrenic nerve in the neck and thorax through a thoracotomy (9,16,22,25,27,28). The initial device consisted of an external battery-powered transmitter with an antenna placed on the skin and a radio receiver placed subcutaneously beneath the antenna (3). See Figure 4.

Successful use of implantable pacemakers for the heart has prompted further interest in development of electrical stimulation of excitable tissues including the diaphragm. Improvements in pacemaker equipment design and intensive-care technology have increased the chances of using diaphragm pacing for the treatment of respiratory failure due to diaphragm paralysis (29). By 2004 approximately 1600 patients worldwide had been implanted with one of these pacing systems during last 35 years (9,22).

In multicenter trials of SCI patients, 98% of patients were liberated from their ventilators with the diaphragm pacing system, which led to US Food and Drug Administration (FDA) approval for this indication in 2008.

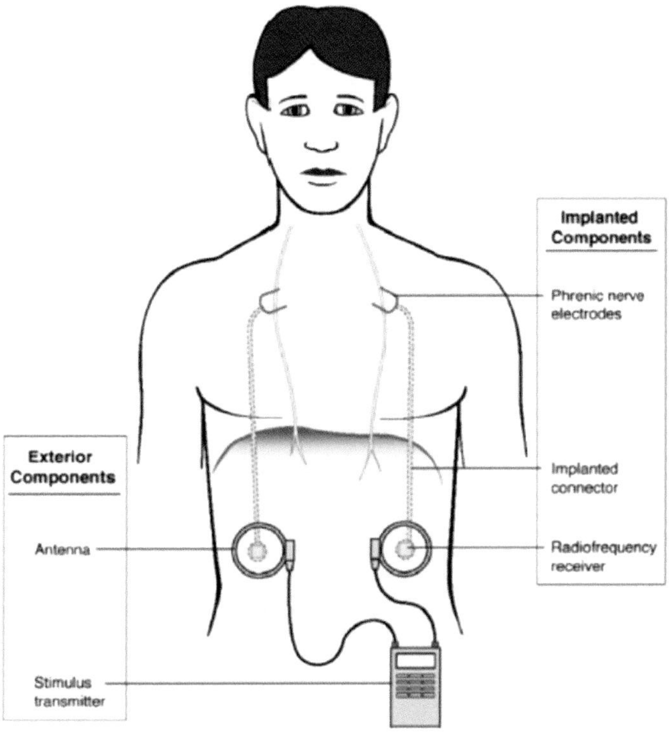

Reproduced with permission by Functional Electrical Stimulation Therapies after Spinal Cord Injury. David Gater et al. NeuroRehabilitation 28 (2011)231-248

Figure 4. Functional electrical stimulation of the diaphragm for respiration

3. Indications

The accepted indications for phrenic nerve pacing are respiratory paralysis after Cervical SCI above the origin of the phrenic nerve neurons (C1-C2) that are ventilator-dependent and the chronic Central Hypoventilation Syndrome associated with central apneas (2,13,23,26,30,31). Diaphragm pacing has also been tried in chronic obstructive pulmonary disease (COPD), ALS (15,32,33) and chronic hiccup (34,35). Glenn et al elaborated on indications for the use of these pacemakers.

A diaphragmatic pacemaker may be considered for:

1. Chronic, respiratory failure requiring invasive mechanical ventilation via permanent tracheostomy on either a temporary, intermittent or continuous basis.
2. A central neurological cause for the respiratory failure such as
   a. Alveolar hypoventilation, either primary or secondary to a brainstem disorder.
   b. Interruption of neuronal conduction at the upper cervical level, above the C3 level
3. Integrity of the intrathoracic section of the phrenic nerve

4. Acceptable pulmonary function
5. Normal level of consciousness (36).

Acquired CAHS has been described with medullary tumors, infection (particularly poliomyelitis), upper cervical trauma, some mitochondrial diseases, degenerative diseases (eg multiple sclerosis), and non-specific ischemic insults (12).

In the case of ALS patients, the goal is to initiate phrenic pacing before tracheostomy is required in order to maintain diaphragm strength. This will help convert diaphragm muscle fibers from the fast-twitch type IIb to slow-twitch type I and perhaps have a trophic effect that allows the phrenic motor neurons to live longer (32).

Diaphragm pacing has also been tried for Arnold Chiari malformation, meningomyelocele, neurofibromatosis, incomplete C3-C4 fractures, C4-C5 fractures with ascending paralysis to C2-C3 level, radiation induced phrenic nerve injury (3).

4. Evaluation

Diaphragm pacing is a costly undertaking, and depending on the specific technique of implantation, variable amounts of risks are associated with the surgical procedure. Therefore, potential candidates should be carefully screened and meet specific eligibility criteria. Initial evaluation should thoroughly assess psychological factors (4,37,38). Some centers will even wait a year after injury to consider diaphragmatic pacemaker implantation (9). Patients with lesions of lower motor neurons, of the phrenic nerve itself or its roots, or with diaphragm weakness not due to disuse atrophy should not be consider for pacing (28,39).

The ideal candidates for phrenic nerve pacing are those with normal phrenic nerves, diaphragms, and lungs (5,21). Pacing may not be effective in patients with lesions involving the segment of the cord C3 and C5 as some or all of the phrenic nerve cell bodies or lower motor neurons may be destroyed (21). Glenn et al reported that of 77 cases selected, 48 patients had defects in respiratory control, and 29 had lesions of the upper motor neurons of the phrenic nerve (21). For patients who do not have intact phrenic nerves, conventional or intramuscular diaphragmatic pacing is not an option (5).

Once suspected, diaphragmatic dysfunction can be confirmed by a number of tests. Chest radiographs may reveal elevated diaphragms and basal subsegmental atelectasis. Sniff tests are not useful to diagnose bilateral diaphragmatic paralysis (2,38). Pulmonary function tests, especially measurements of upright and supine vital capacity, are non invasive and may support or refute the diagnosis(2,14,38). Arterial blood gas values during mechanical ventilation (23,36,38) and a sleep study when possible, add diagnostic information (23).

Maximal static inspiratory pressure and sniff nasal inspiratory pressure have limitations due to patient effort. Both tests are markedly reduced to less than 30% of the predicted value, in those with bilateral diaphragm paralysis, as well as tetraplegia patients (2,6).

Other tests to assess diaphragmatic function could be invasive like transdiaphragmatic pressure (Pdi) or noninvasive like ultrasonography (2). Measurement of Pdi provides the difference between gastric and esophageal pressures during tidal breathing, maximal sniff maneuvers (sniff Pdi), maximal inspiratory efforts against a closed glottis (Pdi max), or transcutaneous electrical or magnetic stimulation of the phrenic nerve (twitch Pdi) (2,25,38).

A twitch Pdi greater than $10cmH_2O$ with unilateral phrenic-nerve stimulation or greater than 20 cmH_2O with bilateral phrenic-nerve stimulation also rules out clinically significant weakness. Ultrasonography of the diaphragm at its zone of apposition with the rib cage shows thickening of the diaphragm reflecting shortening during inspiration. Loss of thickening is diagnostic of diaphragmatic paralysis (2). Ultrasonography is ideal in children because it is noninvasive, painless, safe and portable. Image quality is superior in children compared with adults because of the small body size and lower body fat (40).

Electromyography (EMG) of the diaphragm during tidal breathing or after phrenic nerve stimulation is limited by technical issues of electrode placement, "crosstalk" from adjacent muscle groups, and variable distance of electrodes to muscle related to subcutaneous thickness when electrodes are placed at standardized places like seventh and ninth intercostal spaces (4,18).

Phrenic nerve integrity must be demonstrated by EMG twitch of diaphragm contraction in response to electrical stimulation prior to considering diaphragmatic pacemaker insertion. This is tested by cervical magnetic stimulation and/or electrical stimulation of the phrenic nerve in the neck (20,21,36,38,39). However a recent French series which looked at long term outcomes, found benefit in phrenic nerve pacing even in patients who had injuries dating back several years. (20,39). EMG response of the diaphragm is considered normal if the latency was within normal range between 5.5 and 6.5 ms for cervical magnetic stimulation, and between 6.5 and 8 ms for electrical stimulation. In patients on prolonged mechanical ventilation, due to diaphragm atrophy, conduction times may be prolonged (4,5,20). Fluoroscopic evaluation of diaphragm movement during phrenic nerve stimulation, is useful to exclude both false-positive and false-negative results of phrenic nerve stimulation. The diaphragm should descend at least 3 to 4 cm during stimulation as visualized fluoroscopically (4,23). Phrenic nerve function can also be assessed by measurements of transdiaphragmatic pressure Pdi (4,39). See Figure 5.

5. Surgical implantation techniques

The goal of any diaphragmatic pacing system is to provide safe and effective activation of the diaphragm, sufficient to provide adequate ventilation to meet metabolic requirements (4).

In the past the pacemaker electrodes were placed at the cervical area (25); but is presently discouraged for several reasons. Cervical phrenic nerve stimulation may result in incomplete diaphragm activation in the presence of an accessory branch from a lower segment of the cervical spinal cord that joins the main trunk of the phrenic nerve in the lower neck region or thorax.(4).

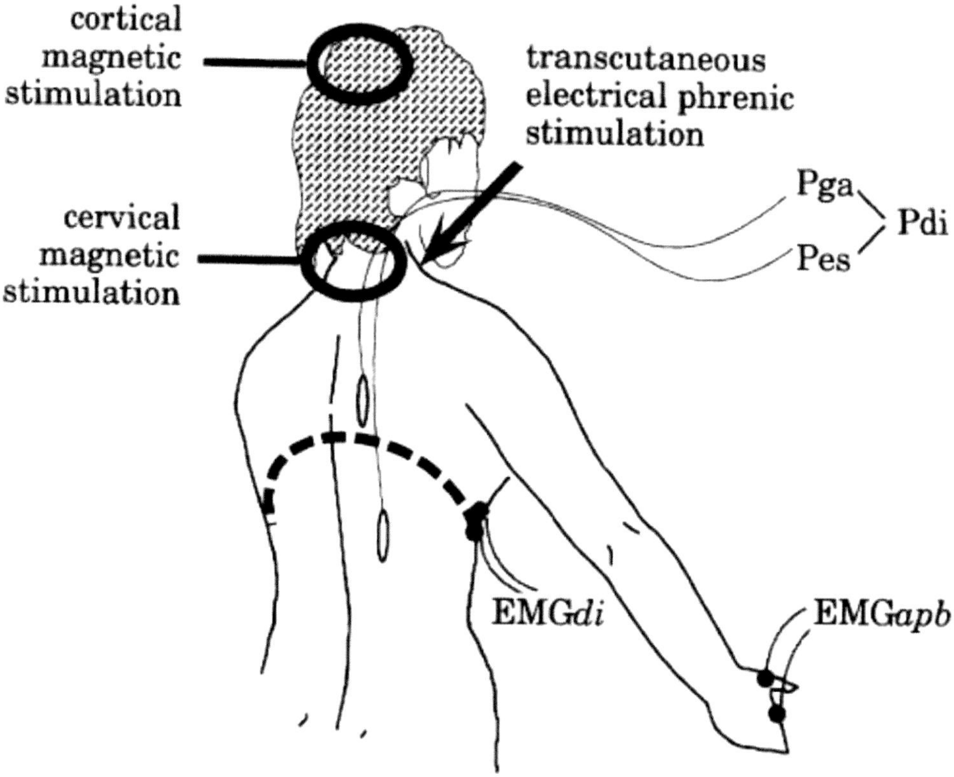

Reproduced with permission. Assessment of the Motor Pathway to the Diaphragm using Cortical and Cervical Magnetic Stimulation in the Decision-making process of phrenic Pacing. Thomas Similowski et al. Chest 1996; 110:1551-57

Figure 5. Schematic representation of the experimental setup used to study the patients. Diaphragmatic EMG (EMGdi), esophageal pressure (Pes), and gastric pressure (Pga) were measured in response to cortical and cervical magnetic stimulation, and to transcutaneous electrical stimulation of the phrenic nerve in the neck. Pdi was derived from Pes and Pga. An EMG ofthe APB (EMGapb) was used as control in some patients.

In Glenn's series, bilaterally thoracotomy procedures were performed 10 to 14 days apart. Once phrenic nerves were exposed surgically the platinum electrodes were placed directly in contact with the perineurium of the nerve in a tunnel behind the nerve that was large enough to allow free movement of the electrode within it. Then, the electrodes were connected to the receiver in the subcutaneous pocket were it was tested prior to skin closure (21).

Le Pimpec-Barthes et al successfully used Video-assisted thoracic surgery (VATS) for the implantation. The endoscopic camera was inserted in the pleural space through a second intercostal space incision. Careful dissection of the phrenic nerve was carried out in front of the vena cava on the right and in the pulmonary hilum on the left. Then quadripolar electrodes were implanted in both sides, 2 above and 2 below the nerve. Each Teflon patch was sutured to pleura or pericardium to prevent dislodgement. Then wires were brought out through a mini-thoracotomy, and tunneled under the pectoralis major muscle to a subcutaneous pocket. The wires were then connected to the subcutaneous radiofrequency receivers on each side. Intraoperative testing confirmed correct placement. No nerve injury or other significant intraoperative complications were observed (20). Robotic surgical placement has also been tested successfully including in patients with tetraplegia (4).

Another minimally invasive approach advocated intramuscular placement of the stimulating electrodes in the diaphragm laparoscopically (5,9). In this method, identification of motor points of the phrenic nerves was done by a mapping procedure which involved electrical stimulation each hemidiaphragm with a probe at several locations. Two electrodes were placed in each diaphragm to stimulate all branches of the phrenic nerve maximally at the point where stimulation evoked the best motor response of the diaphragm (5,9,11). After testing all 4 wires are brought out through the epigastric port, and then tunneled to the chest where they were connected to the transcutaneous exiting wires. Onders emphasized that the accurate identification of motor points is crucial for successfully pacing the diaphragm (9). DiMarco et al described further improvement of the technique with coarse mapping and direct visualization of diaphragmatic contraction (4,15). A significant difference was noted in patients with ALS whose diaphragms had weaker contractions with the typical mapping stimulation.-Nevertheless, the laparoscopic procedure can be safely performed at multiple independent hospital sites for ventilator-dependent tetraplegia and ALS (11). Laparoscopic approach has cost and simplicity advantages and can be performed on an outpatient basis. In addition there is no manipulation of the phrenic nerve by itself (17).

Assouad et al have tried placing the electrodes through a cervical incision thoracic endoscopic surgery (CITES). Here a mediastinoscopy is followed by bilateral pleurotomies, and then a gastroscope is used in the pleural space to locate the phrenic nerve penetration points at the dome of the diaphragm. Finally needle and electrode hooks were placed close to the entry point of the phrenic nerves (19).

There are three commercially available diaphragmatic pacing systems depicted in table 1: a) Avery Biomedical Devices, b) Atrotech OY, and c) Medimplant systems. Each system is designed for lifetime use (4)

6. Settings

After surgical implantation, a period of 2 weeks should elapse before initiation of diaphragm pacing (20,28,35). The diaphragm is weakened from prolonged mechanical ventilation, therefore, at the beginning a process of conditioning is carried through gradual lengthening of periods of stimulation (28,38). Thus, a strategy of minimizing diaphragm fatigue during pacing should involve the gradual conditioning with low-frequency stimulation and a slow respiratory rate (29). Diaphragmatic conditioning is a process by which the fast-contracting fibers (anaerobic, highly glycolytic fibers), which are highly susceptible to get fatigued, are converted to slow-contracting fatigue-resistant (aerobic oxidative fibers), which enable permanent ventilatory support using diaphragmatic pacing (4,36).

Device	AVERY I-107A (superceded)	AVERY I-110A	ATROTECH	MEDIMPLANT
Receiver size (mm)	46 (diam) x 16	30 (diam) x 8	49 (diam) x 8.5	56 x 53 x 14
Battery life (hr)	160	100	160-320 (12V) 8 (9V)	24
Controller + battery weight (kg)	3.6	0.54	0.45 + 0.6 (12V) 0.45 + 0.045 (9V)	0.8 + 0.62
Controller size (mm)	179 x 114 x 97	146 x 140 x 25	185 x 88 x 28	170 x 130 x 51
Breaths/min	10-50	6-24	8-35	5-60
Pulse interval (ms)	35-170	40-130	10-100	25-170
Pulse width (microsec)	150	150	200	100-1000
Sigh possible	yes	yes	yes	yes
Electrodes	Monopolar; bipolar	Monopolar; bipolar	Quadripolar	Quadripolar
No. of receivers to stimulate both hemidiaphragms	2	2	2	1

Reproduced with permission. Electrical Stimulation to Restore Respiration. Journal of Rehabilitation Research and Development. Vol 33. N 2. April 1996: 123-132

Table 1. Technical features of phrenic nerve stimulators

While on mechanical ventilation, many patients are generally maintained with large tidal volumes. Diaphragmatic pacing is likely to generate smaller tidal volumes leading to respiratory acidosis therefore ventilator adjustments are needed initially (4).

Glenn initiated 5 minutes per hour of stimulation with low frequency stimulation (11Hz) at slow rate (8 to 10 per minute). Tidal volumes at the beginning and end of each stimulation period were measured. Once tidal volumes at the end of stimulation period were at least 75% of the beginning volumes, the length of pacing was progressively increased by one to two minutes per hour until the diaphragm was paced 30 minutes per hour. After that, periods of pacing were increased by 5 minute per hour daily. Mechanical ventilation was discontinued during pacing once minute volume was adequate (>5L/min in adults). Diaphragm conditioning is performed during daytime. Each hour of pacing with good minute volume is followed by an hour of rest on the ventilator. Pacing duration is incrementally increased by 15 minutes per session until 6 hours are reached. These periods are progressively extended to 8, 10 and 12 hours. When pacing on each side has been extended to 12 hours, while producing satisfactory minute volumes and normal arterial blood gases, the patient can be completely removed from mechanical ventilation. This weaning process usually takes 2 to 3 months, which is the time frame required for diaphragmatic fiber recovery (21,28,36,38,41). A considerably longer period of conditioning is required in children because of immaturity of respiratory components (21). Every few weeks the pulse frequency and respiratory rate are decreased until the lowest values were reached at which ventilation was still adequate (41). Once the maximal stimulation time has been established, several schedules for maintenance can be followed. For patients who respond normally to stimulation of either side of the diaphragm, they recommended pacing each side alternately, 12 hours at the time (28). The voltage required to effect minimal (threshold) and maximal diaphragm motion during pacing was confirmed or adjusted about once a month (41). Alternatively uninterrupted simultaneous pacing of both hemidiaphragms, using a low-frequency stimulation (7-8 Hz) with a respiratory rate of 5 to 9 per minute may be appropriate for adult patients (41). In general the transition from mechanical ventilation to chronic full-time pacing must be individualized for each patient (4). Occasionally this weaning process can be performed with a home-based ventilator weaning and conditioning program (22,42).

Until full-time pacing is achieved, a tracheostomy needs to remain in place, even after discontinuation of positive pressure ventilation to facilitate intermittent suctioning. This also serves as a back up to resume mechanical ventilation in case of pacemaker failure or other issues like the lack of coordination between the paced diaphragm, the upper airway muscles, and the accessory respiratory muscles in tetraplegics (28,34).

In patients with CAHS, upper airway resistance is augmented by diaphragmatic contraction or diminished upper airway muscle activity and may be induced by diaphragm pacing during sleep (34,43). In this population without muscle paralysis, pacing can be more aggressively initiated, 8 to 10 hours nightly by the third week postoperatively. Moreover, CAHS patients should have baseline sleep study with and without pacing to assure adequacy of pacing and identify any upper airway obstruction (21).

ALS patients begin conditioning programs by five 30-min pacing sessions a day. If ALS patients develop hypoventilation, the amount of time paced can be increased and then used at night. Continuous positive airway pressure (CPAP) or noninvasive positive-pressure ventilation may still be needed to maintain a patent upper airway (11).

Pacemaker function should be monitored on a routine basis and emergently in situations in which patients complain of difficulty breathing. Tidal volumes can be easily measured by spirometry; both electrodes stimulating each diaphragm can be independently evaluated. Pulse oxymetry as well end-tidal PCO_2 should also help to assess ventilation (4).

7. Benefits

Ventilation by phrenic nerve pacing appears to provide both health and lifestyle advantages to the user. Freedom from positive-pressure ventilator reduces the risks of ventilator-associated problems like tracheomalacia, infections, bleeding, barotraumas, and tracheo-esophageal fistulas (4,22,23).

Other ventilator-related disasters are also prevented like sudden death from accidental disconnection from ventilator, or mechanical ventilation device failure (23).

Olfaction was altered because nasal fossae were bypassed during positive-pressure ventilation on tracheostomy patients. Thus, improved speech and sense of smell recovery contribute to a better perception of quality of life in patients with successful diaphragmatic pacing (8,23,44).

Phrenic nerve pacing allows negative-pressure ventilation, leading to a decrease in respiratory infections, in addition to improved patient comfort (8).

Liberation from ventilation also leads to reduced weight of their wheelchair and simplified transfers as well as elimination of social embarrassment associated with ventilator dependency (4,7).

Additionally, patients with pacing systems felt an overall improvement in their well being by reducing fatigue, depressed mood state and sleep disruptions that result from prolonged mechanical ventilation(7). A case report has demonstrated clinical evidence of improvement in right heart failure from pacing, and a fall in red cell volume and pulmonary artery pressures (33). Better ventilation of the posterior lobes minimizes atelectasis and improves cardiac function by increasing venous return (7).

Interestingly, in patients with ALS, diaphragmatic pacing significantly reduced the rate of decline of FVC from 2.4% preimplant to 0.9% per month postimplantion extrapolating to a 24-month improvement in survival (32).

8. Complications

A major complication is the iatrogenic injury to the phrenic nerve during operative implantation of phrenic nerve electrode and subsequent pacemaker failure (4,30). In patients with thoracoscopic pacemaker implantation the most feared complication is phrenic nerve entrapment (36).

In addition to complications common to all surgical procedures, laparoscopy may be associated to pneumothorax, capnothorax (CO_2 tracking from the pressurized abdomen to the pleural space) and subcutaneous emphysema. Right shoulder pain may result from stimulation of phrenic nerve afferents (11,27,28,45). All surgical procedures involving implantation of a foreign body carry some risk of infection, with rates of approximately 3% in case of phrenic nerve pacing (4).

Phrenic pacing can worsen or induce upper airway obstruction with central alveolar hypoventilation; therefore a patent tracheostomy is necessary during sleep (4,29). Similarly in ALS patients that have severe bulbar weakness the upper airway can collapse during inspiration, thus needing a tracheostomy or CPAP treatment (15).

DiMarco reported one subject developed intermittent aspiration of food during meals, due to large negative airway pressure generated during diaphragmatic contraction (27).

Potential long-term complications related to pacing include electrode dislodgement and breakage that will result in device malfunction (22,27).

Pacemaker failure due to technical problems is always a possibility. Strong magnetic fields, such as magnetic resonance imaging can override the electronic system of diaphragmatic pacemakers (4).

9. Outcomes

Diaphragmatic pacing can allow patients the benefits of negative pressure breathing. They have been used safely up to 19 years post injury in individuals with tetraplegia (7). All of these patients were able to tolerate outpatient surgery without perioperative morbidity.

Retrospective assessments have indicated a correlation between excess mortality and neurological level of injury, older age at injury, and injury at earlier calendar years (5).

The problems associated with bilateral phrenic nerve pacing in infants and children are related more to cor pulmonale, as result of hypoventilation, than the mechanics of pacing itself, which can lead to uncertain outcomes (13).

It has been shown to improve quality of life and to extend survival in patients with advanced respiratory muscle weakness (12).

Carefully selected patients should undergo phrenic nerve pacemaker placement by experienced surgeons. They need to have individualized monitored pacing regimens with close follow up for best outcomes (25,37).

The cost savings could be significant. The average cost of ventilator-dependent patient is three times that without a ventilator. During 2004 available phrenic nerve pacing devices with the hospitalization cost more than $120,000. One of the patients in that series who was nursing homebound was able to save $13,000 a month to Medicaid, because he no longer needed to be in a ventilator unit (9). Another series demonstrated that the first year investment for diaphragmatic pacing is paid off after three years. When costs of a respiratory infection are incorporated in the cost analysis, the diaphragm pacing becomes more cost effective in 1 year. (18).

Overall, patients with SCI treated with phrenic nerve pacing instead of standard mechanical ventilation experienced less airway infections, had reduced costs for single use airway equipment, had improved the quality of speech, had improved quality of life, and probably derived a mortality benefit (18).

Although the number of patients who may benefit from this technology is small, the potential improvement in quality of life is substantial (46,47).

Garrido-Garcia and colleague found the mortality to be 22.7% (36). The problems associated with bilateral phrenic nerve pacing in infants and children are related more to cor pulmonale, as result of hypoventilation, than the mechanics of pacing itself (13).

Diaphragmatic pacemakers are safe to use in patients with cardiac pacemakers.

Patient satisfaction in recipients of diaphragm pacing was very high particularly in tetraplegic patients on ventilators (20).

10. Conclusion

Over the last fifty years, significant progress has been made in diaphragmatic pacing. Improvement in surgical techniques have reduced procedural complication during implantation Research in this field has relatively lagged behind other pacemakers such as cardiac devices presumably due to less financial motivation. Ideally a diaphragmatic pacemaker should synchronize with electrical signals from the central nervous system, and adapt to changing metabolic demands. Further development of such devices promises hope for patients with chronic respiratory failure for improved quality of life and possible mortality benefit at a reasonable cost.

In conclusion this technique is efficient in liberating selected ventilator-dependent patients with respiratory paralysis and treating alveolar hypoventilation syndromes. Future clinical trials will increase acceptance of this method as an alternative form of treatment for respiratory failure in selected patients.

Author details

Jorge F. Velazco[1,2], Shekhar Ghamande[1,2] and Salim Surani[1,*]
Texas A&M University, Texas, USA
Scott & White Hospital, Temple, Texas, USA

11. References

[1] Neuromuscular adaptations to respiratory muscle inactivity. Carlos B. Mantilla; et al. Respir Physiol Neurobiol. 2009 Nov 30; 169(2): 133-140.
[2] Dysfunction of the Diaphragm. F. Dennis McCool, M.D; et al. N Engl J Med 2012; 366:932-942.
[3] Diaphragmatic Pacemaker. Salim Surani, MD. Modern Pacemakers - Present and Future. In-Tech. 2011.453-470.
[4] Inspiratory Muscle Pacing in Spinal Cord Injury: Case Report and Clinical Commentary. Anthony F. DiMarco,MD; et al. J Spinal Cord Med 2006; 29:95-108.
[5] Respiratory Dysfunction and Management in Spinal Cord Injury. Robert Brown, MD; et al. Respir Care. 2006 Aug; 51(8): 853-870.
[6] Effect of Spinal Cord Injury on the Respiratory System: Basic Research and Current Clinical Treatment Options. M. Beth Zimmer, PhD; et al. J Spinal Cord Med. 2007; 30:319-330.
[7] Diaphragm Pacing Stimulation System for Tetraplegia in Individuals Injured During Childhood or Adolescence. Raymond P. Onders, MD; et al. J Spinal Cord Med. 2007; 30:S25-S29.
[8] Multicenter analysis of diaphragm pacing in tetraplegics with cardiac pacemakers: Positive implications for ventilator weaning in intensive care units. Raymond P. Onders, MD; et al. Surgery 2010; 148:893-898.
[9] Mapping the phrenic nerve motor point: The key to a successful laparoscopic diaphragm pacing system in the first human series. Raymond P. Onders, MD; at al. Surgery 2004; 136:819-826.
[10] Delayed diaphragm recovery in 12 patients after high cervical spinal cord injury. A retrospective review of the diaphragm status of 107 patients ventilated after acute spinal cord injury. T Oo; et al. Spinal Cord (1999) 37:117-122.
[11] Complete worldwide operative experience in laparoscopic diaphragm pacing: results and differences in spinal cord injured patients and amyotrophic lateral sclerosis patients. Raymond P. Onders; et al. Surg Endosc (2009) 23:1433-1440.

* Corresponding Author

[12] Ondine's curse: anesthesia for laparoscopic implantation of a diaphragm pacing stimulation system. Ahtsham U. Niazi, MBBS; et al. Can J Anesth/J Can Anesth (2011); 58:1034-1038.
[13] Congenital central hypoventilation syndrome: A report of successful experience with bilateral diaphragmatic pacing. Michael Coleman; et al. Arch Dis Child. 1980 Nov; 55(11): 901-903.
[14] Diaphragm plication in adult patients with diaphragm paralysis leads to long-term improvement of pulmonary function and level of dyspnea. Michel I.M. Versteegh; et al. European Journal of Cardio-thoracic Surgery 32 (2007):449-456.
[15] Laparoscopic diaphragmatic pacer placement – a potential new treatment for ALS patients: a brief description of the device and anesthetic issues. Clifford A. Schmiesing MD; et al. Journal of Clinical Anesthesia (2010) 22, 549-552.
[16] Radio-Frequency Electrophrenic Respiration Long-Term Application to a Patient With Primary Hypoventilation. John P. Judson, MD; et al. JAMA Mar 18, 1968;203(12):129-134.
[17] Phrenic Nerve Pacing in a Tetraplegic Patient via Intramuscular Diaphragm Electrodes. Anthony F. DiMarco; et al. Am J Respir Crit Care Med 2002; 166:1604-1606.
[18] Mechanical ventilation or phrenic nerve stimulation for treatment of spinal cord injury-induced respiratory insufficiency. S Hirschfeld; et al. Spinal Cord (2008); 46:738-742.
[19] Minimally invasive trans-mediastinal endoscopic approach to insert phrenic stimulation electrodes in the human diaphragm: a preliminary description in cadavers. Jalal Assouad; et al. European Journal of Cardio-thoracic Surgery 40 (2011) e142-e145.
[20] Intrathoracic phrenic pacing: A 10-year experience in France. Francoise Le Pimpec-Barthes, MD; et al. J Thorac Cardiovasc Surg 2011;142:378-383.
[21] Diaphragm Pacing by Electrical Stimulation of the Phrenic Nerve. William W.L. Glenn, MD; et al. Neurosurgery 17:974-984, 1985.
[22] Functional electrical stimulation therapies after spinal cord injury. David R. Gater, Jr; et al. NeuroRehabilitation 28 (2011) 231-248.
[23] Electrical stimulation to restore respiration. Creasey, Graham, MD; et al. Journal of Rehabilitation Research and Development; Apr 1996; 33:123-132.
[24] Lung function in diaphragm pacing S.W. Epstein, MD; et al. CMA Journal Jun 9,1979; 120:1360-1367.
[25] Diaphragm pacing. John Moxham; et al. Editorial. Thorax 1988; 43:161-162.
[26] Central Hypoventilation; Long-term Ventilatory Assistance by Radiofrequency Electrophrenic Respiration. William W. L. Glenn, M.D et al. Annals of Surgery, Oct 1970; 172(4): 755-773.
[27] Phrenic Nerve Pacing Via Intramuscular Diaphragm Electrodes in Tetraplegic Subjects. Anthony F. DiMarco, MD; et al. Chest 2005; 127:671-678.
[28] Long-Term Ventilatory Support by Diaphragm Pacing in Quadriplegia. William W.L. Glenn, MD; et al. Ann Surg 1976; 183(5): 566-577.
[29] Problems Associated with Diaphragm Pacing. Takashi Nishino. Respiration 2002; 69:12-13.

[12] Ondine's curse: anesthesia for laparoscopic implantation of a diaphragm pacing stimulation system. Ahtsham U. Niazi, MBBS; et al. Can J Anesth/J Can Anesth (2011); 58:1034-1038.

[13] Congenital central hypoventilation syndrome: A report of successful experience with bilateral diaphragmatic pacing. Michael Coleman; et al. Arch Dis Child. 1980 Nov; 55(11): 901-903.

[14] Diaphragm plication in adult patients with diaphragm paralysis leads to long-term improvement of pulmonary function and level of dyspnea. Michel I.M. Versteegh; et al. European Journal of Cardio-thoracic Surgery 32 (2007):449-456.

[15] Laparoscopic diaphragmatic pacer placement – a potential new treatment for ALS patients: a brief description of the device and anesthetic issues. Clifford A. Schmiesing MD; et al. Journal of Clinical Anesthesia (2010) 22, 549-552.

[16] Radio-Frequency Electrophrenic Respiration Long-Term Application to a Patient With Primary Hypoventilation. John P. Judson, MD; et al. JAMA Mar 18, 1968;203(12):129-134.

[17] Phrenic Nerve Pacing in a Tetraplegic Patient via Intramuscular Diaphragm Electrodes. Anthony F. DiMarco; et al. Am J Respir Crit Care Med 2002; 166:1604-1606.

[18] Mechanical ventilation or phrenic nerve stimulation for treatment of spinal cord injury-induced respiratory insufficiency. S Hirschfeld; et al. Spinal Cord (2008); 46:738-742.

[19] Minimally invasive trans-mediastinal endoscopic approach to insert phrenic stimulation electrodes in the human diaphragm: a preliminary description in cadavers. Jalal Assouad; et al. European Journal of Cardio-thoracic Surgery 40 (2011) e142-e145.

[20] Intrathoracic phrenic pacing: A 10-year experience in France. Francoise Le Pimpec-Barthes, MD; et al. J Thorac Cardiovasc Surg 2011;142:378-383.

[21] Diaphragm Pacing by Electrical Stimulation of the Phrenic Nerve. William W.L. Glenn, MD; et al. Neurosurgery 17:974-984, 1985.

[22] Functional electrical stimulation therapies after spinal cord injury. David R. Gater, Jr; et al. NeuroRehabilitation 28 (2011) 231-248.

[23] Electrical stimulation to restore respiration. Creasey, Graham, MD; et al. Journal of Rehabilitation Research and Development; Apr 1996; 33:123-132.

[24] Lung function in diaphragm pacing S.W. Epstein, MD; et al. CMA Journal Jun 9,1979; 120:1360-1367.

[25] Diaphragm pacing. John Moxham; et al. Editorial. Thorax 1988; 43:161-162.

[26] Central Hypoventilation; Long-term Ventilatory Assistance by Radiofrequency Electrophrenic Respiration. William W. L. Glenn, M.D et al. Annals of Surgery, Oct 1970; 172(4): 755-773.

[27] Phrenic Nerve Pacing Via Intramuscular Diaphragm Electrodes in Tetraplegic Subjects. Anthony F. DiMarco, MD; et al. Chest 2005; 127:671-678.

[28] Long-Term Ventilatory Support by Diaphragm Pacing in Quadriplegia. William W.L. Glenn, MD; et al. Ann Surg 1976; 183(5): 566-577.

[29] Problems Associated with Diaphragm Pacing. Takashi Nishino. Respiration 2002; 69:12-13.

[30] Twenty Years of Experience in Phrenic Nerve Stimulation to Pace the Diaphragm. William, W. Glenn, MD; et al. PACE (1980) Vol 9. pp 780-784.
[31] Eight-Year Follow-Up Study of a Patient with Central Alveolar Hypoventilation Treated with Diaphragm Pacing. Fumihiko Yasuma et al. Respiration 1998; 65:313-316.
[32] Amyotrophic lateral sclerosis: the Midwestern surgical experience with the diaphragm pacing stimulation system shows that general anesthesia can be safely performed. Raymond P. Onders, M.D; et al. The American Journal of Surgery (2009) 197, 386-390.
[33] Diaphragm pacing in ventilatory failure. S Lozewicz; et al. BMJ 1981, Oct 17; 283:1015-1016.
[34] The Swedish Experience in Phrenic Nerve Stimulation. Harald Fodstad. PACE, 10, January-February, Part II, 1987:246-251.
[35] Transesophageal Diaphragmatic Pacing for Treatment of Persistent Hiccups. David W. Andres, M.D; et al. Letter to Editor. Anesthesiology 2005; 102:483.
[36] Treatment of chronic ventilatory failure using a diaphragmatic pacemaker. H Garrido-Garcia; et al. Spinal Cord (1998) 36:310-314.
[37] Long-Term Follow-Up of bilateral Pacing of the Diaphragm in Quadriplegia. John F. Elefteriades, MD; et al. Letter to the Editor. N Engl J Med 1992; 326:1433-1434.
[38] Transdiaphragmatic pressure in quadriplegic individuals ventilated by diaphragmatic pacemaker. Honesto Garrido-Garcia; et al. Thorax 1996; 51:420-423.
[39] Assessment of the Motor Pathway to the Diaphragm Using Cortical and Cervical Magnetic Stimulation in the Decision-making Process of Phrenic Pacing. Thomas Similowski, MD; et al. Chest 1996; 110:1551-1557.
[40] Ultrasound evaluation of piglet diaphragm function before and after fatigue. Keith C. Kocis; et al. J Appl Physiol 83:1654-1659, 1997.
[41] Ventilatory Support by Pacing of the Conditioned Diaphragm in Quadriplegia. William W.L. Glenn, MD; et al. N Eng J Med 1984; 310:1150-1155.
[42] Lo stimolatore frenico, valido supporto ventilatorio per l'assistenza domiciliare dei pazienti tetraplegici. Caso clinico. A. M. Giglio; et al. Minerva Anestesiol 2002; 68:567-571.
[43] Conditioning of the diaphragm by phrenic nerve pacing in primary alveolar hypoventilation. Pearce G Wilcox; et al. Thorax 1988; 43:1017-1018.
[44] Diaphragm pacing restores olfaction in tetraplegia. D. Adler; et al. Eur Respir J 2009; 34: 365-370.
[45] Chest Pain and Diaphragmatic Pacing after Pacemaker Implantation. John L. Jefferies, MD; et al. Texas Heart Institute Journal. Volume 32, Number 1, 2005:106-107.
[46] Diapham pacing. Gerhard A Baer; et al. Correspondence. Thorax 1988; 43:743-744.
[47] Efficacy of Combined Inspiratory Intercostal and Expiratory Muscle Pacing to Maintain Artificial Ventilation. Anthony F. DiMarco; et al. Am J Respir Crit Care Med 1997; 156:122-126.